Karl Hörmann • Thomas Verse

Surgery for Sleep Disordered Breathing

Second Edition

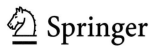 Springer

Prof. Dr. Karl Hörmann
Universitätsklinikum Mannheim
Hals-Nasen-Ohrenklinik
Theodor-Kutzer-Ufer 1-3
68167 Mannheim
Germany
karl.hoermann@umm.de

Prof. Dr. Thomas Verse
Asklepios Klinik Harburg
Abteilung HNO
Eißendorfer Pferdeweg 52
21075 Hamburg
Germany
t.verse@asklepios.com

ISBN: 978-3-540-77785-4   e-ISBN: 978-3-540-77786-1

DOI: 10.1007/978-3-540-77786-1

Springer Heidelberg Dordrecht London New York

Library of Congress Control Number: 2009926259

© Springer-Verlag Berlin Heidelberg 2010, 2005

Cover design: eStudio Calamar, Figueres/Berlin

Printed on acid-free paper

Springer is part of Springer Science+Business Media (www.springer.com)

Nasal continuous positive airway pressure ventilation is the gold standard in the treatment of obstructive sleep apnea. Long-term compliance rates are about 60%. Therefore, several alternative treatment options are of special interest. Beside conservative therapies, various surgical concepts exist. The field of surgery for sleep disordered breathing has rapidly grown with new instrumentation and surgical techniques in the last 10 years. Surgeons in these fields have to attend scientific meetings, participate in workshops, and read the literature to stay up to date.

In our sleep laboratories we conduct 30 polysomnographies each night. Each year, we perform almost 1,000 surgical procedures for sleep disordered breathing apart from numerous other conservative and apparative treatment modalities. Referring to our experience and the present literature, we tried to give new information on surgical techniques in this second edition.

The chapters are grouped in different anatomical fields of interest. We wanted to give general advice and specific new hints for the surgery of sleep disordered breathing so that the reader learns basic techniques followed by more advanced surgery. In addition to the illustrated surgical descriptions, the chapters contain informations about indications and contraindications of each surgical procedure and the postoperative care.

Special interest has been dedicated to evidence-based medicine. So in each chapter, there is a table of references summarizing the effectiveness of the procedure and EBM grade.

The enclosed DVD version of the book contains video files of elected procedures explained in the book. The reader has first the possibility to read the chapter text and then to reinforce his learning experience by reviewing the actual video of the procedure. The result is a complete illustrated information of the surgical procedure.

We hope that the second edition of this book will help training surgeons with special interest in modern sleep medicine.

Mannheim and Hamburg,   Prof. Dr. Karl Hörmann
December 2009   Prof. Dr. Thomas Verse

Contents

1 Sleep Disordered Breathing 1
Kerstin Rohde and Thomas Verse

2 General Aspects of Therapy 5
Thomas Verse

  2.1 Conservative Treatment 6
  2.2 Apparative Treatment 7
  2.3 Fundamental Reflections Regarding the Treatment Decision 8
    2.3.1 Pediatric SDB 8
    2.3.2 Daytime Symptoms 9
    2.3.3 Patient Expectations 10
    2.3.4 Site(s) of Obstruction 10
    2.3.5 Severity of SDB 10
  2.4 Concept of Continuous Narrowing of the Upper Airway 11

3 Identifying the Site of Obstruction 19
Joachim T. Maurer and Thomas Verse

  3.1 Pressure Measurements 20
  3.2 Flexible Endoscopy 21
  3.3 Analysis of the Respiratory Sounds During Sleep 22
  3.4 Further Imaging Procedures 22

4 Nasal Surgery 25
Thomas Verse and Wolfgang Pirsig

  4.1 Effectiveness of Treatment 26
    4.1.1 Effectiveness of conservative treatment 26
    4.1.2 Effectiveness for Simple Snoring 26
    4.1.3 Effectiveness for OSA 27
  4.2 Postoperative Care and Complications 28
  4.3 Indications and Contraindications 29
  4.4 Impact of Nasal Surgery on Nasal CPAP Treatment 30
  4.5 Conclusion 31

5   Nasopharyngeal Surgery...   33
       Thomas Verse and Wolfgang Pirsig

       5.1 Effectiveness of Treatment   34
             5.1.1 Corticosteroids...   34
             5.1.2 Nasopharyngeal Tubes   34
       5.2 Surgical Treatment...   35
       5.3 Postoperative Care and Complications   35
       5.4 Indications and Contraindications..   36

6   Palatal Surgery   37

       6.1 Tonsils   39
             6.1.1 Tonsillectomy and Adenotonsillectomy.....................................   39
                     Thomas Verse
                     6.1.1.1 Children   40
                     6.1.1.2 Postoperative Care and Complications.......................   43
                     6.1.1.3 Adults..   44
                     6.1.1.4 Postoperative Care and Complications.......................   44
                     6.1.1.5 Indications and Contraindications   45
             6.1.2 Tonsillotomy..   47
                     Thomas Verse
                     6.1.2.1 Surgical Technique   47
                     6.1.2.2 Effectiveness for Simple Snoring...............................   48
                     6.1.2.3 Effectiveness for OSA   48
                     6.1.2.4 Postoperative Care and Complications.......................   49
                     6.1.2.5 Indications and Contraindications   50
             6.1.3 Interstitial Radiofrequency Treatment (RFT)............................   51
                     Boris A. Stuck and Thomas Verse
                     6.1.3.1 Principles of Interstitial Radiofrequency Surgery   52
                     6.1.3.2 Surgical Technique   53
                     6.1.3.3 Effectiveness for SDB   54
                     6.1.3.4 Postoperative Care and Complications.......................   55
                     6.1.3.5 Indications and Contraindications   56
       6.2 Uvulopalatopharyngoplasty (UPPP)   59
             Wolfgang Pirsig and Thomas Verse
             6.2.1 Surgical Technique...   60
             6.2.2 Effectiveness for Simple Snoring...   63
                     6.2.2.1 Comparison of Different Soft Palate Surgical Techniques...........   64
             6.2.3 Effectiveness for OSA...   65
             6.2.4 Postoperative Care and Complications   66
             6.2.5 Indications and Contraindications..   71
       6.3 Recent Modifications of Uvulopalatopharyngoplasty..........................   75
             Wolfgang Pirsig and Thomas Verse
             6.3.1 Surgical Technique...   75
                     6.3.1.1 Uvuloplatal Flap   75
                     6.3.1.2 Lateral Pharyngoplasty   78

6.3.2   Effectiveness for SDB 79
6.3.3   Postoperative Care and Complications 82
        6.3.3.1 Uvulopalatal Flap 82
        6.3.3.2 Other Techniques 83
6.3.4   Indications and Contraindications... 83
        6.3.4.1 Extended Techniques 84
6.4 Laser-Assisted Uvulopalatoplasty (LAUP)... 87
Thomas Verse and Wolfgang Pirsig
6.4.1   Surgical Techniques 88
6.4.2   Effectiveness for Simple Snoring.. 90
        6.4.2.1 Lupp.. 92
        6.4.2.2 Laup 92
        6.4.2.3 Raup 94
6.4.3   Effectiveness for OSA.. 94
6.4.4   Postoperative Care and Complications 96
        6.4.4.1 Pain 99
6.4.5   Indications and Contraindications... 99
6.5 Radiofrequency Surgery.. 103
6.5.1   Interstitial Radiofrequency Treatment (RFT).......................... 103
        6.5.1.1 Surgical Technique 103
        6.5.1.2 Effectiveness for Simple Snoring 106
        6.5.1.3 Effectiveness for OSA 107
        6.5.1.4 Postoperative Care and Complications....................... 108
        6.5.1.5 Indications and Contraindications 109
6.5.2   Radiofrequency-UPP.. 111
        6.5.2.1 Surgical Technique 111
        6.5.2.2 Effectiveness for Simple Snoring 112
        6.5.2.3 Effectiveness for OSA 112
        6.5.2.4 Postoperative Care and Complications....................... 113
        6.5.2.5 Indications and Contraindications 114
6.6 Palatal Implants 115
Joachim T. Maurer and Thomas Verse
6.6.1   Surgical Technique... 115
6.6.2   Effectiveness for Simple Snoring.. 116
6.6.3   Effectiveness for OSA.. 117
6.6.4   Postoperative Care and Complications 119
6.6.5   Indications and Contraindications... 119
6.7 Other Soft Palate Procedures... 121
Thomas Verse
6.7.1   Uvulectomy 121
6.7.2   Palatal Stiffening Operation 122
        6.7.2.1 Surgical Technique 122
        6.7.2.2 Effectiveness for Simple Snoring 124
        6.7.2.3 Effectiveness for OSA 124
        6.7.2.4 Indications, Complications, and Postoperative Care 125

6.7.3   Injection Snoreplasty.. 126
        6.7.3.1 Surgical Technique 126
        6.7.3.2 Effectiveness for Simple Snoring and OSA 127
        6.7.3.3 Indications, Complications, and Postoperative Care.................... 127
6.7.4   Transpalatal Advancement Pharyngoplasty...................................... 128

7   Lower Pharyngeal Airway Procedures 131

7.1 Interstitial Radiofrequency Treatment (RFT).. 133
    Boris A. Stuck and Thomas Verse
    7.1.1   Surgical Technique.. 133
    7.1.2   Effectiveness for Simple Snoring.. 136
    7.1.3   Effectiveness for OSA.. 137
    7.1.4   Postoperative Care and Complications 139
    7.1.5   Indications and Contraindications... 141
7.2 Hyoid Suspension... 143
    Nico de Vries and Thomas Verse
    7.2.1   Introduction: Hyoid Suspension Alone and As Part
            of Combined Treatment.. 143
    7.2.2   Surgical Technique 144
            7.2.2.1 Original Surgical Technique (1986), Historical
                    Perspectives, and Nomenclature 144
            7.2.2.2 First Modification (1994)....................................... 145
            7.2.2.3 Hörmann's Modification (2001)................................. 147
    7.2.3   Effectiveness for SDB.. 150
    7.2.4   Postoperative Care and Complications 151
    7.2.5   Indications and Contraindications... 151
7.3 Tongue Base Resection.. 153
    Joachim T. Maurer and Thomas Verse
    7.3.1   Surgical Technique... 154
    7.3.2   Effectiveness for OSA.. 158
    7.3.3   Postoperative Care and Complications 159
    7.3.4   Indications and Contraindications... 160
7.4 Tongue Suspension... 161
    Boris A. Stuck and Thomas Verse
    7.4.1   Surgical Technique... 161
    7.4.2   Efficiency for Simple Snoring.. 163
    7.4.3   Efficiency for OSA.. 164
    7.4.4   Postoperative Care and Complications 164
    7.4.5   Indications and Contraindications... 165

8   Maxillofacial Surgeries 167

8.1 Genioglossus Advancement (GA).. 169
    Thomas Verse
    8.1.1   Surgical Technique... 169
            8.1.1.1 Effectiveness for OSA 171
    8.1.2   Postoperative Care and Complications 171
    8.1.3   Indications and Contraindications... 172

8.2 Maxillomandibular Advancement (MMA) 175
  Thomas Hierl
  8.2.1 Surgical Technique 176
      8.2.1.1 Surgery on the Upper Jaw 176
      8.2.1.2 Surgery on the Lower Jaw 177
  8.2.2 Efficiency of Maxillomandibular Advancement for OSA 178
  8.2.3 Postoperative Care and Complications 179
  8.2.4 Indications and Contraindications 180
8.3 Distraction Osteogenesis (DOG) 183
  Thomas Hierl
  8.3.1 Mandibular Distraction Osteogenesis 184
      8.3.1.1 Surgical Technique 185
  8.3.2 Maxillary-Midfacial Distraction Osteogenesis 186
      8.3.2.1 Surgical Technique 186
      8.3.2.2 Efficiency of DOG for OSA 187
      8.3.2.3 Complications and Postoperative Care 188
      8.3.2.4 Indications and Counter Indication 189

9 Laryngeal OSA 193
  Thomas Verse

  9.1 Pediatric Laryngeal OSA 193
      9.1.1 Surgical Techniques 194
      9.1.2 Efficiency for SDB 197
      9.1.3 Postoperative Care and Complications 197
      9.1.4 Indications and Contraindications 198
  9.2 Adult Laryngeal OSA 199
      9.2.1 Surgical Techniques 200
      9.2.2 Efficiency for SDB 200
      9.2.3 Postoperative Care and Complications 201
      9.2.4 Indications and Contraindications 201

10 Multilevel Surgery 203
  Thomas Verse

  10.1 Surgical Concepts 204
      10.1.1 Effectiveness of Minimally Invasive
             Multilevel Surgery for Mild-to-Moderate OSA 204
      10.1.2 Effectiveness of Multilevel Surgery
             for Moderate-to-Severe OSA 205
  10.2 Postoperative Care and Complications 210
  10.3 Indications and Contraindications 211
      10.3.1 Multilevel Surgery in Children 212

11 Tracheotomy 215
  Thomas Verse and Wolfgang Pirsig

  11.1 Surgical Technique 215
  11.2 Effectiveness for OSA 216

11.3   Postoperative Care and Complications 217
11.4   Indications and Contraindications 218

12 Bariatric Surgery 221
Helge Kleinhans and Thomas Verse

12.1   Techniques 222
        12.1.1 Adjustable Gastric Banding 222
        12.1.2 Vertical Banded Gastroplasty 222
        12.1.3 Sleeve Gastrectomy 223
        12.1.4 Intragastric Balloon 224
        12.1.5 Jejunal Bypass 224
        12.1.6 Biliopancreatic Diversion 224
        12.1.7 Roux-en-Y Gastric Bypass 224
12.2   Effectiveness for OSA 226
12.3   Indications and Contraindications 227
12.4   Postoperative Care and Complications 229

13 Anesthesiologic Airway Management 231
Harald V. Genzwuerker

13.1   Implications in Patients with OSA 231
13.2   Strategies for Intubation in Patients with a Known or
        Suspected Difficult Airway 232
13.3   Life-Threatening Situations 236
13.4   Extubating the Difficult Airway 237
13.5   Negative Pressure Pulmonary Edema 238
13.6   Postoperative Care 238
13.7   Documentation 239

References 241

Index 291

About the Authors 297

Contributors

Karl Hörmann, MD
Department of Otorhinolaryngology
Head and Neck Surgery
University Hospital Mannheim
68135 Mannheim, Germany

Thomas Verse, MD
Department of Otorhinolaryngology
Head and Neck Surgery
Asklepios Clinic Harburg
Eissendorfer Pferdeweg 52
21075 Hamburg, Germany

Alexander Baisch, MD
Otorhinolaryngologist
Am Leimengraben 32
69168 Wiesloch, Germany

Harald V. Genzwuerker, MD
Department of Anesthesiology
and Intensive Care Medicine
Neckar-Odenwald Clinic
Dr. Konrad-Adenauer-Strasse 37
74722 Buchen, Germany

Thomas Hierl, MD, DDS
Department of Oral and
Maxillofacial Plastic Surgery
University of Leipzig, Germany

Kerstin Huber, MD
Department of Otorhinolaryngology
Head and Neck Surgery
Asklepios Clinic Harburg
Eissendorfer Pferdeweg 52
21075 Hamburg, Germany

Helge Kleinhans, MD
Department of Otorhinolaryngology
Head and Neck Surgery
Asklepios Clinic Harburg
Eissendorfer Pferdeweg 52
21075 Hamburg, Germany

Joachim T. Maurer, MD
Department of Otorhinolaryngology
Head and Neck Surgery
Sleep Disorders Center
University Hospital Mannheim
68135 Mannheim, Germany

Wolfgang Pirsig, MD
Department of Otorhinolaryngology
Head and Neck Surgery
Mozartstrasse 22/1, 89075 Ulm
Germany

Boris A. Stuck, MD
Department of Otorhinolaryngology
Head and Neck Surgery
University Hospital Mannheim
68135 Mannheim, Germany

Nico de Vries, MD, PhD
Department of Otolaryngology
Saint Lucas Andreas Hospital
PO Box 9243, 1006AE Amsterdam
The Netherlands

Sleep Disordered Breathing

1

Kerstin Rohde and Thomas Verse

Core Features

> In the case of primary snoring, the patient does not suffer from hypersomnia, excessive daytime sleepiness, or sleep disruption attributable to snoring or airflow limitation.
> In adult obstructive sleep apnea, the patient complains of daytime sleepiness, unrefreshing sleep, fatigue, or hypersomnia. Polysomnography recordings show five or more scoreable respiratory events per hour of sleep.
> In pediatric obstructive sleep apnea, the caregiver reports snoring, labored, or obstructed breathing. Paradoxical inward rib-cage motion during inspiration, morning headaches, secondary enuresis, hyperactivity, or aggressive behavior may occur. Excessive daytime sleepiness is seen less commonly in children than in adults with OSA. Polysomnography recordings show one or more scoreable respiratory events per hour of sleep.

In our modern competitive society, nonrestorative sleep is acquiring an increased significance. The international classification of sleep disorders includes 95 different diagnoses of possible causes for nonrestful sleep [12]. A subgroup with a comparatively high incidence rate is formed by the so-called sleep-related breathing disorders (SRBD; synonyma: sleep disordered breathing (SDB)). These are further divided into disorders with central sleep apnea (CSA), obstructive sleep apnea (OSA), sleep related hypoventilation syndromes, and other SRBDs. OSA syndromes are separated into adult OSA and pediatric OSA. The term upper airway resistance syndrome (UARS) is subsumed under this diagnosis because the pathophysiology does not significantly differ from that of OSA. Primary snoring is included in a different subgroup, namely isolated symptoms, apparently normal variants, and unresolved issues.

Snoring is a respiratory sound generated in the upper airway during sleep; it typically occurs during inspiration. Primary snoring occurs without episodes of apnea or hypoventilation. The intensity of snoring may vary and often will disturb the bed partner's sleep and even awaken the patient. Primary snoring does not cause symptoms of daytime sleepiness or hypersomnia [13].

K. Hörmann, T. Verse, *Surgery for Sleep Disordered Breathing*,
DOI: 10.1007/978-3-540-77786-1_1, © Springer Verlag Berlin Heidelberg 2010

In contrast to primary snoring, adult OSA has an adverse effect on the daytime life quality. The most frequent symptoms of OSA are intermittent snoring (94%), daytime sleepiness (78%), and diminished intellectual performance (58%). Further symptoms are personality changes (48%), impotence in men (48%), morning headaches (36%), and enuresis nocturna (30%) [253].

OSA is a widespread disorder affecting up to 10.9% of the male and up to 6.3% of the female population [331, 841]. OSA is associated with serious adverse consequences, such as myocardial infarction [311], stroke [166], hypertension [555], and traffic accidents [737], for the afflicted individuals.

In the case of OSA, an imbalance exists between forces dilating and occluding the pharynx during sleep. The muscle tone supporting the pharyngeal lumen is too low, and the inspiratory suction force and the pressure of the surrounding tissue narrow the pharynx and are situated too high [561, 596]. This disorder occurs only during sleep because of a physiological loss of muscle tone of the pharyngeal muscles in this state. The effects are complete cessation of breathing (apneas) or reduced breathing phases (hypopneas). Both events trigger, if sustained long enough, an emergency situation for the body. The body reacts with a central arousal that disturbs the physiological sleep by a release of catecholamines. The latter lead to a strain upon the cardiovascular system via an increase of the tone of the sympathetic system. However, the frequency of apneas and hypopneas during sleep correlates poorly with daytime symptom severity and impact on quality of life. It is possible for any severity level of OSA to occur with any degree of symptomatic sleepiness and, in cases, with no subjective complaints.

The major predisposing factor for OSA is excess body weight. The risk of OSA increases as the degree of additional weight increases, with an extremely high prevalence of OSA with morbid obesity. Patients with normal body weight are more likely to have upper airway obstruction due to localized structural abnormality such as a maxillomandibular malformation or adenotonsillar enlargement.

In other words, primary snoring is merely an irritating annoyance, whereas OSA represents a disease with a significant morbidity and mortality. This implies that distinct therapy goals are warranted. Therefore, we consider it as vital that a precise diagnosis is established before the initiation of any therapy. The necessary diagnostic work-up includes an anamnesis using standardized questionnaires, a physiological and otolaryngological assessment, and a sleep lab evaluation. For details, see the relevant literature [14–16, 19, 200].

Pediatric OSA is characterized by prolonged partial upper airway obstruction and obstructive apnea or hypopnea that disrupts normal ventilation during sleep. Children with OSA may demonstrate several different breathing patterns during sleep. Some children have cyclic episodes of obstructive apnea, similar to that of adults with the syndrome [12, 248]. However, some patients, particularly younger children, have a pattern of obstructive hypoventilation, which consists of long periods of persistent partial upper airway obstruction associated with hypercarbia and arterial oxygen desaturation. Most children with OSA present with a history of breathing difficulties during sleep. Snoring is usually loud and may be punctuated by pauses and gasps, with associated movements or arousal from sleep. However, some patients, particularly infants and those who are weak, may not snore. Children have a very compliant rip cage. As a result, paradoxical breathing is a prominent sign of these patients. Children may sleep in unusual positions, such as seated or with their neck hyperextended. Excessive daytime sleepiness may be present, especially in older children, but is seen less commonly in children than in adults with OSA [178]. Although studies have shown that children with OSA generally have larger tonsils and adenoids than do other children, the size of the tonsils and adenoids does not predict disease in individual patients. The prevalence of OSA is approximately 2% in otherwise-normal young children with a peak incidence in the preschool age [12]. For details in necessary diagnostic work-up see the relevant literature [178, 248].

Take Home Pearls

> A diagnosis differentiating between primary snoring on the one hand and OSA on the other hand including sleep studies is crucial before making a treatment decision in modern sleep medicine.
> Definitions of disease and treatment modalities substantially differ in adult and pediatric patients.

General Aspects of Therapy

2

Thomas Verse

Core Features

> Treatment options for SDB are either conservative, apparative, or surgical.
> The decision regarding which treatment fits for which patients depends on several parameters. The most important criteria are severity of SDB, daytime symptoms, comorbidities, age (especially children or adults), BMI, site(s) of obstruction, and of course, the preferences of the patient.
> Today, guidelines, statements, and reviews that summarize scientific data according to evidence-based medicine criteria are available. This book highlights the data for each chapter according to the Oxford Criteria of EBM.
> Focussing on surgical treatment, the authors define five main areas of indication for surgery for SDB. These are (a) improvement of nasal breathing to support ventilation therapy (nasally applied CPAP), (b) minimally-invasive surgery for primary snoring and (very) mild OSA, (c) invasive surgery for mild and moderate OSA, (d) multilevel surgery for moderate and severe OSA as secondary treatment after failure or definitive interruption of ventilation therapy, and (e) adenotonsillectomy or adenotonsillotomie in pediatric OSA.

In the meantime, a multitude of treatment options for SDB exists. They can be classified into conservative, apparative, and surgical methods. While this book focuses solely on surgical therapies, for the competent surgeon, it is necessary to be familiar with the conservative and apparative treatment options in order to be able to define the ideal therapy concept for every patient. What follows is, therefore, a concise discussion of the most important nonsurgical treatment options. We point the interested reader to readable surveys of the topic. Even when aware of the complete array of treatment options, the decision regarding which treatment is the best for which patient is not always easy. For years, the authors have been leading clinical seminars on this topic in the context of the German Academy for Otolaryngology, Head and Neck Surgery. The experiences from these courses are presented in the second part of this chapter.

K. Hörmann, T. Verse, *Surgery for Sleep Disordered Breathing*,
DOI: 10.1007/978-3-540-77786-1_2, © Springer Verlag Berlin Heidelberg 2010

2.1
Conservative Treatment

Conservative methods include weight reduction, optimizing of sleeping hygiene, conditioning in respect of the avoidance of certain sleep positions, and drug treatments.

Obesity is considered the main risk factor for SDB. But most patients are not able to reduce their weight sufficiently and consistently [570]. Yet, even in those cases in which healing is initially achieved merely through weight reduction, a symptomatic SBD may occur again later even though the weight is kept on a low level. This fact may be interpreted as indicating that SDB is a multi-factored event, in which obesity plays a significant role in the pathogenesis of many patients. But in the case of obese patients, other factors also usually play a role, which, together with the adiposity, contribute to the development of OSA. Nevertheless, a weight reduction is of essential importance and simplifies every other OSA therapy; however, weight reduction in itself is only rarely able to resolve an OSA without further therapy.

A new field in the treatment of SDB is surgical weight reduction, the so-called bariatric surgery. Chapter 12 highlights this issue.

The maintenance of a certain level of sleeping hygiene (avoidance of alcohol and sedatives, reduction of nicotine and other noxious substances, observance of a regular sleep rhythm, etc.) is part of the standard recommendations in the treatment of SDB. Obviously, no controlled long-term studies exist relating to these measures.

In the case of positional OSA, apneas and hypopneas occur predominantly or solely only in supine position. In these cases, one should always consider the existence of a primarily retrolingual obstruction site. In supine position, the tongue, in accordance with gravity, falls backward because of the physiological muscle relaxation. As a result of the lower mass, this effect apparently plays a lesser role in the case of the soft palate. As minimal criterion for a positional OSA, it is necessary that the AHI in supine position is at least twice the value of the AHI in lateral position. Similarly, there are incidents of primary snoring wherein socially disruptive respiratory noises are only manifest in supine position.

In order to prevent supine position, the following methods have been used: verbal instructions, a "supine position alarm", a ball sewed into the back of the pyjama, or a vest, or backpack. Backpack and vest reliably prevent supine position; verbal instructions are only successful in 48% of cases. On average, the AHI could be reduced by 55%. Unfortunately, no long-term results exist for these methods, yet there are several controlled studies. All in all, data of 69 patients exist. The average success rate lies at 75% [447]. In a randomized cross-over study [335], a significantly better AHI was found with CPAP than with the backpack; however, daytime sleepiness and productivity were identical with either treatment.

Avoidance of supine position makes sense in the case of positional sleep apnea. It can also help in optimizing the results of a ventilation therapy or a surgical treatment.

In 1998, a survey was published, which assessed the efficacy of 43 drugs in the treatment of SDB [273]. Yet currently, there is no drug that can be considered viable in the treatment of SDB. Similarly, a Cochrane review on the topic of drug treatment of OSA found that the existing data do not support the efficacy of medication for OSA [690]. Therefore, a drug therapy cannot be recommended.

2.2
Apparative Treatment

Apparative treatment options include respiratory treatment with continuous positive airway pressure (CPAP) with its various modifications, oral appliances, and electrostimulation.

The CPAP ventilation therapy, according to Sullivan [728], which for the most part is nasally applied, splints the upper airway pneumatically from the nares to the larynx (Fig. 2.1).

Concerning the implementation of CPAP therapy and its diverse modifications, we refer to the specialized literature [158]. CPAP ventilation reduces or removes snoring, daytime symptoms, and the cardiovascular risk. Two excellent studies demonstrate the efficacy of the method [37, 330], as does a systematic Cochrane review [815]. With a primary success rate of 98%, CPAP therapy is, alongside tracheotomy, the most successful therapy modality available. Only these two treatment modalities achieve sufficient cure rates in cases of extreme obesity and severe OSA. With respect to quality of life and risk of traffic accidents, the cost effectiveness of a CPAP therapy was recently corroborated [29]. As an example of many new insights, we refer to the work of Drager et al. [162], which demonstrated that already after 4 months of CPAP therapy (compared to no therapy) significant changes of intima thickness, pulse wave speed, C-reactive protein, and catecholamines in the serum occured. A new review [258] demonstrates the efficacy of CPAP in comparison to placebo on arterial hypertonia under reference to 572 patients of 12 randomized studies.

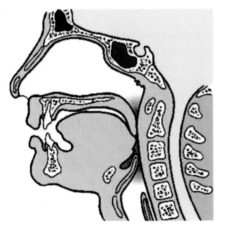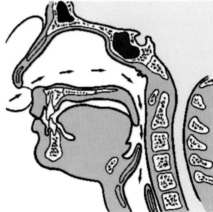

Fig. 2.1 Method of pneumatic stenting of the upper airway with CPAP. (*Left*) Airway collapse. (*Right*) Stabilization with continuous positive airway pressure

Therefore, nasal CPAP therapy is considered to be the gold standard in the treatment of OSA. All other therapies for OSA must be measured against this method. Unfortunately, the long-term acceptance rate of CPAP therapy lies below 70% [453]. The acceptance rate of CPAP therapy especially decreases the younger the patient is, and the less his subjective ailments improve with a CPAP therapy [328, 416]. As a consequence, many patients with moderate and severe OSA in need of treatment have to be secondarily guided into another therapy. Often surgery is successful in these cases [699].

Among the oral devices, the mandibular advancement devices have established themselves. For mild to moderate severe OSA, success rates of 50–70% have been reported (new survey in [99]). The compatability of the mandibular advancement devices is given as between 40 and 80% [193]. Main side effects in up to 80% of the patients are hypersalivation, xerostomy, pain in the jaw, dental pain, and permanent teeth misalignments with malocclusion [542]. Oral devices are recommended for the treatment of simple snoring and mild and medium OSA.

Recently, the playing of digeridoos has been added as a curiosity to the list of OSA therapies. A first randomized study [583] demonstrates a significant effect on AHI and daytime sleepiness for 25 sleep apnea patients after 4 months of digeridoo playing in comparison to zero therapy. The playing of digeridoos allegedly strengthens the floor of the mouth and tongue muscles, comparable to electrical stimulation therapy. However, the latter has only been shown to have a limited effect on the AHI [588, 589, 779]; therefore, this form of therapy has not established itself as an isolated treatment option. As supplemental therapy, the strengthening of the muscles of the upper airway is certainly valuable.

2.3
Fundamental Reflections Regarding the Treatment Decision

If a patient is transferred for treatment of sleep disordered breathing (SDB), there are basically several factors that have to be taken into account to make a proper treatment decision (Table 2.1).

2.3.1
Pediatric SDB

As stated in Chap. 1, the medical conditions vary substantially in children compared to adults. For children, already more than 2 breathing pauses per hour of sleep are considered pathologic. We refer here to an engaging current survey [261]. Since the sleep-medical anamnesis and diagnosis of children are much more difficult and elaborate, the question is which children should be examined more closely. Concerning this question, several new results exist, of which the following will be discussed as examples. The anamnesis in children can be supported with specific questionnaires. For instance, the Pediatric Sleep

Table 2.1 Criteria for treatment decisions in sleep disordered breathing

Criteria for treatment decisions
Adults or children?
Daytime symptoms?
Does the patient prefer surgical or nonsurgical treatment?
Site(s) of obstruction
Severity of disease (AHI, symptoms, concommitant diseases)
Special shapes of OSA
Only in supine position
Complex malformations
Laryngeal OSA

Questionnaire (22 items) was successfully used in a longitudinal study of 159 children before and 1 year after an adenotonsilectomy [108]. Other authors use their own questionnaires [478, 730]. In any case, obese children should be examined. Obesity and increase of the BMI are considered to be primary risk factors [839]; however, they also count as secondary risk factors for the recurrence of an OSA after an initially successful adenotonsilectomy [21]. Further risk factors for OSA are trisomy 21, tonsilhyperplasy, low social status, and low weight at birth [536, 672, 700, 838].

Treatment of pediatric OSA is dominated by the removal or reduction of adenoids and tonsils and will be discussed in Chaps. 5, 6.1.1 and 6.1.2. For very young children, special postoperative conditions exist, which will be discussed in Chap. 13.

2.3.2
Daytime Symptoms

Most frequent symptoms of OSA are arhythmic snoring, unquite sleep, daytime sleepiness, and reduction of intellectual vigor. In contrast, the significantly higher risk of morbidity and mortality (in comparison with the healthy population) is not directly noticeable for a sleep apneic, but remains a hypothetical risk. For treatment success of an aid, for instance, nCPAP therapy or oral appliances, a consistent use of the aid is neccessary. Herein often lies the problem. Today, it is known that especially patients who initially experience a significant improvement of their daytime symptoms after starting the use of their aid show a high long-term compliance. In these cases, the subjective advantage (finally restorative sleep) stands in a good relation to potential inconveniences which the long-term use of these aids includes. On the other hand, it is often the patients who experience little subjective advantage from the therapy who will discontinue a genuinely effective therapy. Included in this group are of course those patients who already have experienced few or no daytime symptoms before the therapy. This group is particularly suited for surgical therapy since after the perioperative phase, a special therapy compliance is not needed.

2.3.3
Patient Expectations

Frequently, patients will already have had contact to self-help groups or friends and family, or have informed themselves through other means. Our daily practice has shown us that the patients often already come to a consultation with a specific therapy notion. Specifically, there are patients who do not want to undergo surgery under any circumstances;others do not want to use an intrusive appliance which they will have to use their whole life. In the framework of the therapy principles described here, we always attempt to take into account the wishes of the patients, unless serious reasons indicate that it is neccessary to counter a patient's expectation. We have found that being aware of a patient's wishes helps us in guiding our patients.

2.3.4
Site(s) of Obstruction

For CPAP therapy it is irrelevant where exactly the site(s) of obstruction is (are) located in the upper airway, because the whole upper airway is being pneumatically aligned. For the treatment decision for oral devices and especially for the customized surgical therapy, a thorough knowledge of the site(s) of obstruction is neccessary. The following Chap. 3 discusses the scope of topodiagnosis.

2.3.5
Severity of SDB

The severity of SDB is crucial in deciding which therapy is most suitable for which patient. The simple snorer is not ill. Therefore, the goal of treatment in the case of primary snoring lies in the reduction of both the duration and the intensity of snoring to a socially acceptable level. In principle, it needs to be kept in mind (1) that a treatment should not harm the patient, (2) that a treatment should only be carried out if the patient has explicitly articulated such a wish, and (3) that after any treatment, nasal ventilation therapy should remain possible [17]. This last aspect is of importance due to the fact that the incidence of OSA increases with age [427]. Many cases have been described in which nasal ventilation therapy was no longer possible due to the development of a nasopharyngeal insufficiency or stenosis [485], especially after aggressive soft palate surgery. These cases have in many places seriously impaired the trust in soft palate surgery.

In the case of OSA, the goal of treatment consists in a complete elimination of all apneas, hypopneas, desaturations, arousals, snoring, and other related symptoms in all body positions and all sleep stages. Of course, here it also has to be stressed that a treatment should in principle not harm the patient. But it must be pointed out that in the case of OSA, a disease with corresponding symptoms is already manifest. Therefore, in order to achieve the therapy goal, one will be less reluctant to consider a more invasive therapy with heightened morbidity and complication rate, a decision which would not be defensible in the case of harmless primary snoring.

In general, the severity of OSA is classified according to the apnea hypopnea index (AHI; equals the number of apneas plus the number of hypopneas per hour of sleep). Unfortunately, especially in the case of the mild forms of SDB, the AHI is not necessarily correlated to the clinical symptoms of the patients. Furthermore, the AHI is age-dependent. Concerning adults, the updated version of the International Classification of Sleep Disorders (ICSD) [12] uses the following distinction for OSA:

Mild OSA	$5 \leq AHI < 20$
Moderate OSA	$20 \leq AHI < 40$
Severe OSA	$40 \leq AHI$

The term upper airway resistance syndrome (UARS) is subsumed under the diagnosis OSA because the pathophysilogy does not significantly differ from that of OSA. It needs to be taken into account that the above values are applicable to 30-year olds. In the case of a 70 year old, an AHI of maximally 15 is still not necessarily in need of treatment if the patient does not have any daytime symptoms.

Apart from the AHI, the ailments of the patient play a role. That is, a patient with a low AHI suffering from intense daytime sleepiness may already be in need of treatment, whereas an older patient with an AHI of 15 may be fine without treatment. The concomitant diagnoses also need to be taken into account. Since SDB constitutes risk factors for myocardial infarction, arterial hypertension, and strokes, patients with a corresponding anamnesis need to be sufficiently treated early on. One should also take special note of traffic accidents in the anamnesis, as these are frequently a result of sleepiness behind the wheel, which again suggests the existence of an SDB [121, 230, 268, 537].

In younger but not in middle-age groups, OSA has been reported to be more prevalent in African Americans compared with Caucasians. The prevalence of OSA in Asia patients with craniofacial features that predispose them to developing OSA may be high in spite of their having a BMI in comparison with Caucasian patients.

2.4
Concept of Continuous Narrowing of the Upper Airway

Modern concepts regard primary snoring on the one hand and OSA on the other hand as different manifestations of the same pathophysiological disorder (Fig. 2.2) [479]. We agree with this conception and have made it the foundation for our therapeutic decisions.

From Fig. 2.2 two important therapy principles can be inferred. On the one hand, a surgical therapy, if it is to produce recovery from SDB, has to be performed more aggressively the more severe the SDB is. Surgical procedures are performed both in the case of primary snoring and at all severity levels of OSA. For the treatment of primary snoring, minimally invasive techniques with a low complication rate should be preferred. In the case of higher level OSA, surgery is only secondarily indicated after an unsuccessful nasal CPAP-therapy. For a primary surgical treatment, an AHI of approximately 30 and a BMI lower 30 kg/m^2 are considered as threshold value [768].

Fig. 2.2 Continuous narrowing of upper airway modified after Moore [479]

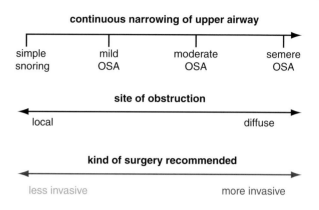

The second therapy principle entails the notion that SDB is more and more considered as a disorder of the entire upper airway. For many years, ENT surgeons, by only assuming two sites of obstruction, pursued a concept which from our perspective is too mechanistic. Fujita, for example, classified OSA patients into those with an obstruction solely behind the soft palate (type I), those with an obstruction solely behind the tongue (type II), and those with an obstruction both behind soft palate and tongue (type III) [227]. The following Chap. 3 will discuss more specifically the established techniques of this topodiagnosis. Yet up to now, this topodiagnosis has not been conductive in, for instance, raising the success rate of soft palate surgery significantly above 50%. Therefore, we now assume that this simplified classification into a retropalatal and a retrolingual site of obstruction is only applicable for primary snoring and, to a certain extent, in the case of mild OSA. In these patient groups, we perform an individually selected surgery based on the findings of our topodiagnosis. We call this selection calculated surgery. Starting with moderate OSA, i.e., from an AHI of approximately 20, there is a need, in accordance with our experiences and assessments, for a surgical treatment of both of the two mentioned, potential sites of obstruction along the lines of the so-called multilevel surgery. Also, in this case, the appropriate combination depends upon the severity and the anatomical disposition, but always addresses at least the level of the soft palate and the level of the hypopharynx (see Chap. 10 multilevel surgery). The following algorithm (Fig. 2.3) tries to summarize our thoughts discussed above in a flow-chart.

Figure 2.4 illustrates the indications for the surgical techniques preferred by us, in dependence of the severity of the SDB. The following chapters will discuss these techniques in detail.

Nasal surgery seldomly affects the severity of OSA and is of use only in the lesser half of patients with primary snoring. Nevertheless, we see an indication as adjuvant therapy especially to facilitate a nasal ventilation therapy. Currently, we do not see an indication for the following procedures: uvulectomy, injection snoreplasty, cautery assisted palatal stiffening operation, transpalatal advancement pharyngoplasty, and tongue suspension procedures.

In the following, the surgical methods are discussed according to their anatomical position, beginning with the nose and ending with the stomach. Insofar these surgical techniques are not part and parcel of surgery primers; the techniques favored by the authors and some important techniques of other authors are elucidated.

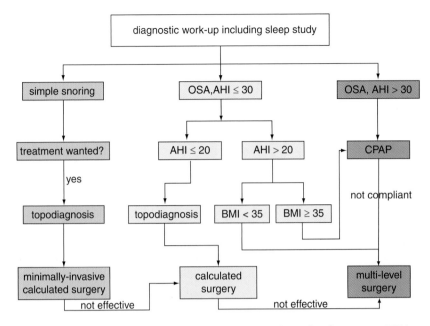

Fig. 2.3 Algorithm for treatment decision in adult SDB. *OSA* obstructive sleep apnea; *AHI* Apnea Hypopnea Index; *CPAP* continuous positive airway pressure; *BMI* body mass index

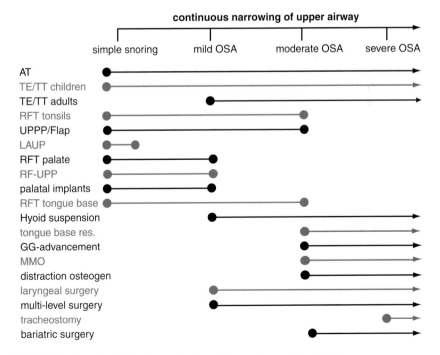

Fig. 2.4 Indications for different surgeries depending on the severity of SDB

Table 2.2 Oxford Centre for evidence-based medicine levels of evidence (May 2001)

Level	Therapy/prevention, etiology/harm	Prognosis	Diagnosis	Differential diagnosis/ symptom prevalence study	Economic and decision analyses
1a	SR (with homogeneity[a]) of RCTs	SR (with homogeneity[a]) of inception cohort studies; CDR[b] validated in different populations	SR (with homogeneity[a]) of Level 1 diagnostic studies; CDR[b] with 1b studies from different clinical centers	SR (with homogeneity[a]) of prospective cohort studies	SR (with homogeneity[a]) of Level 1 economic studies
1b	Individual RCT (with narrow Confidence Interval[c])	Individual inception cohort study with ≥80% follow-up; CDR[b] validated in a single population	Validating[d] cohort study with good[e] reference standards; or CDR[b] tested within one clinical center	Prospective cohort study with good follow-up[f]	Analysis based on clinically sensible costs or alternatives; systematic review(s) of the evidence; and including multiway sensitivity analyses
1c	All or none[g]	All or none case-series	Absolute SpPins and SnNouts[h]	All or none case-series	Absolute better-value or worse-value analyses[i]
2a	SR (with homogeneity[a]) of cohort studies	SR (with homogeneity[a]) of either retrospective cohort studies or untreated control groups in RCTs	SR (with homogeneity[a]) of Level >2 diagnostic studies	SR (with homogeneity[a]) of 2b and better studies	SR (with homogeneity[a]) of Level >2 economic studies
2b	Individual cohort study (including low quality RCT; e.g. <80% follow-up)	Retrospective cohort study or follow-up of untreated control patients in an RCT; Derivation of CDR[b] or validated on split-sample[j] only	Exploratory[d] cohort study with good[e] reference standards; CDR[b] after derivation, or validated only on split-sample[j] or databases	Retrospective cohort study, or poor follow-up	Analysis based on clinically sensible costs or alternatives; limited review(s) of the evidence, or single studies; and including multiway sensitivity analyses
2c	"Outcomes" Research; Ecological studies	"Outcomes" Research		Ecological studies	Audit or outcomes research

Level					
3a	SR (with homogeneity[a]) of case-control studies	SR (with homogeneity[a]) of 3b and better studies	SR (with homogeneity[a]) of 3b and better studies	SR (with homogeneity[a]) of 3b and better studies	SR (with homogeneity[a]) of 3b and better studies
3b	Individual Case-Control Study		Non-consecutive study; or without consistently applied reference standards	Non-consecutive cohort study, or very limited population	Analysis based on limited alternatives or costs, poor quality estimates of data, but including sensitivity analyses incorporating clinically sensible variations
4	Case-series (and poor quality cohort and case-control studies[k])	Case-series (and poor quality prognostic cohort studies[c])	Case-control study, poor or nonindependent reference standard	Case-series or superseded reference standards	Analysis with no sensitivity analysis
5	Expert opinion without explicit critical appraisal, or based on physiology, bench research, or "first principles"	Expert opinion without explicit critical appraisal, or based on physiology, bench research, or "first principles"	Expert opinion without explicit critical appraisal, or based on physiology, bench research, or "first principles"	Expert opinion without explicit critical appraisal, or based on physiology, bench research, or "first principles"	Expert opinion without explicit critical appraisal, or based on economic theory or "first principles"

Produced by Bob Phillips, Chris Ball, Dave Sackett, Doug Badenoch, Sharon Straus, Brian Haynes, Martin Dawes since November 1998

Users can add a minus-sign "−" to denote the level that fails to provide a conclusive answer because of:

· EITHER a single result with a wide Confidence Interval (such that, for example, an ARR in an RCT is not statistically significant but whose confidence intervals fail to exclude clinically important benefit or harm)

· OR a Systematic Review with troublesome (and statistically significant) heterogeneity

· Such evidence is inconclusive, and therefore, can only generate Grade D recommendations

[a] By homogeneity, we mean a systematic review that is free of worrisome variations (heterogeneity) in the directions and degrees of results between individual studies. Not all systematic reviews with statistically significant heterogeneity need be worrisome, and not all worrisome heterogeneity need be statistically significant. As noted above, studies displaying worrisome heterogeneity should be tagged with a "−" at the end of their designated level

[b] Clinical Decision Rule (these are algorithms or scoring systems which lead to a prognostic estimation or a diagnostic category)

[c] See note 2 for advice on how to understand, rate, and use trials or other studies with wide confidence intervals

[d] Validating studies test the quality of a specific diagnostic test, based on prior evidence. An exploratory study collects information and trawls the data (e.g., using a regression analysis) to find which factors are "significant"

(continued)

Table 2.2 (continued)

^e*Good* reference standards are independent of the test, and applied blindly or objectively to all patients. *Poor* reference standards are haphazardly applied, but still independent of the test. Use of a nonindependent reference standard (where the "test" is included in the "reference", or where the "testing" affects the "reference") implies a level 4 study

^fGood follow-up in a differential diagnosis study is >80%, with adequate time for alternative diagnoses to emerge (e.g., 1–6 months acute, 1–5 years chronic)

^gMet when *all* patients died before the Rx became available, but some now survive on it; or when some patients died before the Rx became available, but *none* now die on it

^hAn "Absolute SpPin" is a diagnostic finding whose Specificity is so high that a *Positive* result rules-*in* the diagnosis. An "Absolute SnNout" is a diagnostic finding whose Sensitivity is so high that a *Negative* result rules-*out* the diagnosis

ⁱBetter-value treatments are clearly as good but cheaper, or better at the same or reduced cost. Worse-value treatments are as good and more expensive, or worse and the equally or more expensive

^jSplit-sample validation is achieved by collecting all the information in a single tranche, then artificially dividing this into "derivation" and "validation" samples

^kBy poor quality *cohort* study we mean one that failed to clearly define comparison groups and/or failed to measure exposures and outcomes in the same (preferably blinded) objective way in both exposed and nonexposed individuals and/or failed to identify or appropriately control known confounders and/or failed to carry out a sufficiently long and complete follow-up of patients. By poor quality *case-control* study we mean one that failed to clearly define comparison groups and/or failed to measure exposures and outcomes in the same (preferably blinded) objective way in both cases and controls and/or failed to identify or appropriately control known confounders

^lBy poor quality prognostic cohort study we mean one in which sampling was biased in favor of patients who already had the target outcome, or the measurement of outcomes was accomplished in <80% of study patients, or outcomes were determined in an unblinded, nonobjective way, or there was no correction for confounding factors

^{‡‡}Good, better, bad, and worse refer to the comparisons between treatments in terms of their clinical risks and benefits

Table 2.3 Levels of evidence

A	Consistent level 1 studies
B	Consistent level 2 or 3 studies *or* extrapolations from level 1 studies
C	Level 4 studies *or* extrapolations from level 2 or 3 studies
D	Level 5 evidence *or* troublingly inconsistent or inconclusive studies of any level

"Extrapolations" are where data are used in a situation which has potentially clinically important differences than the original study situation

For each case, we present the results concerning the effectiveness of the particular technique for primary snoring and OSA separately. In isolated cases we discuss the issue separately for children and adults.

In any case we tried to summarize the relevant data in tables. Each table displays the grading of the particular study according to the Oxford Centre for Evidence-based Medicine Levels of Evidence [535] (Table 2.2). Depending on the level of the single studies, the level of evidence for each surgical treatment can be determined as shown in Table 2.3. This level of evidence is stated in the last row of each table in the effectiveness part of each chapter.

A third chapter deals with the postoperative care and potential complications. We give pointers toward postoperative supervision and a survey of potential complications of the specific method. Finally, indications and contraindications are specified.

Identifying the Site of Obstruction

3

Joachim T. Maurer and Thomas Verse

Core Features

> In order to reduce pre- and postoperative risk and morbidity, sleep surgeons try to do as much as necessary and contemporaneously as few as possible. Therefore, the identification of the site(s) of obstruction in SDB is very important.

> Pressure measurements with one or more sensors, flexible endoscopy in the awake and during sedation, analysis of sounds during sleep, and various imaging techniques are used to identify the site of obstruction and/or the origin of breathing sounds.

For a long time, strong emphasis was laid on the importance of the topodiagnosis of the collapse site(s) in the upper airway, especially before choosing an adequate surgical treatment method. [663, 665]. An initial classification stems from Fujita, who differentiated the patient pool into three types in accordance with retrovelar, retrolingual, or a combined collapse site [227]. But, especially, CT investigations during sleep have demonstrated that this classification oversimplifies the dynamic processes occurring in the pharynx [321]. Yet still today, some studies advocate a rigorous preoperative topodiagnosis [529], but this postulate can no longer be held without reservations. This is due to the fact that the pharyngeal obstruction site is not determined once and for all. It can change first between wakefulness and sleep, second between the different sleep stages, third depending on body position, fourth postoperatively after upper airway surgery, and finally in dependence of a person's age [182, overview in 777]. Nevertheless, as surgical success has to be improved and should be far more predictable than today, topodiagnosis is still a matter of discussion and research. Therefore, the most important techniques of topodiagnosis will be discussed here censoriously.

3.1
Pressure Measurements

Increased respiratory effort in both children and adults can be recognized with the help of simple esophagus pressure measurements [745]. If these measurements are combined with the registration of the oro-nasal air flow, it is then possible to differentiate between central, mixed, and obstructive respiratory events [752]. Together with the demonstration of frequent arousals in polysomnography, the esophageal pressure probe provides the essential tool in the verification of respiratory effort-related arousals (RERA) [710].

Initially, single flexible pressure sensors were pulled through the pharynx in order to identify a pharyngeal collapse site [304]. As this method turned out to be too time-consuming, catheters with up to six pressure sensors were developed. With these sensors, it is also possible to measure nasal as well as oral airflow and to identify several collapse sites during a whole night recording. The multichannel pressure measurements using catheters of a diameter of 2 mm are well tolerated [521], affecting neither sleep structure [684] nor breathing during sleep [751]. Moreover, it could be demonstrated that the placement of the oropharyngeal sensor at the free margin of the soft palate under visual control was sufficient to differentiate between "upper" and "lower" obstructions. The distribution of the collapse sites during sleep could be reproduced in 90% of the individuals during a second night if there were less than 40% or more than 60% palatal obstructions [621]. However, "lower" obstructions cannot be differentiated into tongue base and epiglottic obstructions. Furthermore, when comparing the levels of obstruction as defined during simultaneous drug-induced sleep endoscopy, there seem to be relevant differences [679].

Skatvedt recommends pressure probes in the selection of patients for laser-assisted uvulopalatopharyngoplasty (UPPP) even though there was only minimal impact on the reduction of upper hypopneas [683]. In a very small sample of 14 patients, Osnes found a significantly better outcome after UPPP in the subgroup of 11 patients with mainly "upper" obstructions [533]. Tvinnereim attests pressure recordings before Coblation assisted upper airway procedures a better outcome even though there is no control group [753]. Other study groups are more cautious in regard to the predictive value, because postoperative shifts of the collapse site into a different pharynx level, both toward cranial and caudal, have been observed [303, 461, 663, 686]. In summary, pressure recordings are reliable, but evidence concerning their impact on surgical outcome is limited.

Several reasons have been discussed for the conflicting results of topodiagnosis with pressure measurements in regard to the selection of patients for palatal surgery. On the one hand, pressure probes are incapable of recognizing segments that are already severely constricted but not yet totally collapsed [831]. Suratt et al. [731] observed a shift of the obstruction site during a single apnea phase toward caudal. Furthermore, other authors have registered such a high number of retrolingual obstructions that they in principle recommend the inclusion of the tongue base into the surgery concept along the lines of the so-called multilevel surgery [685, 830].

3.2
Flexible Endoscopy

A fiberoptic endoscopy of the upper airway can be administered without difficulty on the awake patient in sitting and supine positions. But it must be said that the results do not correlate with the results gained during sleep [296]. Sleep videoendoscopy is a very sophisticated procedure and has to be restricted to specific indications [61, 567, 620]. Disadvantages of the method are, among other aspects, the reduction of the cross-section of the airway by the endoscope, arousal reactions due to the mechanic stimulus, visual obstruction by the phlegm, the simultaneous assessment of only one level of the airway, and the personnel-intense aspects of the procedure [296]. The Müller maneuver consists in the endoscopic observation of the upper airway during intensified inspiratory respiration with closed nose and closed mouth. While older studies considered the Müller maneuver as an identification method for the velar collapse type, and therefore recommended it as selection criterium for a successful UPPP [666], nowadays, this investigation is no longer regarded to have that value [60, 613, 825].

The flexible endoscopic assessment of the upper airway during pharmacologically induced sleep was first suggested for children [131], and later also for adults [130]. In addition to the disadvantages of an endoscopy during sleep already mentioned above, the employment of this procedure is further restricted by the fact that pharmacologically induced sleep cannot simply be equated with natural sleep [133, 435, 586]. Differences in collapse sites according to different sleep phases have already been mentioned. However, there is some evidence that at least breathing during pharmacologically induced sleep is not relevantly altered compared to natural sleep [636]. Furthermore, sleep endoscopy is able to convincingly display different patterns and sites of obstruction to surgeon and patient. Recent data suggest that the treatment plan may change in 40–75% of the cases if drug-induced sleep endoscopy is performed before treatment [280, 446]. In fact, it continues to be recommended for preoperative topodiagnosis [278]. Chisholm and Kotecha achieved a high success rate (90%) of LAUP eventually with tonsillectomy in 20 patients with moderate to severe OSA who were selected only if they demonstrated palatal or oropharyngeal obstruction during drug-induced sleep nasendoscopy [110]. Sleep endoscopy with gentle mandibular advancement was shown to be a good selection tool before mandibular advancement device therapy [332]. Yet we do not know of any study which was able to convincingly demonstrate that the surgical success can actually be improved by virtue of such a preoperative diagnosic procedure.

According to our own experience, videoendoscopy under sedation is helpful in assessing laryngeal obstructions. There is no other tool that can clearly show impaired breathing due to supraglottic or glottic collapse.

Another development is the digital analysis of fixated endoscopic images of the soft palate with the help of appropriate software. In an initial study, morphological differences were described in a pool of 121 primary snorers, 79 patients after LAUP, and 51 healthy control subjects [592]. It remains to be seen whether this concept will foster a viable method for the clinical routine.

3.3
Analysis of the Respiratory Sounds During Sleep

In principle, a differentiation between the retropalatal and retrolingual collapse site can be established with the help of a recording of the respiratory sounds during sleep using Fast Fourrier Transfer (FFT) analyses [646]. It was possible to raise the on-target rate of the UPPP from 52.6% [665] to approximately 75% [646]. However, results regarding other interventions such as LAUP are not unanimous [68, 431]. In addition, snoring sound analysis could only identify pure tongue base snoring and not distinguish between different levels of obstruction as seen during drug-induced sleep endoscopy [643].

In the U.S. such a diagnostic option for the clinical routine exists in the form of the so-called SNAP procedure [790]. The investigator has the possibility to send in an audio cassette with snoring sounds for both an FFT analysis and an acoustic evaluation by an experienced listener. The analytic criteria of the system are not open and the surgeon has to blindly trust the company. In Europe the working group of Osman et al. developed the so-called Glan Clwyd Snoring Box, an instrument to differentiate between palatal from nonpalatal snoring [529, 532]. There are some other systems on the market now, but none of them has proven its superiority over simple clinical examination as far as surgical outcome is concerned. Nevertheless, continuous research is performed in order to clarify the role of sound analysis as a preoperative diagnostic procedure.

3.4
Further Imaging Procedures

Many studies have attempted to establish the collapse site with the help of somnofluorscopy, radiocephalometry, computer tomography, and magnetic resonance imaging. Overall, the mentioned imaging procedures are only of limited use in predicting the surgical success of a UPPP [39]. Body mass and AHI continue to be decisive parameters.

Radiocephalometry is more successful in determining a retrolingual than a retropalatal collapse site [545, 601]. Accordingly, in the case of therapy failures after UPPP, it is possible to determine a more constricted retrolingual airway and a hyoid bone situated lower in relation to the mandible [602]. Both parameters also influence the success rate of nasal surgery in regard to the AHI in patients with mild OSA [659]. While radiocephalometry cannot generally be recommended as a routine form of diagnosis, it is certainly of use in patients with malocclusion or suspected retrolingual collapse site, and in patients who need to undergo surgery. An absolute indication is given before a planned maxillomandibular osteotomy [39, 284].

Fluoroscopy, rapid computer tomography, and functional magnetic resonance tomography have not been able to become part of the clinical routine, as they are too cost-intensive and cover a too short period of sleep. Another instrument in this context is acoustic reflectometry. A probe generates a noise signal and measures the reflecting sound using a microphone [181]. As the probe is flexible, it already has proven feasibility in sleeping sleep

Table 3.1 Techniques for objective localization of upper airway narrowing

Technique	During sleep	Quantification	Disadvantages	Clinical routine
Pressure measurements in the upper airway	+	+	SE, limited life-span of the expensive probes	+
Flexible nasopharyngoscopy	+	(+)	SE, mom	+
Analysis of the respiratory sounds	+	+	SE	(+)
Cinefluoroscopy	+	+	Rad, mom	−
Rapid CT scans	+	+	Rad, mom	−
Radiocephalometry	−	+	Rad, mom	+
Acoustic reflexions	+	+	SE, not commercially available	−
Rapid MRI scans	+	+	Mom (up to 1 h)	−

SE special expert knowledge necessary; *mom* detects only short periods of sleep; *Rad* exposure to radiation

apneics [183]. Unfortunately, the system is not commercially available any longer. These procedures remain reserved for specific lines of research [567].

Table 3.1 summarizes once more the advantages and disadvantages of the diagnostic procedures described above. Even though all these procedures have relevantly increased our understanding of and insight into the pathophysiology of OSA, their significance for daily practice is limited. We have essentially made the decision that in addition to the otorhinolaryngological evaluation, we only perform an endoscopy during wakefulness and sometimes a radiocephalogram. All of the other procedures outlined above are available in our center, but are in need of a specific indication. More research is strongly needed in order to specify their potential benefits.

Take Home Pearls

> Pressure recordings are reliable, but evidence concerning their impact on surgical outcome is limited.
> Videoendoscopy under sedation is helpful in assessing laryngeal obstructions. There is no other tool that can clearly show impaired breathing due to supraglottic or glottic collapse.
> Analysis of breathing sounds during sleep has not yet proven its superiority over simple clinical examination as far as surgical outcome is concerned. More research is requested in this field.
> Various imaging procedures have relevantly increased our understanding of and insight into the pathophysiology of OSA. However, their significance for daily practice is limited.
> We only perform an endoscopy during wakefulness and sometimes a radiocephalogram. All of the other procedures outlined above are available in our centers, but are in need of a specific indication.

Nasal Surgery

4

Thomas Verse and Wolfgang Pirsig

Core Features

> A clearly defined connection between nasal breathing or nasal resistance and sleep-disordered breathing does not exist; instead, the relationship is a very complex one.

> It is difficult to measure snoring objectively. The available measurement methods are cost-intensive.

> Many nasal appliances are available. But in contrast to the advertised promises, all of them have virtually no influence on the severity of obstructive sleep apnea (OSA) and are only partially successful in the case of primary snoring.

> The studies for primary snoring have not been standardized. Usually, the success is measured with the help of questionnaires filled out by the bed partner. The success rate is estimated to be about 40%. In the case of OSA, the success rate of isolated nasal surgery (correlated with the severity measured with the AHI) is approximately 10%. The subjective success rate in relation to sleep quality and daytime symptoms is significantly higher.

> Surgery improving the nasal air passage can improve the success of continuous positive airway pressure (CPAP) therapy; and in some cases, CPAP therapy is only made possible if this kind of surgery is performed.

Already in the ancient world, it was known that impaired nasal airflow may lead to sleep-disordered breathing. Hippocrates (de morbis, Liber II Sect V) described snoring, besides enlargement of the lateral nasal walls and croaky voice, as symptom of nasal polyposis. In 1581, Levinus [394] reported that mouth breathing in supine position causes restless sleep. In 1886, Krieg [372] successfully performed a submucous septal resection under cocaine anesthesia in an 8-year-old girl with obstructed nose, snoring, and attacks of suffocation during sleep. In 1892, Cline [113] published a first case study of relief of excessive daytime sleepiness following nasal surgery. In 1898, Wells [807] reported an increase of daytime vigilance in 8 of 40 patients after nasal surgery.

Still today, ENT physicians are often confronted with the expectation that the restoration of the nasal airway leads to an elimination or reduction of sleep-related breathing

K. Hörmann, T. Verse, Surgery for Sleep Disordered Breathing,
DOI: 10.1007/978-3-540-77786-1_4, © Springer Verlag Berlin Heidelberg 2010

disorders. But the relation between nasal airway and SDB is very complex and, at present, still not completely understood in every detail. Several excellent review articles summarize the current state of knowledge in regard to the role of the nose in the pathophysiology of SDB [590, 625, 778]. From these reviews, it can be concluded that nasal obstruction may have a negative impact on sleep quality; however, it can only be considered as a cofactor in the pathophysiology of SDB.

4.1
Effectiveness of Treatment

4.1.1
Effectiveness of conservative treatment

Currently, no scientific data exist in regard to the multitude of nasal oils, which are mainly offered over the Internet [460]. What have been researched are antiinflammatory nose drops [351], nasal corticosteroids [77, 128, 359], and nasal dilators [overviews in 625, 778]. The objective data are inconsistent. Some series reported a significant reduction of the respiratory arousals or of the AHI; but most series did not produce a significant effect. Djupesland et al. [157] even reported a significant increase of the AHI from 9.3 without dilators to 12.2 with dilators in 18 patients with UARS.

The subjective data present a more consistent picture. For the most part, improvements in subjective sleep quality, daytime sleepiness, quality of life, and nonapneic snoring are reported [overview in 590, 625, 778].

4.1.2
Effectiveness for Simple Snoring

Up to now, no long-term results exist concerning the effectiveness of nasal surgery in the treatment of SDB. Present data are mostly based on noncontrolled and nonrandomized studies, and do maximally fulfill a grade B of recommendation according to the criteria of evidence-based medicine. Some working groups provide subjective data regarding the impact of nasal surgery on simple snoring.

Summarizing these very inhomogeneous data which usually lack polygraphic or polysomnographic investigation, a noteworthy reduction or disappearance of snoring is reported in a few studies (Table 4.1).

Furthermore, Illum [316] reported that of the 50 patients who underwent septoplasty and conchal surgery 58% were snoring preoperatively and 41.5% complained of snoring 5 years postoperatively. From these few examples (often cited) and similar publications it is virtually impossible to estimate a success rate percentage of nasal surgery in primary snorers.

Nasal surgery may reduce the sound intensity of snoring by 5–10 dB [645]. Nasal surgery improves nasal ventilation, sleep quality, and daytime vigilance [202].

Table 4.1 Effect of nasal surgery for simple snoring

Author	N	Follow-up (months]	Method	Cessation of snoring (%)	Reduction of snoring (%)	EBM
Fairbanks [188]	13	12	Q	53.8	38.5	4
Fairbanks [187]	47	No data	Q		76.6	4
Ellis et al. [169]	126	6–24	Q	31.0	57.1	4
Low [425]	30	4–12	VAS (0–10)	50.0		3b
Woodhead and Allen [821]	29	1.5	VAS (0–10)		69.0	3b
Grymer et al. [245]	26	3–6	Q	50.0		3b
Elsherif and Hussein [171]	96	6–9	Q	50.0	39.6	4
Bertrand et al. [50]	8	12	VAS (1–4)		87.5	3b
All	375	1.5–24		41.9	85.3	B

VAS Visual Analogue Scale; *Q* questionnaire; *EBM* Evidence based-medicine

4.1.3
Effectiveness for OSA

Only few case reports exist on cures of OSA after nasal surgery [163, 272, 677]. On the other hand, already in 1977, Simmons et al. [675] reported about cases with no significant AI reduction despite considerable subjective improvement of nasal breathing and sleep quality.

Up to the year 2008, 14 studies on nasal surgery for OSA have been found which provide data on pre and postoperative AI or AHI (Table 4.2). Altogether, 272 patients were included in the studies. For the entire group the postoperative AHI showed hardly any changes compared to baseline. The follow-up periods were for the most part short and lasted from 1 [629] to 50 months [770]. In only two studies [361, 629], a statistically significant improvement of the severity of OSA after nasal surgery alone was found. In four other studies with a total of 30 patients, an increase in the severity of OSA was noticed postoperatively (Table 4.2), which was not statistically significant in all studies. We recorded a noticeable worsening of OSA in two patients with polyposis nasi after paranasal sinus surgery [771]. Despite the reconstitution of nasal breathing, the AHI rose from 14.0 before to 57.7 after surgery. Both patients developed excessive daytime sleepiness and required nasal continuous positive airway pressure (CPAP) therapy. Similar cases after septorhinoplasty have been reported by Dagan [132] and Balcerzak et al. [36].

Lavie et al. [388] reported on 14 patients with OSA who all underwent only septoplasty. OSA severity did not change after surgery, but 12 of their 14 subjects showed improved sleep quality in the polysomnography and reported less daytime fatigue.

In our prospective study including 26 patients we did not observe any significant change in AHI as well [770]. In contrast, nasal resistance (anterior rhinomanometry at 150 Pa) was significantly reduced after surgery ($p = 0.0089$) and daytime sleepiness decreased as well. The Epworth Sleepiness Scale (ESS) was ranked 11.9 before surgery and fell to 7.7 after nasal surgery ($p = 0.0004$). Despite a reduced nasal resistance, the severity of OSA increased in four patients. Using Sher's criteria [665] (reduction of AHI > 50% and to values <20), only 3 of 19 patients with OSA (15.8%) were classified as cured after isolated nasal surgery.

Table 4.2 Effect of nasal surgery on the severity of obstructive sleep apnea

Author	N	Follow-up	AHI pre	AHI post	p-Value	EBM
Rubin et al. [629]	9	1–6	37.8*	26.7*	<0.05	4
Dayal and Phillipson [138]	6	4–44	46.8	28.2	n.s.	4
Caldarelli et al. [89]	23	No data	44.2*	41.5*	n.s.	4
Aubert-Tulkens et al. [28]	2	2–3	47.5*	48.5*	–	4
Sériès et al. [658]	20	2–3	39.8	36.8	n.s.	4
Sériès et al. [659]	14	2–3	17.8*	16*	n.s.	4
Utley et al. [760]	4	No data	11.9	27	–	4
Verse et al. [771]	2	3–4	14	57.7	–	4
Friedman et al. [221]	22	>1.5	31.6	39.5	n.s.	4
Verse et al. [770]	26	3–50	31.6	28.9	n.s.	4
Kim et al. [361]	21	1	39	29	<0.0001	4
Balcerzak et al. [36]	22	2	48.1	48.8	n.s.	4
Nakata et al. [490]	12	No data	55.9	47.8	n.s.	4
Virkkula et al. [785]	40	2–6	13.6	14.9	n.s.	4
Koutsourelakis et al. [367]	49	3–4	31	31	n.s.	4
All	272	1–50	33.0	31.8		C

AHI Apnea Hypopnea Index; *n.s.* not statistically significant; *EBM* level of evidence-based medicine; *Apnea Index

Other studies report cure rates of nasal surgery for OSA between 0 [28, 771] and 33% [138]. In the literature, raw data for 76 patients with OSA are available. Using Sher's criteria the cure rate of these patients is only 17.5%.

To sum it up, patients may be allocated to two groups. With the vast majority of patients, the normalization of nasal resistance leads to a positive impact on the well-being and the sleep quality, however not on the severity of OSA. Even a worsening of the condition has been described. In a smaller number of patients, an improvement, in some cases even healing, of an existing OSA can be achieved. Reliable criteria to identify responders have not yet been found. Therefore, the prediction of success of a rhinosurgical treatment for an individual with sleep-disordered breathing is currently not possible.

4.2
Postoperative Care and Complications

A discussion of the complications and the specific postoperative follow-up treatment after rhinosurgery lies beyond the scope of this book. For this, we refer the reader to the specialized rhinological literature.

Yet in connection with SDB the issue of nasal packing needs to be addressed. In the case of primary snoring and mild OSA, nasal packing usually does not present a problem [84]. However, in the elderly patient with moderate-to-severe OSA (AHI > 30), the AHI may increase if nasal packing is used for epistaxis or after surgery. In older publications, even vital complications have been reported [93, 812]. The danger is especially prevalent in the first 6 h postoperatively [46]; therefore, the patient needs to be postoperatively monitored during this phase. Yet in the opinion of the authors, a monitoring in an intensive care unit, even in the case of severe sleep apnea after multiple surgeries on the upper airway with nasal packings in situ, is only necessary in individual cases. For the specific anesthesiological procedures in the case of sleep-apneics, see Chap. 13.

If patients with a preoperatively existent CPAP-obligatory OSA receive nasal packing postoperatively, then it is recommended that the continuation of the CPAP ventilation should be done either via a combined mouth nose mask (fullface) or via an oral mouthpiece. Dorn et al. [161] investigated the use of such an oral CPAP application in a pilot study including five patients with severe OSA (mean AHI = 54.5) whose noses were packed after nasal surgery. Oral CPAP ventilation proved to be effective and safe.

4.3
Indications and Contraindications

Unfortunately, we as yet do not know any factors which can predict success. Low [425] did not find any influence of either preoperative severity of nasal obstruction, preoperative intensity of snoring, preoperative collapsibility of the soft palate, or degree of reduction of nasal obstruction on the postoperative result. In seven of 14 patients with mild OSA, Sériès et al. [659] found that a radiocephalometry revealed narrowing of the airway space behind the tongue (PAS) and an increased distance from the mandible to the hyoid bone. Three months after nasal surgery, a comparison of those with and without anatomical abnormalities showed that those with normal anatomy experienced a significant improvement in sleep and respiratory parameters (AHI, Arousal Index). In patients with pathological radiocephalometric findings however, both indices remained unchanged after surgery. The authors conclude that the presence of craniomandibular abnormalities makes it unlikely that nasal surgery will improve mild obstructive sleep apnea.

In our hand the following approach has proved its feasibility. Dealing with simple snorers the prescription of a nasal appliance, in other words an internal or external dilator, may help to identify those patients who benefit from nasal surgery in regard to snoring. If the appliance helps the surgery will probably do as well [185].

In case of OSA we only perform nasal surgery if the patient subjectively suffers from impaired nasal breathing, and we inform the patient preoperatively that nasal surgery alone seldom cures OSA. Apart from that nasal surgery frequently is necessary to facilitate or enable nasal CPAP treatment.

Otherwise, palatal surgery seems to influence nasal patency and resistance. Antila et al. [24] described a tendency of higher postoperative values of midnasal volume in baseline and decongestion recordings indicating that the conchal area is more patent after laser-assisted uvulopalatoplasty. Using rhinomanometry, other authors found a significantly lower nasal resistance 3–6 months [347] and 18 months [805] following UPPP.

4.4
Impact of Nasal Surgery on Nasal CPAP Treatment

There are only a few papers reporting on the effect of nasal surgery on the requested CPAP. Apart from several case reports [452, 612, 817], Series et al. [658] reported on seven patients who needed nasal operations before they were able to tolerate the nCPAP treatment.

Powell et al. [578] designed a prospective, randomized, double-blind, placebo-controlled clinical study in 22 patients comparing the effect of an interstitial radiofrequency treatment (RFT) of the nasal turbinates vs. a sham operation. Both, nasal breathing and the self-reported CPAP adherence ($p = 0.03$) was statistically superior in the verum group 4 weeks after surgery.

Table 4.3 summarizes the current knowledge about the effect of isolated nasal surgery on effective CPAP. Because of the limited number of patients, the data have to be regarded as preliminary. However, there is a trend that surgical improvement of nasal breathing is able to reduce the required CPAP.

Convenient results were reported by Biermann [52] who retrospectively compared the charts of each 35 severe sleep apneics with and without septoplasty and turbinoplasty. All patients were on nasal CPAP ventilation. In the group of patients who underwent a nasal operation, the requested CPAP was 1.5 mbar lower ($p < 0.01$), and the mean duration of daily use was 0.8 h longer ($p < 0.01$) as compared to the control group. Similar results were reported in a prospective Spanish study including 182 nCPAP users with septal deformities [179]. Either medical or surgical therapy was offered to these patients. The outcome was that patients treated with septoplasty became more compliant with their nCPAP than those medically treated.

The influence of an increased nasal resistance on initial acceptance of nCPAP in treatment for SDB has been shown by two prospective studies using active anterior rhinomanometry [490, 727]. Sugiura et al. [727] studied 77 patients with OSAS who received nCPAP. The CPAP therapy was accepted by 56 patients. BMI, AHI, and ODI were significantly higher ($p < 0.01$) and nasal resistance was lower ($p = 0.003$) in patients who accepted nCPAP than in those who did not. Logistic regression analysis, with patient age, BMI, ESS score, AHI, ODI, and nasal resistance before CPAP treatment as explanatory variables, showed that nasal resistance (NR + 0.1 Pa/cm³/s: 1.48; $p = 0.002$) and AHI (NR + event/h: 0.93; $p = 0.003$) were significant factors for CPAP nonacceptance.

Table 4.3 Effect of nasal surgery on effective continuous positive airway pressure (CPAP)

Author	N	CPAP pre (cm H$_2$O)	CPAP post (cm H$_2$O)	p-Value
Mayer-Brix et al. [452]	3	9.7	6.0	No data
Friedman et al. [221]	6	9.3	6.7	<0.05
Dorn et al. [161]	5	11.8	8.6	<0.05
Masdon et al. [441]	35	9.7	8.9	n.s.
Nakata et al. [490]	5	16.8	12.0	<0.05
Zonato et al. [845]	17	12.4	10.2	<0.001
All	71	11.0	9.1	

n.s. not significant

Nakata et al. [490] performed nasal surgery in 12 males who were refractory to treatment with nCPAP. 41 OSA patients with nCPAP were used as control. Nasal surgery resulted in a significant decrease in nasal resistance and in a significant reduction of ESS score.

All cited reports agree that the requested nasal CPAP can be statistically significantly reduced by nasal surgery. In several cases, nasal surgery improves the patients' compliance regarding a necessary CPAP treatment. Therefore today, in most sleep medical centers nasal surgery is included in a comprehensive treatment concept of OSA [221].

4.5
Conclusion

Nonsurgical or operative reduction of nasal resistance significantly improves the well-being, daytime fatigue, and sleep quality of the persons concerned; moreover, the number of arousals can be reduced. The number of apneas and hypopneas hardly alters within the group of patients.

Recapitulating the rhinosurgical data of patients with SDB, the authors would like to make the following conclusions. The success rate of only nasal surgery for simple snoring is not available and the success rate for OSA seems to be much less than 20%. The reasons for the low success rates have been articulated by Hoffstein et al. [286]: "Neither the site of obstruction during apneas nor the site of generation of snoring is in the nose." As a consequence, we perform nasal surgery only in patients who complain of nasal obstruction and impaired nasal breathing either during wakefulness or during sleep.

Nevertheless, rhinosurgery occupies a valid position in sleep medicine in those cases where it is necessary to optimize a CPAP therapy, or to make it available to the patient in the first place.

Take Home Pearls

> For only about 40% of the patients, nasal surgery reduces snoring to a socially acceptable level. Nasal appliances may help to identify appropriate candidates for surgery.

> In patients with OSA, surgical improvement of nasal breathing has hardly any effect on the number of apneas and hypopneas and on snoring. On the other hand, sleep quality and daytime fatigue frequently improve after nasal surgery. This is why any nasal surgery requires postoperative sleep studies to determine the severity of OSA.

> Nasal surgery is commonly used to optimize a necessary nasal CPAP treatment. The reduction of nasal resistance increases compliance of nasal CPAP ventilation. Therefore nasal surgery should be included in a comprehensive treatment concept of OSA.

Nasopharyngeal Surgery

5

Thomas Verse and Wolfgang Pirsig

Core Features

> (Adeno)tonsillar hypertrophy and its surgical removal will be discussed in Sect. 6.1.1 in Chap. 6.

> In children, apart from enlarged adenoids, antral choanal polyps are the main cause for nasopharyngeal obstruction. In adults, case reports describe various tumors of the nasopharynx as the cause of obstructive sleep apnea (OSA).

> Topical nasal steroids have proven to be helpful in children with enlarged adenoids. Nasopharyngeal tubes are effective as well but are afflicted with minor compliance rates. Surgical removal of adenoids or other nasopharyngeal tumors is the treatment of choice.

> In adults, complete obstruction of the nasopharynx rarely occurs. The treatment is mainly surgery.

Cephalometric analysis of patients with obstructive sleep apnea (OSA), simple snorers, and normal controls does not show any significant differences concerning nasal structures [42]. In contrast, Donnelly et al. [159] found significantly reduced nasopharyngeal patency and significantly enlarged adenoids in 16 young sleep apneics as compared to 16 age-matched controls. In childhood, adenoidal hypertrophy is a common feature predisposing SDB. Pediatric OSA is equally common in both sexes [507, 799]. Today, there is evidence that the relative adenoid size strongly correlates with the severity of OSA in children [74, 261, 323]. A positive correlation between snoring and adenoid size was already described more than 20 years ago [281, 451, 695].

Apart from enlarged adenoids [836], antral choanal polyps (ACP) may cause snoring or even OSA in children. Only a few cases have been described with snoring of children as a symptom of ACP [103, 374, 528], and only three well-documented cases of pediatric OSA caused by ACP exist in the literature [66, 618, 638]. Crampette et al. [129] reported on two children with snoring suffering from sphenochoanal polyps. Gong et al. [238] described an 11-year-old girl with retropharyngeal lipoma with OSA (AHI = 13.9) and

K. Hörmann, T. Verse, *Surgery for Sleep Disordered Breathing*,
DOI: 10.1007/978-3-540-77786-1_5, © Springer Verlag Berlin Heidelberg 2010

growth reduction (BMI = 16.9 kg/m^2). Six months after successful surgery, BMI increased to 18.9 kg/m^2 (no postop PSG).

In adults, however, a complete obstruction of the nasopharynx rarely occurs. Piccin and Sorrenti [562] report on a 73-year-old female with OSA (AHI = 43, ESS = 15), obesity (BMI = 32), and nCPAP incompliance. Her retropharyngeal lipoma was operated. After 1 month, all symptoms disappeared (AHI = 12, ESS = 4). They cite three other cases with OSA because of a retropharyngeal lipoma in a 36-year-old man [5], in a 56-year-old man [152], and in a 64-year-old man [285]; all were cured of OSA after tumor removal.

5.1
Effectiveness of Treatment

5.1.1
Corticosteroids

Intranasal corticosteroids have been demonstrated to reduce adenoid size, independent of the individual's atopic status [77, 510]. To sum it up, there seems to be some evidence of an improvement in the severity of OSA in children treated with intranasal corticosteroids, but further studies are needed before such therapy can be routinely recommended.

5.1.2
Nasopharyngeal Tubes

Already in 1981, Afzelius et al. [2] reported about two patients with severe OSA cured by self-intubation with a nasopharyngeal tube during sleep. The tubes were individually fitted under fiberoptic visualization with a 3.0–4.0 mm uncuffed latex pediatric endotracheal tube that extended from the nares to a level 5 mm above the epiglottis. Within 6-months follow-up, no complications were found.

Nahmias and Karetzky [488] treated 44 patients with OSA with nasopharyngeal tubes. At 4-months follow-up, 44% of the patients still tolerated their tubes. The AI was reduced by 62.3%. Responder rates were given as 36.4%, which is higher than the rhinosurgical success rates. The reason for this high responder rate might be the splinting of the nasopharynx, which is not affected by rhinosurgery.

Masters et al. [442] described the successful use of a modified nasopharyngeal tube to relieve upper airway obstruction in nine infants with Pierre-Robin sequence, isolated micrognathia, Down's syndrome, and idiopathic generalized hypotension. The well-tolerated tube allows simultaneous use of oxygen prongs. The tube was required for a median of 6 months in children with Pierre-Robin sequence ($N = 6$) and for up to 15 months for the other infants. Apart from three infants who experienced regurgitation of feeds into the nasopharyngeal tubes in the initial period, no other complication occurred.

5.2
Surgical Treatment

Khalifa et al. [358] have reported that enlarged adenoids may be associated with ventilatory impairment which is reversible after adenoidectomy. However, the correlation between adenoid hypertrophy and OSA is not as obvious. Data on the not-always-sufficient efficacy of isolated adenoidectomy in cases of pediatric OSA have been reported by Nieminen et al. [507] in a controlled, prospective, nonrandomized clinical trial. Fifty-eight snoring but otherwise healthy children aged 3–10 years with symptoms suggestive of OSA underwent polysomnography twice, namely before and 6 months after surgery. A second group of 30 nonsnoring, healthy children served as controls. Twenty-one children with an obstructive AHI greater than 2 underwent adenotonsillectomy. Seventy-three percent of the children operated on (16/21) had had previous adenoidectomies, which had not resolved the obstructive symptoms, or the symptoms had begun after the adenoidectomy. The epipharynx was checked intraoperatively during the adenotonsillectomy, and none of the children appeared to have substantial regrowth of the adenoidal tissue. In other words, an isolated adenoidectomy does neither seem to be as effective as an isolated tonsillectomy nor as a combined adenotonsillectomy for OSA. Nevertheless, isolated adenoidectomy has been shown to improve mental performance in children [538].

In the cited cases of ACP, OSA resolved after paranasal sinus surgery. However, this origin of OSA is too rare to recommend paranasal sinus surgery as standard procedure for OSA.

5.3
Postoperative Care and Complications

This issue will be discussed in context with combined adenotonsillectomies in Sect. 6.1.1 in Chap. 6. Apart from the evidence stated there, no reports exist of OSA-related problems after isolated adenoidectomy within the peri- and postoperative period. Adenoidectomy is usually performed on an outpatient basis, the documentation of a standardized bleeding history prior to surgery is strongly recommended before adenoidectomy [651]. Most problems occur after adenoidectomy in early life and in obese children [261, 313, 444].

For pain control, diclofenac turned out to be superior to paracetamol in small children [33]. We have good first-hand experience with diclofenac, and with ibuprofen.

5.4
Indications and Contraindications

As stated in Sect. 6.1.1 in Chap. 6, children with severe OSA show reduced neurocognitive performance, which is reversible after combined adenotonsillectomy [209]. In the treatment of OSA, adenoidectomy alone is not as effective as combined adenotonsillectomy. Therefore, we prefer and recommend the combined procedure if OSA has been diagnosed. This applies also to children younger than 3 years, even though the incidence of postoperative complications is higher after tonsillectomy in this age group. This fact means that children under 3 years require more intensive postoperative monitoring.

Less is known about children who snore but do not suffer from severe upper airway obstruction. Recently, two controlled studies indicated that, compared to normal controls, children who snored but were otherwise healthy showed reduced neurocognitive and academic performance [57, 758]. In these cases without any other clinical symptoms of sleep-disordered breathing apart from regular snoring we perform an isolated adenoidectomy in our pediatric patients.

Take-Home Pearls

> Adenoidectomy is a highly effective treatment for pediatric snoring and OSA, justifying its use as first-line treatment. Often it is combined with tonsillectomy or tonsillotomy (Sects. 6.1.1 or 6.1.2 in Chap. 6).
> Postoperative risk after adenoidectomy is much less than after tonsillectomy, justifying its use for simple snoring.

Palatal Surgery

Tonsils

6.1

Core Features

> (Adeno)tonsillar hypertrophy occurs much more frequently in children than it does in adults. Therefore, this issue is discussed separately.

> Concerning simple snoring, only a few studies investigate the influence of adenotonsillectomy (ATE) on breathing sounds. Data originate in part from controlled studies; these studies document an efficiency of ATE for simple snoring.

> (Adeno)tonsillar hypertrophy is the most common etiology for pediatric obstructive sleep apnea (OSA). Accordingly, (adeno)tonsillectomy is often performed as first-line treatment of OSA in children. Cure rates are high.

> With tonsillotomy (TT) and interstitial radiofrequency treatment (RFT), less invasive surgical alternatives for ATE are available (see Sects. 6.1.2 and 6.1.3).

> Substantial tonsillar hypertrophy is a rare condition in adulthood. Data for simple snoring do not exist. In contrast, a strong correlation between tonsillar hypertrophy and severity of OSA has recently been described.

6.1.1
Tonsillectomy and Adenotonsillectomy

Thomas Verse

It seems certain that one of the main reasons for obstructive sleep apnea (OSA) in children is obstructive tonsillar hypertrophy [382, 765, 837]. It has been demonstrated previously that adenotonsillectomy (ATE) during childhood cures OSA with high efficiency. In adults, a strong correlation between tonsillar hypertrophy and the severity of OSA has been demonstrated as well [220, 846, 847]. However, it is not as clear to what extent tonsillectomy (TE) is effective in these latter cases. For this reason, the issue will be discussed separately for children and adults.

Furthermore, surgical techniques such as tonsillotomy (TT) [309], intracapsillary TE, and different interstitial thermal ablation techniques [495] have recently been (re)

K. Hörmann, T. Verse, *Surgery for Sleep Disordered Breathing*,
DOI: 10.1007/978-3-540-77786-1_6.1, © Springer Verlag Berlin Heidelberg 2010

introduced into the field of sleep surgery. These new developments give this issue new topicality. As interstitial radiofrequency surgery is a completely different operative technique, it will be discussed separately in Sect. 6.1.3.

6.1.1.1
Children

Effectiveness of Treatment

Effectiveness for Simple Snoring

Surprisingly, there are only a few studies focusing on the efficacy of tonsilar surgery for simple snoring. This might be due to the reason that sleep studies are much more difficult to perform in children than in adults. Many studies do not precisely differentiate between simple snoring and OSA. Another problem consists in the lack of established and validated objective measurement techniques to analyze snoring sounds. Table 6.1.1 summarizes the data and quality of studies focusing on (adeno)tonsillectomy for simple snoring (Table 6.1.1).

What to be mentioned especially is the work by Hultcranz and colleagues [309] who, in a randomized study, investigated the efficacy of TT compared to TE. In both study arms, snoring had not reappeared in the majority of children postoperatively after a year. Only two of the children continued snoring after the TT, both 6 and 12 months postoperatively. This would seem to point to an advantage of the conventional TE compared to TT. But the

Table 6.1.1 Efficiency of pediatric tonsillar surgery for simple snoring

Author	N	Follow-up [months]	Surgery	Method	No more snoring	EBM
Ahlquist et al. [4]	85	1–12	TE	Q	90.5%	4
Swift [732]	20	1	ATE	Q	95%	4
Agren et al. [3]	20	12	ATE	Q	95%	4
Hultcrantz et al. [309]	20	12	TT (N = 21) vs. TE (N = 20)	Interview	All: 95.1% 90.5% vs. 100%	2b
Helling et al. [274]	99	2–24	Laser-TT	Q	88%	4
Coticchia et al. [125]	10	1	ATE (N = 10) vs. AT + RFT tonsils (N = 13)	VAS 0–10	VAS pre: 7.4 VAS post: 1.0	2b
All	254	1–24			91.0	B

ATE combined adenotonsillectomy; *TE* tonsillectomy; *TT* tonsillotomy; *Q* questionnaires; *VAS* visual analog scale

difference was not statistically significant. Yet the postoperative morbidity rate in children who underwent TT was significantly lower in comparison with those who received conventional surgery.

Coticchia et al. [125] compared TE with interstitial radiofrequency treatment (RFT) of the tonsils, both groups combined with adenoidectomy (AT). Results in regard to snoring were similar, but the TE group suffered from significantly more postoperative pain and body weight loss

In a third controlled study, Stradling et al. [711] examined 61 children before and 6 months after ATE, as well as 31 healthy, age-matched children at the beginning of the study and 6 months later. In the group of the children having received surgery, the oxygen saturation and the movement time during sleep, as well as various subjective parameters, were normalized to the level of the untreated, healthy children. An improvement of intellectual performance and – in the case of a preexisting developmental deficiency – an acceleration of the maturing process were also found [107, 247].

Interesting in this context is the finding of Tzifa and colleagues [753] that TE during childhood does not reduce the likelihood of becoming an adult snorer.

Effectiveness for OSA

The number of childhood adenotonsillectomies performed in Europe and the United States has declined over the last two decades. At the same time, the indications for ATE have undergone a transition: while fewer operations have been performed for recurrent inflammation, there has been a percentual increase in ATE performed for relief of obstructive symptoms [627, 628]. The spontaneous resolution of OSA secondary to adenotonsillar hypertrophy without surgery has been reported at only 9% [4] within a 1-year observation period [4].

Therefore, ATE is the most common major surgical procedure performed on children [364, 544]. The number of papers providing data of sleep studies as well pre as postoperatively are to many to abstract them well arranged in a table. Various recent reviews underline the importance of ATE as first-line treatment for pediatric OSA [67, 391, 470, 668]. In the first edition of this book we calculated the mean surgical success rate in otherwise healthy children with pediatric OSA as 85.8%.

In 2003, in the form of a Cochrane evidence-based medicine (EBM) review [415], Lim and McKean reviewed 196 references concerning ATE for OSA in children. They did not find one single randomized trial, which means that they could not verify any results. Today there is more information; Table 6.1.2 summarizes all controlled studies available (deadline 1.1.08).

All in all, we found raw data of 356 otherwise healthy children who underwent ATE as an isolated procedure for OSA. All selected studies showed significant improvements in respiratory parameters postoperatively. In mean the apnea hypopnea index (AHI) fell from 12.3 to 2.7 after surgery. Apart from the data assembled in Table 6.1.2, it has been shown that craniofacial deformities are common in children with adenotonsillar hypertrophy, and improve significantly with surgical treatment of the airway obstruction [3]. Görür et al.

Table 6.1.2 Controlled trials investigating the effect of ATE on the severity of obstructive sleep apnea (OSA) in children

Author	N	Follow-up [months]	Age (years)	surgery	AHI pre	AHI post	Success (AHI < 5)	EBM grade	Control group
Stradling et al. [711]	61	6	2–14	ATE	3.6	1.5	No data	3b	N = 31 no treatment
Ali et al. [8]	12	3–6	6–12	ATE	3.0	1.4	No data	3b	N = 11 no treatment
Nieminen et al. [507]	27	6	2–10	ATE	6.9	0.3	77.8	3b	N = 30 no treatment
Montgomery-Downs et al. [477]	19	4	4.4	ATE	10.1	1	100	2b	N = 19 no treatment
Chervin et al. [107]	78	12	5–13	ATE	7.3	1.1	No data	3b	N = 27 no treatment
Coticchia et al. [125]	10	3	2.6–12.5	ATE	7.7	0.3	No data	2b	N = 13 RFT tonsils + AT
Tauman et al. [735]	110	1–15	1–16	ATE	22	6	71	3b	N = 20 no treatment
Mitchell and Kelly [472]	39	5.1	3.1–15.6	ATE	17.1	2.4	72.0	3b	N = 33 obese ATE
All	356	1–15	1–15.6	ATE	12.3	2.7	75.0	B	

AHI apnea hypopnea index; *EBM* evidence-based medicine; *RFT* interstitial radiofrequency treatment; *AT* adenoidectomy

[239] illustrated that adenotonsillary disease with OSA symptoms leads to right and/or left ventricular enlargement and hypertrophy which resolved after ATE. In addition, ATE was shown to have a long-term effect on quality of life in pediatric patients with sleep disordered breathing (SDB) (review worth reading: [229, 473]).

Guilleminault et al. [249] compared different pediatric surgeries for OSA in a retrospective investigation of 400 consecutively seen children. ATE turned out to provide the best results.

However, in those studies in Table 6.1.2 that provide corresponding figures, the success rate of isolated ATE is "only" 75%. Risk factors for persisting OSA are high baseline AHI [669, 735], overweight [471, 669, 735], and other morbidities like Prader Willi syndrome [549].

In some children, obstructive symptoms reoccur years later. Postoperative increase of body mass index (BMI) and overweight were recently identified as risk factors for recurrent disease [21]. In this context, Guimaraes et al. [254] described increased lingual tonsils after prior TE. In a follow-up study performed after an average 7.5 years, Guilleminault found radiocephalometric evidence of anatomic anomalies, particularly behind the tongue

(PAS) and in the mandible, as an explanation for recurrence of OSA [247]. Another reason contributing to the recurrence of OSA may be AT in conjunction with unilateral TE. In these cases, the remaining tonsil may undergo hyperplasia, as adenoids may regrow [671]. Guilleminault [251] reported recurrent OSA during the pubertal growth spurt in adolescents who as children had undergone ATE for relief of adenotonsillar hyperplasia and OSA and who had been free of obstructive symptoms over several years.

These findings show that children treated successfully with ATE for OSA should continue to be monitored, particularly those in families with a history of bite abnormalities, which reach their full manifestation during puberty.

6.1.1.2
Postoperative Care and Complications

In general, TE seems to be a procedure with low morbidity in the otherwise healthy child [810]. However, there are some reports suggesting that there may be an increased perioperative morbidity in some children with OSA after ATE [392, 455, 628, 640]. Risk factors are obesity, age below 3 years, Down's syndrome, congenital heart defect, asthma bronchiale, craniofacial anomalies, and cerebral deficiencies [669, 691, 701, 715, 733]. These children require intense postoperative monitoring for at least 24 h [392, 455, 626]. In some of these cases, a postoperative bilevel positive airway pressure ventilation within the immediate postoperative period has been shown to avoid the risk of reintubation and mechanical ventilation [220].

As minor complications, laryngospasm, nasopharyngeal hemorrhage, and transient airway obstruction have been described after ATE for OSA in children [631].

Indications and Contraindications

After several studies have demonstrated that children who suffer from snoring perform weaker in school than their nonsnoring peers [57, 240, 470, 758], and that these deficits can be eliminated with an ATE [108, 209, 210, 471, 477], a reevaluation process has begun in relation to when an ATE is indicated. Today, we receive far more referrals for an ATE than several years ago.

Based on the available data, we continue to regard ATE principally indicated for children with primary snoring.

In the treatment of pediatric OSA, TE, often in combination with adenotomy, belongs to the most successful surgical procedures, despite a lack of sufficiently large randomized studies. The cure rate of ATE as an isolated procedure in normal weight children lies at approximately 85–95%. We consider surgical indication given in the case of verified OSA even if no clinical evidence of hypertrophy of tonsils and/or adenoids impresses, since the clinical findings correlate only weakly with the extent of the functional obstruction [4, 72, 387]. Children with OSA suffering from trisomy 21 [436] or sickle-cell anemia [639] also profit from an ATE.

In a retrospective analysis of 400 cases of pediatric OSA persistent SDB was found in 14.5% after various treatment modalities [249]. Adenotonsillectomy was performed in only 68% of the cases, but showed the best results. Nevertheless, after ATE, there also remained some nonresponders. In a second prospective survey, the same working group [250] proved that multidisciplinary evaluations of the anatomic abnormalities (i.e., mandibular deficiencies, etc.) before surgery lead to better overall treatment results.

6.1.1.3
Adults

Effectiveness for Simple Snoring

Still no sufficient data exist in the literature documenting any positive effect of isolated TE on simple snoring in adults. Fairbanks reported one single case of complete resolution of snoring in an adult patient [188]. On the other hand, Tzifa et al. [754] considered whether TE could affect snoring, no matter what age and the indication of surgery are. One thousand people took part in their study and filled out questionnaires. The prevalence of snoring was 12.5–48% depending on age, mainly in men. In 19.8% of the cases, TE had already been performed, usually in childhood. TE did not at all reduce the likelihood of becoming an adult snorer.

Effectiveness for OSA

Since substantial hypertrophy of the palatine tonsils is rare in adults, there are only a few studies available (Table 6.1.3).

All of the studies listed in Table 6.1.3 are case series and furnish raw data. All in all, there are 95 complete sets of data of sleep apnea patients who exclusively underwent TE. Counting all ten studies together, the average number of breathing events per hour of sleep sank from preoperative 49.5 to postoperative 7.8. This difference is statistically highly significant ($p < 0.0001$). In accordance with the success criteria of Sher [665], this amounts to a healing rate of 80.0% in this selected patient pool.

Although the EBM grade of recommendation is low, it can be inferred from these data that a massive tonsillar hyperplasia is rarely seen in adults, but if it exists, TE for the treatment of OSA is almost as successful as in childhood.

6.1.1.4
Postoperative Care and Complications

TE is a standard procedure. The complications and the specific aftercare are sufficiently described in otolaryngological surgery handbooks. Specific aspects in the peri and postoperative management of patients with SDB will be discussed in Sect. 13.

Anyway one problem is worth mentioning. TE patients suffer from substantial pain within the first 10 days after surgery. Therefore, a sufficient pain treatment is mandatory.

Table 6.1.3 Effect of TE on the severity of OSA in adults

Author	N	Follow-up (months)	AHI pre	AHI post	Success (%)	EBM grade
Orr and Martin [526]	3	1–30	55.5[a]	9.8[a]	100	4
Rubin et al. [629]	5	2–6	50.9[a]	26.6[a]	40	4
Aubert-Tulkens et al. [28]	2	1–15	31.1[a]	18.9[a]	50	4
Moser et al. [486]	4	2–43	20.1[a]	7.5[a]	75	4
Houghton et al. [297]	5	1–3	54.6	3.6	100	4
Miyazaki et al. [474]	10	No data	14.0	3.0		4
Verse et al. [769]	9	3–14	46.6	10.1	88.9	4
Martinho et al. [440]	7	3	81.0	23.0	85.7	4
Nakata et al. [491]	30	6	69.0	30.0	No data	4
Nakata et al. [489]	20	6	55.7	21.2		4
All	95	1–43	49.5	7.8	80.0	C

AHI apnea hypopnea-index
[a]These study used the apnea index (AI)

In this context, Thorneman and Kervall [744] showed significant advantages of a basic oral pain treatment with paracetamol (750 mg × 6) and diclofenac (50 mg × 3) compared to a regimen in which patients received analgetics only on demand. On the other side, a potentially increased risk of postoperative hemorrhage after TE is discussed with the use of nonsteroidal anti-inflammatory drugs (NSAID). Recently, Krishna et al. [373] published a meta-analysis concerning this topic. Data of seven prospective, controlled trials including 1,368 patients were analyzed. Apart from aspirin there appeared no significant increased risk of postoperative bleeding for nonaspirin NSAIDs in this meta-analysis.

6.1.1.5
Indications and Contraindications

As already mentioned, unfortunately no evidence exists in the literature for the efficiency of TE in the treatment of primary snoring. Nevertheless, every otolaryngological surgeon is familiar with individual cases, in which a socially disruptive snoring has disappeared after solitary TE. In contrast to this stands a significant postoperative morbidity. Our own analyses have shown that on average our patients need analgetics for 12 days after a conventional TE. The literature reports a risk of postoperative bleeding of up to 6.1% [819]. We have become extremely cautious with the indication of conventional TE in the case of primary snoring as radiofrequency surgery and TT procedures with a lower morbidity rate are available today.

In adulthood, a massive tonsillar hyperplasia is rare. If it does occur, a TE (without any additional procedures) will be helpful in any case. From the presented data, we have come to the conclusion that we *always* recommend a TE in the case of a medium-to-severe form of OSA. Also, in the case of mild OSA, we see an indication for a tonsillar procedure if one site of obstruction on the level of the oropharynx is suspected.

Take Home Pearls

> ATE is a highly effective treatment for pediatric snoring and OSA, justifying its use as first-line treatment.

> Main risk factors for persistent or recurrent disease are substantial overweight, Down's syndrome, craniofacial deformities, and age below 3 years. This patient population requires intense follow-up care and postoperative monitoring.

> In adults with OSA, TE is always indicated if the site of obstruction is suspected to be at the level of the soft palate.

> In adults suffering from simple snoring, less invasive surgical procedures are recommended in order to minimize postoperative morbidity and complication rates.

6.1.2
Tonsillotomy

Thomas Verse

Core Features

> With tonsillotomy (TT), a less invasive surgical alternative to ATE is available.
  Terms such as partial tonsillectomy, intracapsular tonsillectomy, or subtotal
  tonsillectomy describe individual techniques of tonsillotomy.
> The technique employed (laser, radiofrequency, bipolar scissors, cold steel, or
  others) does not seem to be relevant with regard to effectiveness and
  postoperative morbidity.
> In comparison with conventional (adeno)tonsillectomy (ATE), (adeno)
  tonsillotomy (ATT) causes less pain, less postoperative weight loss, and less
  disturbance to quality of life.
> Preliminary results assume comparable effectiveness for both ATE and ATT with
  regard to sleep-disordered breathing.
> The most important and frequent contraindication for ATT is chronic tonsillitis.
  As this condition rarely occurs in young children, TT is of particular interest in
  pediatric SDB.

Within the last 10–15 years, a significant amount of research in tonsil surgery has focused on postoperative pain and recovery times [362]. Of growing interest are the recent reports about tonsillotomy (TT), specifically for those patients suffering from SDB due to adenotonsillar hypertrophy. There is no standard technique for TT so far. Various surgeons recently described their individual surgical technique. All of these techniques require significantly less pain medication and allow the patient to return far more quickly to normal oral feeding as compared with conventional tonsillectomy. Within the following chapter, we abstract the available data using the umbrella term TT.

6.1.2.1
Surgical Technique

The basic principle of all these techniques consists in saving the pseudocapsula of the tonsils by performing the resection strictly within the tonsillar tissue. As a consequence, more or less tonsillar tissue remains in the patient. Technical aids such as bipolar electro-surgical scissors [786], radiofrequency ablation [96, 174, 176, 306], argon-plasma supported monopolar surgery [302], various lasers [138, 149, 274, 308, 315, 322, 756], and the microdebrider [120, 150, 363, 418, 692, 694, 696] have been recommended so far.

Sobol and colleagues [692] compared microdebrider-assisted TT with monopolar electrocautery tonsillectomy. The former turned out to take over 4 min longer (16.9 vs. 20.9 min).

6.1.2.2
Effectiveness for Simple Snoring

Ericsson et al. [174] restudied 92 children 1 and 3 years after radiofrequency-assisted TT ($N = 49$) and conventional tonsillectomy ($N = 43$). The authors describe comparable effects for both techniques with regard to snoring, quality of life, infections, and long-term changes in behavior. After 3 years, two children of the TT group were tonsillectomized, one because of peritonsillitis and the other of increased snoring.

Hultcrantz et al. [307] conducted the first controlled study comparing laser-assisted TT ($N = 21$) with conventional tonsillectomy ($N = 20$) in 41 children with SDB focusing on postoperative pain and effectiveness. Results in respect of snoring and breathing obstruction were almost the same in both groups after a 1-year follow-up. The same patients were reevaluated after 6 years [308]. The number of children who remained free from snoring decreased from 40 after the first year to 25 after 6 years (11 TT vs. 14 TE). The authors conclude that both surgical techniques show comparable results with regard to snoring both in the short and the long term. In a similar controlled study [149], comparable results concerning snoring were achieved 3 months and 2 years after laser-assisted TT and conventional tonsillectomy. Another noncontrolled series of 36 children [315] described a successful release of snoring after laser-assisted TT in 91% of the cases. Follow-up time varied between 4 weeks and 4 years.

Koltai and colleagues [363] conducted a retrospective case series including 107 children after tonsillectomy and 243 children after microdebrider-assisted TT. Both operations turned out to be equally effective in relieving SDB.

6.1.2.3
Effectiveness for OSA

Today there is some evidence that TT increases quality of life in children and in teenagers with OSA both in the short and the long term. Smith et al. [689] used the OSA-18 questionnaire [693] and the Brouilette Score [76] to measure quality of life in 30 age-matched controls and 92 children with OSA before and after adenotonsillectomy (ATE; $N = 30$), isolated adenoidectomy (AT; $N = 30$), and adenotonsillotomy (ATT; $N = 32$) (EBM 3b). Quality of life parameters improved postoperatively in all three patient groups after surgery. ATE and ATT improved quality of life parameters similarly, resulting in a quality of life comparable with the healthy control group. AT, however, was less effective than ATE and ATT in this trial. Ericsson and co-workers confirmed comparable large improvements in quality of life in adolescents and young adults (age 16–25 years) after both tonsillectomy and TT in the short-term as well as in the long-term follow-up [175, 176]. The most recent study used the OSA-18 questionnaire 3 months and 1 year after microdebrider-assisted TT in 50 children [120]. The total and individual domain scores were significantly improved at both postoperative intervals.

Vlastos et al. [786] conducted a 2-year prospective study including 243 children after TT and 780 children after tonsillectomy (EBM 3b). Data on weight, patient satisfaction, and recurrence of obstructive symptoms were studied in each of 60 randomly selected subjects. Short-term satisfaction was comparable in both groups. Interestingly, in the long term the authors found that twice as many children in the TT group developed obstructive symptoms again, resulting in 3.5% of the patients who were offered a tonsillectomy. In this context a regrowth of tonsillar tissue after partial tonsillectomy (tonsillotomy) was recently estimated at 3.2–17% [96, 696, 756] in groups of 42–278 children (all studies EBM 4).

The only study so far [140] to provide polysomnographic data includes 29 normal weight children with OSA (age: 2–9 years). Exclusion criteria were obesity, craniofacial abnormalities, or other pulmonary, cardiac or metabolic diseases as well as a positive history for recurrent tonsillitis. All children underwent a laser-assisted tonsillotomy with adenoidectomy (ATT). The mean AHI decreased from 14.9 ± 8.7 ($\pm$ standard deviation) before surgery to 1.1 ± 1.6 twelve months after surgery. All children fulfilled the criteria of surgical success (AHI <5).

6.1.2.4
Postoperative Care and Complications

In a retrospective analysis the overall major complication rate after TT in 870 children was calculated as 0.009%, whereas the overall major complication rate (0.9%) was much higher in 1,121 children after conventional tonsillectomy [694].

The techniques employed (various lasers, coblation, radiofrequency, cold steel, or others) seem to be secondary factors in relation to the observed lowered postoperative morbidity. It seems assured that TT causes much less pain and weight loss as compared with conventional tonsillectomy in the postoperative period [139, 149, 150, 176, 306, 307, 363, 692, 786]. In this context Lister et al. [418] conducted a prospective, randomized, double-blind, matched pair, clinical trial. In 25 children the authors performed a TT on one side and a conventional tonsillectomy on the other side. There was a 100% correlation between the side of otalgia and the side of conventional tonsillectomy.

Ericsson et al. [177] examined presurgical child behavior ratings and pain management after conventional tonsillectomy and laser-assisted TT. SDB influenced children's behavior, but there was no relation to postoperative pain. The surgical method used predicted pain better than the child's behavior rating did. Interestingly, the nurses underestimated the pain experienced by the child. In this context, the reduction of postoperative morbidity and pain after TT is very important.

It remains to be seen in how far TT also reduces the risk of postoperative hemorrhage. The current trend points in this direction [149, 302, 315, 786].

Helling et al. [274] did not observe severe complications such as scarred tonsillar crypts and tonsillar abscesses in a survey compassing 826 children after laser-assisted TT with a follow-up of up to 11 years.

6.1.2.5
Indications and Contraindications

Yet at present TT is only indicated in the case of noninflammatory tonsillar hypertrophy. Chronic tonsillitis is still considered to be a contraindication [140, 242, 274, 696]. Randomized studies show comparable results with regard to quality of life for both TT and conventional tonsillectomy. The only trial providing polysomnographic data [140] as well points to a comparable success rate of TT measured against conventional tonsillectomy for pediatric OSA.

Apart from those for adolescents and very young adults (age <25 years), no studies exist investigating the effectiveness of TT in adults. Because of this fact TT does not play a significant role in the treatment of adult SDB.

Owing to the advantages mentioned above the author strongly prefers TT over conventional tonsillectomy in pediatric SDB. This applies to both diagnoses: simple snoring and OSA.

Take Home Pearls

> Tonsillotomy (TT) shows a similar effectiveness with regard to pediatric SDB as compared with conventional tonsillectomy.
> The intra- and postoperative morbidity after TT is much less than after conventional tonsillectomy, especially in children.
> Unless the patient's history is unsuggestive for chronic tonsillar inflammation, the author always performs a TT for pediatric SDB.
> Data on the use of TT in adults are rare.
> In adults we prefer conventional tonsillectomy due to the higher incidence of chronic tonsillitis and other affections of the tonsils.

6.1.3
Interstitial Radiofrequency Treatment (RFT)

Boris A. Stuck and Thomas Verse

Core Features

> Interstitial radiofrequency treatment (RFT) uses high-frequency alternating current to induce thermal lesions and tissue necroses. Bipolar and monopolar systems exist.
> In sleep surgery, RFT is used within the nasal turbinates, the soft palate, the base of tongue, and the tonsils. Submucosal scarring results in a stiffening of the soft palate and tongue base. Within lymphatic tissue (tonsils) and within the nasal conchae, RFT achieves an additional reduction in tissue volume.
> RFT of the tonsils can easily be performed under local anesthesia. Sedation and a perioperative antibiotic prophylaxis are recommended.
> RFT of the tonsils achieves a 40–75% reduction of tonsillar volume. Preliminary results are comparable to tonsillectomy in regard to reduction in AHI and subjective snoring.
> Within the first days after surgery, a swelling of the tonsils occurs. Pain killers are needed for 1–2 days. Complications are minimal.
> RFT of the tonsils meet our criteria of minimally invasive surgery.

Radiofrequency techniques use high-frequency alternating current to either cut or coagulate tissue. If used as an interstitial treatment, a needle electrode is inserted submucosally into the soft tissue. By applying radiofrequency energy, a thermal lesion is created followed by scar formation. Depending on the tissue that has been treated, this results in either stiffening or shrinking. To differentiate this kind of surgery from cutting radiofrequency procedures, we will use the term interstitial radiofrequency in the following.

Within the scope of sleep surgery, interstitial radiofrequency treatment (RFT) has been established in the treatment of the inferior turbinates [406, 759], the soft palate [577], and the base of tongue [575, 576]. Little is known about its use in the treatment of tonsillar hypertrophy.

The analysis of the current literature is complicated because of the lack of standardization in surgical techniques and its nomenclature. In terms of surgical approaches to the palatine tonsils, radiofrequency surgery is frequently used not only for interstitial treatment but also for partial (tonsillotomy) or total tonsillectomy (e.g., coblation). Those techniques will be discussed in the corresponding chapter of this book, while in the following sections, only interstitial thermotherapy with radiofrequency energy will be presented.

6.1.3.1
Principles of Interstitial Radiofrequency Surgery

The principle of interstitial radiofrequency surgery lies in the submucousal application of radiofrequency energy (low frequency radio waves) via a mono- or bipolar application needle. This induces thermal lesions and tissue necroses (Fig. 6.1.3.1).

In vivo, this results in a tissue necrosis and a perifocal edema, which can be nicely imaged in the MRI (Fig. 6.1.3.2).

Currently, a limited number of systems is available using different methods of energy application (mono vs. bipolar). The energy application can furthermore be either controlled or uncontrolled. The controlled procedures include among others somnoplasty (temperature controlled – Somnus, Gyrus ENT, Bartlett, IL), the Celon system (resistance controlled – Celon AG Medical Instruments, Teltow, Germany), and the reusable devices provided by Sutter (resistance controlled – Sutter Medizintechnik, Freiburg, Germany).

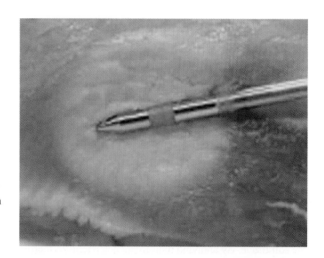

Fig. 6.1.3.1 Interstitial application of radiofrequency energy via a bipolar needle electrode (turkey hen meat). System Celon (RFITT^R, Celon, Teltow, Germany)

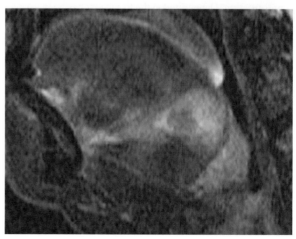

Fig. 6.1.3.2 Radio frequency lesion and perifocal edema in the MRI (TIRM-sequence)

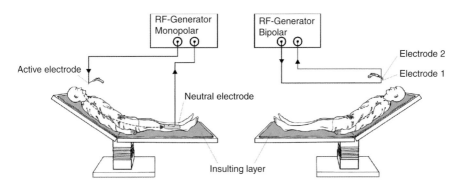

Fig. 6.1.3.3   Mono (i.e., Somnus) and bipolar (i.e., Celon, Sutter) systems for interstitial radiofrequency surgery

The Somnus system is the system that has by far received the most evaluations as it was the first system to be introduced in sleep surgery. Radiofrequency energy is delivered at 465 kHz using a specially constructed needle electrode and monopolar delivery system (Fig. 6.1.3.3). A thermo element is integrated into the tip of the electrode that continuously measures the surrounding tissue temperature. The tissue target temperature is set by the surgeon. While in the case of electrocoagulation, tissue temperatures of above 500°C are reached; with Somnoplasty, it is possible to generate temperatures significantly below 100°C. The lesion size can be regulated via power setting and energy input.

The Celon system regulates the energy input by means of the tissue resistance. It consists of a bipolar system (Fig. 6.1.3.3) with both electrodes in the needle tip, separated by an isolating element (Fig. 6.1.3.1). A neutral electrode is not necessary. With the help of the applied radiofrequency energy (300 kHz to 2 MHz), the water is thrust out of the tissue. As a result, the tissue resistance increases. If the system is used on a high power level, resistance increase rapidly, resulting in a smaller lesion. This means that for larger lesion, e.g. at the tongue base or the tonsils, lower power levels need to be set compared to the nasal concha or the soft palate, where smaller lesions are needed. A comparable method of energy control is used by the reusable bipolar probes of the Sutter system, using two separate probes in one needle.

Furthermore, a multitude of uncontrolled systems are available for interstitial radiofrequency surgery wherein the energy is applied under manual control only. This means that for these systems a certain measure of surgical experience is needed in order to determine the ideal energy input. Popular instances of this type of systems are for example the Plasma Coblation System (ENTec, Arthrocare, USA) or the Ellman system (Ellman International, Oceanside, CA). Unfortunately, almost no studies exist which evaluate the safety level of these systems.

6.1.3.2
Surgical Technique

In adults, surgery is usually performed under local anesthesia as an outpatient procedure (these systems can also be used to treat hypertrophic tonsils in children). Surgery is performed in a sitting position. In order to treat potential complications, an intravenous line is established. The patient may be sedated according to the patients or the surgeons' choice. We prefer Midazolam i.v. for sedation under monitoring with pulse oximetry and ECG.

A superficial disinfection may be performed, and then local anesthesia is executed. We use Prilocaine 2% with suprarenine (1:200,000). According to size, each tonsil is infiltrated with approximately 5 mL local anesthetic. In our opinion, due to the frequent hypersalivation, the use of a surface anesthetic delivered as a spray has not proven to be advantageous.

The technique is similar to that used at other sites. A needle electrode is inserted into the lymphatic tissue of the tonsil. Depending on the size of the tonsil and the technical device used, four to eight lesions are created per side (Fig. 6.1.3.4).

We regularly used the Celon system for tonsil reduction (Celon AG medical instruments) applying 7 W per lesion with a total amount of 4–8 lesions per side.

Regardless of the system used, the amount of swelling in the initial postoperative period exceeds the initial reduction, which means that tonsil size may be equal or larger than the preoperative size. Therefore, we do not recommend using radiofrequency techniques on an outpatient basis in patients with kissing tonsils. Tonsil shrinkage occurs between the first and third week after surgery. A view at 3 weeks postoperatively is shown in Fig. 6.1.3.5.

Like most authors, we perform a single stage procedure, whereas Nelson recommends a second procedure in some cases [495, 496].

6.1.3.3
Effectiveness for SDB

The calculated reduction of the tonsil size is specified as ranging from 51.1 [215] to 75.0% [497]. Pfaar et al. measured tonsil size with sonography and found a volume reduction of 40% [560]. Nelson described improvements in daytime sleepiness (79%), subjective snoring (81%), and in the Epworth Sleepiness Scale (70%) 3 months after surgery in 12 patients. These results remained constant after 6 and 12 months in the same population [496]. In children the same author found an improvement in quality of life parameters up to 1 year after surgery.

Concerning the effectiveness of isolated radiofrequency surgery of the tonsils for obstructive sleep apnea (OSA), only a small number of studies are available.

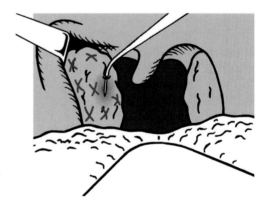

Fig. 6.1.3.4 Application pattern for RFT of the tonsil

Fig. 6.1.3.5   RFT of the tonsils. *Right tonsil*: preoperative situation. *Left tonsil*: situation 3 weeks after surgery

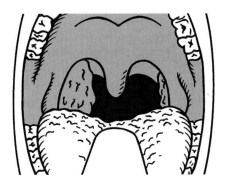

Nelson performed an interstitial RFT of the tonsils, combined with an adenoidectomy, in 10 children [497]. The apnea hypopnea index (AHI) decreased not statistically significant from 8.8 to 4.2 one year after surgery. Additionally, he found improvements in daytime sleepiness and in the obstructive sleep apnea-18 questionnaire score. A recent randomized controlled trial compared effectiveness and postoperative morbidity between temperature-controlled radiofrequency surgery and standard tonsillectomy (in both cases including adenoidectomy) in a group of 23 children with OSA [125]. The authors reported comparable results in terms of clinical efficacy. The mean RDI improved from 7.7 to 0.3 in the tonsillectomy group and from 7.6 to 1.6 in the radiofrequency group (total amount of energy: 13,681 J per treatment). Improvement of daytime sleepiness was comparable in both groups. Postoperative morbidity was less in the radiofrequency group, especially with regard to the return to normal diet.

Fischer et al. [201] performed multilevel interstitial radiofrequency therapy of the soft palate, base of tongue, and tonsils in 15 sleep apneics. All patients received 16 treatment sites with a total dose of 9,750 J (somnoplasty). The AHI significantly decreased from 32.6 to 22.0 after surgery. Using Sher's criteria, 20% were regarded as cured after the procedure. Nevertheless, the specific effect of tonsil reduction in this population can not be established due to the combined approach.

6.1.3.4
Postoperative Care and Complications

To avoid infections, we recommend a perioperative (e.g., cephazolin i.v.) and a postoperative oral antibiotic prophylaxis for 5 days (i.e., penicillin). In some cases, corticosteroids are needed to reduce postoperative swelling; nevertheless, we discourage the regular use of corticosteroids in radiofrequency surgery. There is no specific postoperative care. Patients are recommended to consume ice cream or to suck ice cubes to reduced postoperative swelling. Postoperative morbidity has been estimated by Nelson [495] and by Friedman et al. [215]. The patients reported pain for up to 2 days after surgery. Pain killers were needed for 1–2 days. On average, the patients returned to normal activity within 1–2 days or after 2.4 days respectively. Friedman et al. compared postoperative morbidity of radiofrequency surgery, tonsil coblation, and with standard tonsillectomy in terms of pain days, narcotic-days, and days before return to normal diet and activity and found a substantial reduction in postoperative morbidity in the radiofrequency and coblation group compared to "cold" dissection [215]. In a randomized prospective study of Pfaar et al. [560], postoperative morbidity, blood loss, and procedure time were compared between bipolar interstitial radiofrequency surgery and standard tonsillectomy in a group of 137 patients. The amount of tonsil reduction assessed with sonography was reported as 40%. Postoperative pain, dysphagia, speech problems, and intraoperative blood loss were significantly less in the radiofrequency group compared to the standard tonsillectomy group, and the procedure time was less in the radiofrequency group. Nevertheless, as clinical efficacy was not assessed, the significance of the study is limited.

Interstitial radiofrequency surgery of the tonsils is a safe procedure. Intraoperative blood loss ranges from minimal (<20 mL) to none. Up to now, other working groups and the authors have not seen any postoperative bleedings after radiofrequency of the tonsils [215, 495, 497]. Only Fischer et al. [201] described the formation of a tonsillar abscess. Admittedly, the lymphatic tissue tends to develop postoperative edema and the upper airway may be obstructed immediately after surgery. Therefore, overnight observation is recommended in cases of kissing tonsils and especially in children.

6.1.3.5
Indications and Contraindications

Interstitial radiofrequency surgery of the tonsils is a minimally invasive procedure with low postoperative morbidity resulting in a substantial shrinking of tonsillar tissue. In children, the technique competes with different tonsillotomy techniques. Both techniques, interstitial radiofrequency and tonsillotomy, have to be performed under general anesthesia. Both techniques require overnight observation. Controlled interstitial radiofrequency surgery is still an expensive technique because the majority of applicators are single-use instruments. Therefore, we rarely perform interstitial radiofrequency surgery in children.

In adults, the procedure can easily be performed under local anesthesia on an outpatient basis. According to the underlying anatomy we regularly perform combined procedures on the tonsils, the soft palate and in selected cases the base of tongue in patients with simple snoring and mild OSA.

Exclusion criteria for interstitial radiofrequency procedures are asymmetrical tonsillar hypertrophy with suspected malignancy, a history of peritonsillar abscess, and patients with a clear history of repeated tonsillar infections [215], the latter being a relative contraindication to our understanding. In moderate or severe OSA in adults, interstitial radiofrequency surgery alone is in most cases not sufficient.

> ### Take Home Pearls
>
> › Initial postoperative swelling may lead to upper airway compromise. There RFT of the tonsils should not be performed in kissing tonsils on an outpatient basis.
> › Volume reduction is substantial but less as compared to tonsillectomy and tonsillotomy.
> › Preliminary results in regard to sleep-disordered breathing are promising.

Uvulopalatopharyngoplasty (UPPP)

6.2

Wolfgang Pirsig and Thomas Verse

Core Features

> Since 1963, UPPP has been performed for SDB. Since 1981, it is used to treat OSA.
> The human soft palate has many physiological functions, which need to be preserved by a gentle surgical technique, saving the palatal muscles.
> UPPP is effective for simple snoring. Long-term results (>3 years) show satisfaction rates of more than 70%. However, short-term success rates are even higher. This means that the effect of UPPP in regard to diminishing socially inacceptable snoring ceases within the first year after surgery.
> For OSA, if the tonsils are still present, UPPP always with tonsillectomy is the surgical standard procedure. No other surgical technique has been investigated more intensively so far. As in primary snoring, the effect of UPPP ceases within the first year after surgery. Long-term success rates are about 50%.
> UPPP with and without tonsillectomy causes postoperative morbidity. The pain requires analgetic drugs for a mean of 12 days.
> Various complications have been described after UPPP. Most of them can be avoided by a careful surgical technique preserving the palatal muscles.

No surgical procedure for the treatment of SDB has received more research attention than uvulopalatopharyngoplasty (UPPP). Since the first UPPP for snorers by Ikematsu in 1963 [314] and the introduction of a more radical procedure for OSA by Fujita et al. [224], several modifications that aim at reducing the excessive tissue components of the soft palate mostly combined with tonsillectomy have been published. These early modifications of UPPP were mostly radical, indicated without patient selection, and did not address the often concomitant tongue base level and the lateral velopharyngeal segment collapse. This resulted in unsatisfying outcomes, several long-term side effects, and often a deterioration of the SDB. Recently, the first study of the long-term quality of life outcomes of a group of 49 unselected patients who underwent UPPP between 1980 and 1983 for OSA at Stanford University has been published [235].The details of the various complications and insufficiencies still present 17–20 years after a radical UPPP are rather shocking and will be discussed later.

K. Hörmann, T. Verse, *Surgery for Sleep Disordered Breathing*,
DOI: 10.1007/978-3-540-77786-1_6.2, © Springer Verlag Berlin Heidelberg 2010

In the last two decades of the twentieth century, most UPPP procedures (summary in: [186]) included the resection of too much velar tissue, which is important for functions such as phonation, and nonphonetic functions [199] as swallowing, lubrication, blowing, playing wind instruments, whistling, coughing, gagging, withholding a sneeze, or modifying the resistance of the mouth. To achieve these functions, a complex synergism of the palatal and pharyngeal muscles [300], of muscle spindles in the palatoglossus muscles and tensor palati muscle [375], of an intact sensory innervation of the palatal mucosa, and of small submucosal salivary glands is necessary. The velum with the uvula is especially needed for the transport of the mucus from the nasal septum into the pharynx [312].

In the last 15 years, histological research of the palatal tissues revealed an irreversible polyneuropathy in patients with OSA, and functional studies showed a significant impairment in sensory detection threshold for OSA vs. control subjects in the oropharynx, velopharynx, and at the larynx (summarized in [142, 504]). From these anatomico-pathological and functional data, one can conclude that any type of aggressive surgery to the velum in patients with OSA will enhance the preexisting polyneuropathy.

With this anatomico-pathological and physiological knowledge of the soft palate in mind, a tissue preserving technique of UPPP, partially based on Ikematsu's procedure [314], is presented here, which we have successfully utilized since 1996 in selected patients with SDB and with a minimum of long-term side effects [75, 569]. This is achieved by protecting the anterior palatine arch and the uvula in its muscle containing part.

6.2.1
Surgical Technique

UPPP with or without tonsillectomy is performed under general anesthesia with the patient in the Rose's position (supine with head hanging) and without an infiltration of the soft palate with vasoconstrictive additive and local anesthetic. Partial uvulectomy can be performed at the beginning or at the end of the operation. To do it at the end may mean to shorten a possibly edematous uvula. The uvula tip is grasped and pulled tonguewards. In this way, the muscle bellies can clearly be distinguished, and the excessive mucosa of the uvula tip can be cut off without touching the musculi uvulae. The uvula stump is sewed together with a 3-0 double Vicryl suture (Fig. 6.2.3).

The incision into the mucosa of the anterior pillar is performed with a semicircular movement in the oral fold of the palatoglossus muscle, approximately 2 mm away from the free edge, 1 cm to the uvula base. Then the fibers of the M. palatoglossus are dissected from the tonsil. Tonsillectomy follows, in which the posterior tonsilar pillar is initially preserved (Fig. 6.2.1).

The posterior tonsilar pillar is partially incised (Fig. 6.2.2), precisely at the site of maximum tension of the palatopharyngeus muscle as felt by pulling the posterior pillar with a forceps toward the curvature of the anterior pillar. As a result, the posterior pillar opens up in a "V" shape, which produces a lengthened posterior pillar edge to be

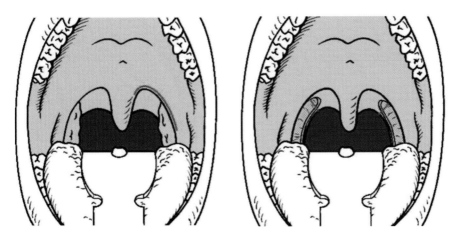

Fig. 6.2.1 Incision along the caudal edge of the left palatoglossus muscle, with scalpel No. 11 (*left*). Situation after tonsillectomy with preservation of the posterior pillar (*right*)

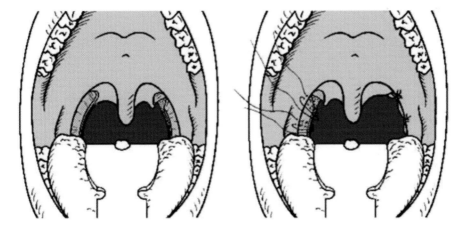

Fig. 6.2.2 Incision of the posterior tonsilar pillar laterally to the uvula (*left*). Suture of both tonsilar pillars with 2-0 absorbable, atraumatic thread (*right*)

sewed together with the anterior pillar (Fig. 6.2.2). Now the two pillars can easily be sutured together without tension. This double suture combines mucosa and musculature of the anterior pillar (1), of the lateral pharyngeal wall (2), and of the posterior pillar (3) with braided, absorbable, atraumatic thread (e.g., VicrylR 2-0 SH or 2-0 SH1 or PolysorbR 2-0 X). Usually three sutures per side are sufficient to close the curvature of the joined pillars leaving open the inferior tonsillar fossa. With these sutures, the posterior tonsilar pillar is moved toward lateral and toward oral. This results in a semi-elliptical soft palate (Fig. 6.2.3) with a functioning uvula. Finally, redundant mucosa on both sides of the uvula is removed, and the mucosal wound is sewed (Fig. 6.2.4).

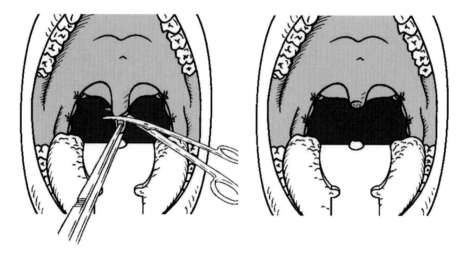

Fig. 6.2.3 Resection of the redundant mucosa of the uvula

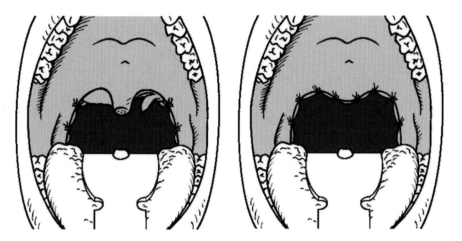

Fig. 6.2.4 Resection of minimal amounts of excessive mucosa on the left posterior pillar (*left*). Final result after adaptive suture (*right*)

Conclusion: This procedure of UPPP with tonsillectomy preserves all velar muscles and sacrifices only a minimum of velar mucosa. The careful adaptation of the mucous membrane folds guarantees a controlled healing of the wound. A less vibrating new velum with a shortened functioning uvula has been created with a lateralized superior posterior pillar and the horizontal edge of the velum more in an anterior position. Together with the tonsillectomy an enlargement of the upper airway caliber at the velopharyngeal level has been achieved without adding more damage to the new velum with its preexisting poly-neuropathy in patients with OSA. With this alternative procedure of UPPP there is no rationale for radical UPPP [568] (Fig. 6.2.4).

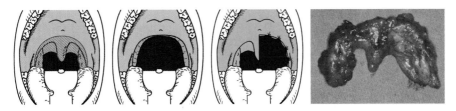

Fig. 6.2.5   Radical or aggressive UPPP technique according to Simmons et al. [676] (*left* and *center*). Specimen resected after Martin et al. [439] (*right*)

In the meantime, UPPP plus tonsillectomy according to the above technique has been performed in Ulm, Mannheim, and Hamburg on more than 600 patients suffering from primary snoring and OSA. As the main postoperative complication, bleeding occurred in 0.7% of the patients. Up to now, no long-term velopharyngeal insufficiency or nasopharyngeal stenosis has been observed. For a bit over 10% of the patients a follow-up nCPAP therapy was necessary. In none of the cases was the therapy impaired by an oral air leakage.

When employing more radical techniques (Fig. 6.2.5), as they have still been suggested since the 1980s, permanent velopharyngeal insufficiencies in up to 24% of cases [257], nasopharyngeal stenoses in up to 4% [344], and nCPAP therapy failures as a result of oral leakage [262, 485] have been described. The permanent subjective complaints as sequelae of these radical UPPP techniques even after 17–20 postoperative years are described by Goh et al. [235] and support our opinion that no indication exists for a radical UPPP today.

6.2.2
Effectiveness for Simple Snoring

Numerous studies have been published regarding the efficacy of isolated UPPP for primary snoring. Here also the definitions of what constitutes surgical success differ immensely; in the following, we therefore have to restrict ourselves to the compilation of studies with long-term data. In our understanding, only follow-ups of at least 3 years can be regarded as long-term data. The existent data are summarized in Table 6.2.1.

Two studies [282, 393] also include short-term results from the identical patient pool. Respectively 87% and 76% were classified as responders. This percentage fell in the long-term follow-up to respectively 46% and 45%. Accordingly Hassid et al. [270] recently described decreasing success rate with increasing follow-up periods.

Combining the values for "snoring reduced" and "no snoring" results in a long-term success rate of 73% for isolated UPPP in the treatment of primary snoring, based on the data of all 868 patients included in Table 6.2.1. But this figure has to be considered with caution, due to the fact that the diverse evaluation criteria are extremely heterogeneous. Accordingly, the success rates vary in the cited studies between 44 and 91%.

It was possible to objectively corroborate a reduction of the alpha-EEG arousals after UPPP in the case of nonapneic snoring [62]. Janson and colleagues [327] found reductions in daytime sleepiness and fatigue in 155 nonapneic snorers following UPPP.

Table 6.2.1   Long-term results of UPPP for primary snoring

Author	N	Follow-up (years)	No more snoring (%)	Snoring reduced (%)	No change (%)	Snoring worse (%)	EBM
Macnab et al. [432]	118	3–7	55	22	20	3	4
Levin and Becker [393]	69	1.5–7	46	11	43	0	4
Chabolle et al. 1998 [97]	39	3–7	44	No data	No data	No data	3b
Hultcrantz et al. [307]	30	5–7	8	77	15	0	4
Hagert et al. [259]	254	1–8	18	73	9	0	4
Pasche et al. [547]	100	4	52	26	22	0	4
Hicklin et al. [282]	201	2–10	19	25	36	19	4
Hassid at al. [270]	57	5	12	68.5	19.5	No data	4
All	868	1.5–10	29.8	43.1	29.4	8.1	C

EBM: evidence-based medicine

6.2.2.1
Comparison of Different Soft Palate Surgical Techniques

Chabolle and colleagues [97] included in the same follow-up study also patients after LAUP. The groups were comparable in regards to age, gender, and BMI. With 44%, the success rate (complete elimination or satisfactory reduction of snoring) was identical in both groups. But the general satisfaction with the surgery was significantly higher in the UPPP group than in the LAUP group. The reasons remained unclear. On average, in the LAUP group 4.2 treatment sessions (UPPP only one) were necessary, and the rate of unwelcome side effects was slightly higher. Nevertheless, the authors conclude that both procedures are suited for the treatment of primary snoring.

An objective analysis of the respiratory sounds during sleep furnished a similar success rate for UPPP and LAUP, both for short-term (2–11 months) and long-term (29–56 months) follow-up assessment [530, 531].

Lysdahl and Haraldson [430] prospectively performed UPPP or LUPP in 121 patients. Both techniques achieved significant improvement of subjective parameters such as snoring, awakenings, apneas, daytime sleepiness, and sleep spells driving at short-term follow-up (3 months). UPPP was superior to LUPP for all clinical effect parameters. Five to eight years after surgery, all subjective parameters except sleep spells while driving worsened with the years, with UPPP again showing better long-term results. Similarly, in the study of Hagert and coworkers [259] the conventional UPPP yielded significantly better results for snoring than LUPP.

6.2.3
Effectiveness for OSA

Only few prospective studies (with the level of evidence 4) exist covering long-term results of up to 9 years after UPPP. As with the other techniques, the comparability of these data is made problematic due to varying success criteria. Almost unanimously, all authors find a discrepancy between adequate subjective improvement of their symptoms and nearly unchanged objective sleep parameters after UPPP. Therefore, a polygraphic or polysomnographic postoperative evaluation is necessary after one to three years.

Every surgeon should study the excellent survey by Sher et al. 1996 [665]. The authors used as success criteria an AHI < 20 and a reduction of the AHI of at least 50% (or analogously: AI < 10 and AI < 50%). For the nonselected patient pool this meta-analysis yielded a surgery success rate of 40.7%. In the selected group with clinically suspected obstruction solely on the level of the soft palate, a success rate of 52.3% was found. For the most part, these data are based on short-term results.

Data concerning long-term success are summarized in Table 6.2.2 (worth reading review in [566]).

Table 6.2.2 impressively demonstrates that the effect of UPPP on the severity of OSA decreases over the years. As a consequence of these findings, we and other study groups infer the necessity of a long-term sleep medical control of the patients after UPPP. The employed success criteria are again heterogeneous. If one combines those data from Table 6.2.2, which use Sher's success criteria [665], this yields a long-term success rate of 49.5% for isolated UPPP including tonsillectomy in the treatment of OSA. Nowadays, one can rightly assume a positive long-term effect of isolated UPPP, possibly in connection with a tonsillectomy.

Recently Maurer [450] published a meta-analysis showing that a simultaneously performed tonsillectomy doubles the success rate of UPPP for OSA. Five studies including 269 patients ($N = 155$ with vs. $N = 114$ without tonsillectomy) were cited in this analysis

Table 6.2.2 Long-term results after UPPP for OSA using Sher's criteria of success

Author	N short	N long	Follow-up short (months)	Follow-up long (years)	Success short (%)	Success long (%)	Criterion of success	EBM
Larson et al. [385]	50	48	6	3.8	60.0	50.0	Sher	4
Lu et al. [426]	13	13	12	7.3	69.2	30.8	Sher	4
Perello-Scherdel et al. [556]		57	6	5 and 10	No data	52.6	AHI <10	4
Janson et al. [326]	25	25	6	4–8	64.0	48.0	Sher	4
Hultcrantz et al. [307]	17	13	3	5–7	82.4	69.2	Sher	4
Boot et al. [60]	38	29	6	1–6.2	42.1	31.6	ODI <50%	4
All	200	185	3–12	3–10	60.5	47.6		C

AHI Apnea Hypopnea Index; *ODI* oxygen desaturation index; *EBM* Evidence-based medicine

Fig. 6.2.6 Long-term survival of patients with OSA and different treatments [271, 349]

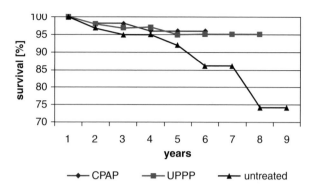

[60, 279, 456, 653, 704]. The surgical success rate was 30% in the patients without tonsillectomy, while it was 59% in the group with concomitant tonsillectomy.

In accordance with these results, in a group of 400 patients with SDB who had received a UPPP or a laser UPP, no increase in mortality was found in comparison to a control group comprising 744 persons [429]. These data may indicate a positive survival effect of UPPP surgery. Keenan et al. [349] contacted their OSA patients treated with either UPPP ($N = 149$) or nasal CPAP ($N = 126$) over a 6-year period to compare long-term survival rates between these two treatments. There was no difference between the two treatment groups (Fig. 6.2.6). Furthermore, UPPP for SDB turned out to improve the patients' stimulated long-term driving performance [265] and decreased the number of car accidents within a 5-year period after surgery [266].

6.2.4
Postoperative Care and Complications

UPPP is one of the most common operations performed for OSA. The anatomic and physiologic abnormalities associated with OSA pose independent risks of complications in the intra- and perioperative periods [135, 438]. Postoperative edema and respiratory depression enhance the risk of reintubation or emergent tracheotomy within the first few hours after surgery [122, 333]. The incidence of lethal complications is given as 0.2–0.03% [90, 356]. Serious cardiorespiratory complications other than death occur in 1.5% of the cases [356].

Intraoperatively, we administer an intravenous single-shot antibiosis with 2 g Cefazolin. Apart from this, antibiotics are only used in the case of relevant inflammatory complications. The severe pain occurring in almost all of the patients in the first postoperative days is treated with diclofenac and metamizol. However, frequently the administration of further, more potent analgesics becomes necessary. At any rate, basic pain treatments with fixed analgetic applications are superior as compared to regimen in which patients received analgetics only on demand [744]. Apart from aspirin there is no significant increased risk of postoperative bleeding for nonaspirin NSAIDs as recently published in a meta-analysis [373].

During the first postoperative day, the patients are fed via infusion, and take in tea and ice-cream as in the case of a tonsillectomy. From the second day on our patients receive

Fig. 6.2.7 Pain after UPPP, UPPP+TE, and LAUP.
x-axis: days postoperative.
y-axis: pain sensation on a visual analog scale (VAS) with the endpoints 0 = no pain, and 10 = unbearable pain

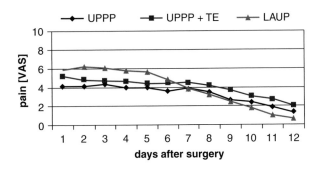

a special tonsillectomy diet. The threads are removed between the 10th and 13th postoperative day. The in-patient time varies between 2 and 5 days, depending on the ability to eat and the extent of pain. Usually, a postoperative intensive care supervision is not necessary after isolated UPPP [82, 464]. Performing the above-mentioned technique of muscle-preserving UPPP, we observed nearly always a pronounced edema of the uvula stump which caused more snoring in the first postoperative nights.

Most patients are able to swallow liquids on the first postoperative day, albeit under pain. For approximately a third of the patients, the pain continues to be rather severe until the fifth day (Fig. 6.2.7); for another third, the pain is comparable to regular tonsillectomy, while the last third of patients receiving surgery experiences virtually no pain on the fifth day. In the context of follow-ups 6 months after UPPP, so far no patient has complained about pain during food intake.

On the whole, postoperative pain after UPPP and LAUP is comparable in respect to duration, intensity, and consumption of pain killers [747, 809]. Much less painful is radiofrequency surgery on the soft palate [623, 718, 748].

Obviously, the new movement pattern of the operated velum during swallowing needs to be trained from scratch. Strongly carbonated beverages may cause gas bubbles to rise into the nasopharynx. Using a technique that removes the oral mucosa of the whole uvula and sews the tip of the uvula muscle into the median soft palate [565] in the long-term, in the case of our own patients after over 4 years, 40% of the patients complained of an increased viscous mucous production in the pharynx because of the loss of the "drip-stone uvula" for transporting nasal secretions. Our more recent technique, described in Fig. 6.2.4, does not lead to an increased mucous production in the pharynx. Clinically, a dry pharynx is often found. Some patients also experience mildly distorted sensations in the area of the soft palate, but no pain.

As with any tonsillectomy, postoperative bleeding during the healing phase is a possibility; though as a result of a careful velum suture, this has become (0.7%) a rare occurrence in our own patient pool. Despite double suture, on the fourth to fifth day the suture often breaks in the descending suture area; yet it remains intact in the horizontal part, which is crucial for the stabilizing scarring. In previous years, we often administered antibiotics (e.g., amoxicillin) over a period of 5–7 days; we repeatedly observed a stomatitis aphthosa in these cases. This has become a very rare occurrence since we have begun applying the antibiotic only perioperatively. Also, the fetid mouth odor setting in with the third postoperative day, which is so typical for tonsillectomy without mucous membrane, is usually absent in our patients.

Fig. 6.2.8 Velopharyngeal incompetence after aggressive UPPP

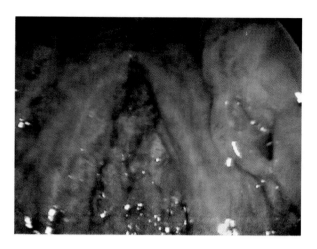

The dreaded velar insufficiency with rhinolalia aperta and/or entrance of food into the nose during swallowing (Fig. 6.2.8) have only been observed when the musculature of the anterior palatine arch is partially resected, which we could see in patients after velar surgery alio loco coming for revision surgery.

Another reason for velopharyngeal insufficiency is a too short and too firm soft palate. Such patients can already be distinguished preoperatively by virtue of the fact that water flows into their nose during the so-called Finkelstein test [199]. Patients are asked to drink water with their heads protruded from under a running faucet. In the case of velum sufficiency no water enters the nose. We use this test pre- and postoperatively in order to document the velar sufficiency of the patient undergoing surgery.

Since OSA cannot be cured by surgery in every case and due to the fact that even after a temporary postoperative normalization SDB can reoccur, soft palate surgery must always be performed in such a way that CPAP therapy remains an option at all times. But if the palate musculature is partially resected during UPPP, then a nasal over pressure respiratory therapy with the help of nasal CPAP can become very difficult, because the air escapes through the mouth. Mortimore et al. [485] discovered that after a UPPP with partial resection of the velum musculature no mask pressure higher than 13 cm water column can be nasally applied through the CPAP mask without creating an air leakage through the mouth. In the case of patients with an intact velum, and also after application of the UPPP technique described here, no air escapes through the mouth, not even in the case of nasal CPAP pressures of 20 cm water column. Han et al. [262] corroborated this observation in a prospective control trial where they found a higher CPAP failure rate because of mouth air leak in the group who underwent a more radical UPPP with removal of all of uvula and part of the soft palate than in the group with a less radical UPPP and the uvula partly preserved.

Equally dreaded is nasopharyngeal stenosis (Fig. 6.2.9). The following are considered as risk factors for the development of a nasopharyngeal stenosis: aggressive surgical technique, extension of surgery to the lateral pharyngeal walls, and postoperative wound infection.

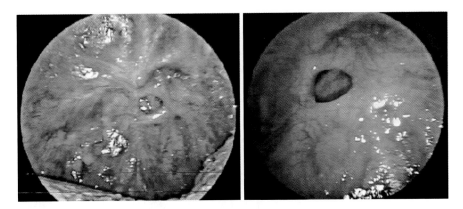

Fig. 6.2.9   Nasopharyngeal stenosis after aggressive UPPP

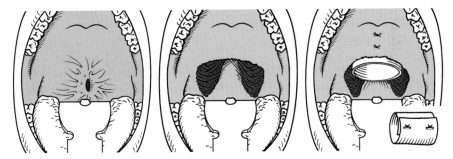

Fig. 6.2.10   Treatment of nasopharyngeal stenosis after UPPP. Stenosis (*left*). Situation after opening (*center*). Situation after insertion of placeholder made of silicon foil (*right*) (see small picture in the *right lower corner*)

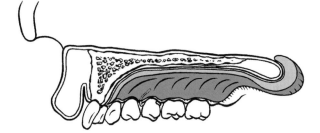

Fig. 6.2.11   Customized palate obturator with nasopharyngeal extension

The surgical treatment of nasopharyngeal stenosis after UPPP is difficult, and unfortunately does not yield positive results in all cases. Often several surgical procedures and intermittent insertion of nasopharyngeal obturators are necessary [231, 369, 370]. We prefer to open the stenosis with scissors as laser surgery may lead to deep thermic lesions and uncontrolled scarring. It is of importance to insert a placeholder in the wound to avoid recurrence of the stenosis. We create such a placeholder out of 1 mm thick silicon foil as shown in Fig. 6.2.10. This has proven to be effective, easy to handle, and cost-effective.

Other authors use other kinds of custom-made nasal obturators (Fig. 6.2.11) [231]. Nowadays, we regard the appearance of a nasopharyngeal stenosis less as an inevitable complication, but as the result of an inadequate surgical technique.

Katsantonis [345] has classified the late-term complications after radical UPPP in descending frequency as follows:

- Pharyngeal dryness and hardening
- Postnasal secretion
- Dysphagia
- Incapability of initiating swallowing
- Prolonged angina
- Taste disorders
- Speech disorders
- Numbness of tongue
- Permanent velopharyngeal incompetence (VPI)
- Nasopharyngeal stenosis

A permanent rhinolalia aperta has not been observed in connection with the muscle-preserving technique described above. Though it must be said that we have observed this sign of a velar insufficiency in the case of patients, who alio loco received too radical surgery (resection of palate musculature and uvula). Several patients, who had received a tonsillectomy with UPPP, reported a positive change in timbre and resonance of their voice. Patients with speech professions (French teacher; radio announcer for Italian and French) and two professional musicians (wind instrument players) experienced no difficulties in resuming their jobs after a 3–4 week interval. Nevertheless, the indication should be made with special restraint for this patient group [75].

Goh et al. [235] published the study with the longest follow-up, namely 17–20 years after a radical UPPP according to the technique of Simmons et al. [676] on 49 unselected patients (now in a mean age of 67.1 ± 10.1 years) who had been operated between 1980 and 1983 for OSA at Stanford University. They investigated the quality-of-life outcomes of these patients by a retrospective chart review and telephone survey. On a visual analogue scale patients graded the clinical benefits and complications of UPPP with tonsillectomy. All patients had improvement of snoring, EDS, and nocturnal arousals after surgery. There was deterioration over time for all three benefits (67.3–40.8% for snoring; 49–34.7% for EDS; 22.4–14.2% for nocturnal arousals). Although the most common complication of UPPP was velopharyngeal insufficiency (28.5%), dry throat (22.4%) tended to cause more significant problems. Complaints of foreign body sensations were reported by 20.4%, swallowing problems by 24.4%, and speech alterations by 16.3% of the patients. Although 43 patients had preoperative sleep studies, only 22 returned for a postoperative sleep study. Of these 22 patients, only one (4.5%) was cured as defined by Riley (RDI < 20) [610]. Six (27.3%) patients had deterioration of sleep study results, whereas 15 (68.2%) were not changed significantly. Of the 21 patients with persistent OSA, 12 (57.1%) developed cardiovascular problems. In the group without postoperative sleep study, 16 of 27

(59.3%) developed cardiovascular consequences, three of them were deceased at the time of study. None of these patients sought or underwent any other medical therapy after UPPP. In this unselected group of OSA patients, 49 patients had a mean BMI of 31.1 ± 5.6 kg/m^2 at time of operation, and 69.8% of 43 had severe sleep apnea according to the preoperative sleep study. We can learn a lot more from Goh's et al. paper which reports on an unselected group of obese patients with mostly a severe OSA who were only treated with a radical UPPP and tonsillectomy.

6.2.5
Indications and Contraindications

Foremost, UPPP can eliminate the snoring sound of the so-called velum snorer. But it is not that easy to recognize with certainty the velum snorer. Clinically, the velum snorer displays characteristic anatomical traits of his or her soft palate, such as a long and/or wide uvula with lateral mucous membrane folds, a salient posterior palatine arch (webbing) (Fig. 6.2.12), a short distance between soft palate and pharyngeal posterior wall, and craniocaudal mucosal folds formation in the mesopharyngeal posterior wall. The velum snorer is especially distinguished by a snoring sound characterized by a base frequency of 25–50 Hz and a multitude of overtones, which results in a regular and harmonic sound pattern [644]. The UPPP has no effect in the case of a "tongue base snorer," whose nighttime respiratory sounds are characterized by loud, hard, metallic, nonharmonic snoring with frequency amplitudes between 1,100 and 1,700 Hz.

The literature provides only few prospective studies for OSA, which suggests the following selection or exclusion criteria for UPPP:

- In general, obesity is a negative selection criterion. The limit for an isolated UPPP appears to lie at a BMI between 28 and 30 kg/m^2.
- A high AHI or ODI is a negative selection criterion for isolated UPPP. The absolute value is disputed; it seems to lie between 20 and 30 per hour. Above an AHI of 25, we pursue a multilevel surgery concept.

Fig. 6.2.12 Soft palate. *Yellow dots*: caudal edge M palatoglossus. *Green dots*: caudal edge M. palatopharyngeus. White line: so-called webbing = distance of the free edge of the posterior palatine arch to the caudal edge of the M. palatopharyngeus

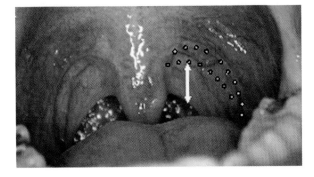

- Large tonsils that are removed with UPPP are a positive selection criterion. If still existing, we always remove tonsils in the context of a UPPP for OSA.
- Contradictory data are produced when radiocephalometric data are used for the selection of patients. A retrognathia or a micrognathia are negative selection criteria. In these cases the obstruction often lies behind the tongue.
- A positive Müller maneuver (provoking of a collapse during inspiration against the artificially closed airway) in the context of the nasopharyngeal videoendoscopy has no predictive values; therefore, we do not employ it.
- Even sleep endoscopy which is able to add to better patient selection in certain cases of SDB does not guarantee a positive outcome of UPPP although the finding of obstruction is found on palate-uvula level [279].

An analysis of the literature data yields the following exclusion criteria for an isolated UPPP, which in principle we already formulated in 1990 based on our own results [774]:

- Chronic heart and/or lung diseases
- Neurological/psychiatric illnesses in need of treatment
- High anesthesia risk
- Obesity; BMI > 30 kg/m^2
- Chronic alcoholism
- Soporific drug abuse
- Severity of OSA; AHI > 25
- Severe bite misalignment
- Narrow pharyngeal airway behind the tongue
- Large distance between lower edge of mandibula to the hyoid
- Certain craniofacial deformities
- Too short soft palate

If indicated, we perform UPPP and T combined with rhinosurgery in the majority of patients. In these cases, the patient is forced to breathe through the mouth during the nasal packing (1–2 days). This leads to a heightened postoperative morbidity; but this is justifiable in the majority of cases. These patients need to be supervised, e.g., in the wake-up room immediately postoperatively (i.e., during the first 3–6 h after surgery). A supervision in an intensive care unit is usually not necessary [464]. Yet the issue of heightened postoperative morbidity should be discussed with the patient preoperatively, since in principle it is of course possible to perform nasal surgery and UPPP separately.

In the case of an AHI of above 25, we no longer perform isolated soft palate surgery. The experience of diminishing success rates with increased initial AHI has shown that in these cases the complete airway is affected by the disease. We therefore prefer a multilevel surgery concept for moderate and severe OSA, in which UPPP or its newer modifications with tonsillectomy play a central role (Chap. 10).

In children, UPPP is indicated only in exceptional cases as, for example, neurologically impaired children, craniofacial deformities, or Down's syndrome [1, 310, 352, 365, 714]. We have only limited but positive experience in individual cases of M. Down and Pierre Robin Sequence.

As until today we have no safe tool to predict the outcome of UPPP in the individual patients they should be informed that UPPP alone can improve, not change or deteriorate their SDB. Therefore a postoperative sleep study is obligatory.

> **Take Home Pearls**
>
> › UPPP is the surgical standard procedure for OSA if the site of obstruction is located at the level of the soft palate. If still present, tonsils need to be removed.
> › For primary snoring less invasive techniques provide comparable results and should therefore be favored.
> › There is no rationale for aggressive UPPP. Aggressive UPPP does not improve surgical success rates but definitely does increase complication rates.
> › Postoperative risk increases with severity of the OSA, BMI and accompanying other diseases. The surgeon must be aware of a possibly difficult intubation.

Recent Modifications of Uvulopalatopharyngoplasty

6.3

Wolfgang Pirsig and Thomas Verse

Core Features

> Modifications of UPPP can be divided in two groups: the so-called uvulopalatal flaps and those techniques extending to lateral pharynx.
> Uvulopalatal flaps are simple techniques that can be performed very quickly. These are used as alternatives to conventional UPPP. Short-term results are comparable to conventional UPPP. Long-term data do not exist so far.
> Techniques addressing the lateral pharynx are recommended as second-line treatments after unsuccessful UPPP. First short-term data are promising.

In our millennium, several modifications of UPPP have been published, some of which have proven to be more effective in reducing pathological sleep parameters of patients with OSA on the short-term follow-up. There is the group performing uvulopalatal flaps [213, 293, 397, 502, 573] and the group including the lateral pharynx in their surgical concepts [87, 88, 540].

6.3.1
Surgical Technique

6.3.1.1
Uvuloplatal Flap

Uvulopalatopharyngoplasty (UPPP) is a relatively time-consuming surgical procedure, even in the case of sufficient surgical experience and practice. This fact has contributed to the interest generated by a modification, the uvulopalatal flap, developed at Stanford [573]. Today, we use a modification of the original technique with lateral extension to the tonsil bed, which impresses by its simple and fast mode of executing [293].

The preparations for surgery are identical to those described for UPPP. Surgery is performed under general anesthesia. The patient lies with reclined head, as in the case of

K. Hörmann, T. Verse, *Surgery for Sleep Disordered Breathing*,
DOI: 10.1007/978-3-540-77786-1_6.3, © Springer Verlag Berlin Heidelberg 2010

Fig. 6.3.1 Situation after tonsillectomy. Bilateral incisions into the soft palate on both sides of the uvula

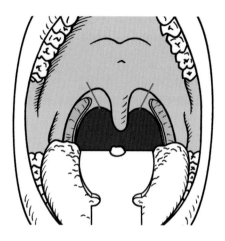

tonsillectomy. In the case of OSA, the first step is always a gentle tonsillectomy (Fig. 6.3.1). In the case of patients who have already undergone tonsillectomy, there is no need for time-consuming opening of the scarring between the anterior and posterior palatine arch as with the UPPP technique. After this, incisions into the soft palate are made bilaterally on both sides of the uvula, as shown in Fig. 6.3.1.

At this point, the classic UPPP technique is left behind. The tip of the uvula is grasped with surgical tweezers, and excessive mucous membrane is resected (Fig. 6.3.2).

The now exposed muscle tip of the uvula is also with the surgical tweezers folded toward cranial. The opening of the velopharyngeal flap is assessed, and the necessary extent of the uvulopalatal flap determined (Fig. 6.3.3). Powell et al. recommend marking the correct position of the uvulopalatal flap on the anterior side of the soft palate with tincture [573]. As a next step, in the marked area, the mucosa of the anterior palatine arch, the fat, and the underlying salivary glands are removed under careful preservation of the muscles (Fig. 6.3.3). The removal of the complete soft tissue above the

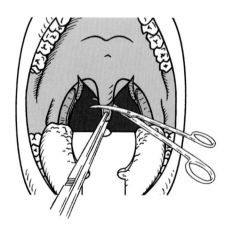

Fig. 6.3.2 Shortening of the uvula

musculature is crucial as only this can prevent the uvulopalatal flap from becoming too thick. A too thick uvulopalatal flap may lead to dysphagia, articulation impediments, and obstructed breathing.

Now, the uvula is loosely folded into the defect and worked in with atraumatic, resorbable suture material. We basically recommend a double suture with a thread thickness of 2.0 or 3.0, depending on the dimension of the soft palate. As a rule, 5 sutures are sufficient. This results in an uvulopalatal flap, which in its thickness is in accordance with the level of the surrounding soft palate (Fig. 6.3.4). Finally, lateralization of the posterior palatine arch is achieved by sewing together of the two palatine arches, comparable to the technique employed for UPPP (Fig. 6.3.4).

The lateralization is achieved by deep intra-muscular sutures (2.0 resorbable thread, atraumatic needle), which are run through the posterior palatine arch (M. palatopharyngeus), through the base of the tonsil bed, and through the anterior palatine arch (M. palatoglossus).

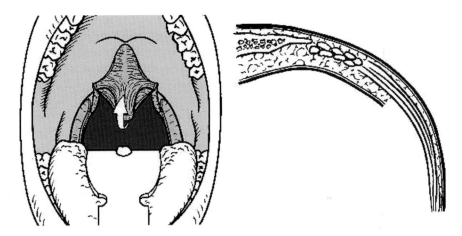

Fig. 6.3.3 Identifying the correct size of the flap by rotating the uvula upwards (*left*). Removal of mucosa, fat, and salivary glands in the estimated area. Lateral aspect of the soft palate (*right*)

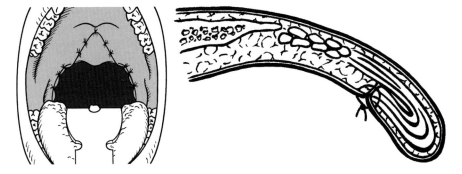

Fig. 6.3.4 Postoperative situation. Frontal aspect (*left*). Soft palate, lateral aspect (*right*)

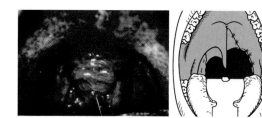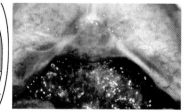

Fig. 6.3.5   Uvulopalatal flap (Mannheim technique). Preoperative finding (*left*). (*Middle*) Diagram comparing preoperative (*left side*) and postoperative (*right side*) situation. (*Right*) Situation 6 weeks postoperatively

We always execute a double suture of the palatine arch; in our experience, a double suture significantly delays a tearing of these sutures. The aim of the lateralization is to prevent a potential traverse folding of the pharyngeal posterior wall. Figure 6.3.5 compares the pre- and postoperative situation.

In 2003, Li et al. [400] published their modification of an extended uvulopalatal flap (EUPF). Under general anesthesia and after bilateral tonsillectomy, the retropalatal space in both the anteroposterior and lateral dimensions is expanded by incisions of the supra-tonsillar fossae. Mucosa and submucosal fat are removed with preservation of the muscle, and the tip of the uvula is excised. From a point in the midline approximately 5–10 mm below the posterior end of the hard palate, a V-shaped incision is made to the upper poles of the bilateral tonsillar fossae. The denuded uvula and soft palate now comprise the EUPF, which is imbricated and sutured to the residual mucosa of the soft palate using 2-0 Vicryl. The new tonsillar fossa is closed to decrease the dead space. The anterior and posterior pillars are approximated using mattress sutures with maximal lateralization.

For treating patients with SDB and with those who had their tonsils already removed, Friedman et al. [213] presented the Z-palatoplasty (ZPP) in 2004. After outlining two adja-cent flaps on the palate – together they look butterfly-shaped – only the mucosa of their anterior aspect is removed. Then, the two flaps are separated from each other by splitting the palatal segment down the midline. A two-layered closure brings the midline all the way to the anterolateral margin of the palate. The final result creates 3–4 cm of distance between the posterior pharynx and the palate. In addition, the lateral dimension of the palate is usually doubled to approximately 4 cm. A uvula-similar structure is not visible although both the uvula muscles are preserved within the new palate. In addition, all patients also underwent tongue base radiofrequency with the application of a total of 4,500 J in monthly intervals.

6.3.1.2
Lateral Pharyngoplasty

In 2003, Cahali [88] introduced the lateral pharyngoplasty (LP) procedure for treating OSA in adults with the intention to splint the lateral pharyngeal muscular walls. These regions, thick-ened and exceedingly collapsible during respiration in these patients, have a key role in the pathophysiology of OSA. After bilateral tonsillectomy the superior pharyngeal constrictor muscle within the tonsillar fossa (outer pharyngeal muscular layer) is sectioned and sutured to the anterior pillar to provide support to the lateral pharyngeal wall. Then, a Z-plasty between the lateral free margin of the soft palate and the palatopharyngeus muscle is performed, thus providing lateral support to the soft palate. In addition, a partial uvulectomy is done. Therefore, the LP supports the pharynx through postoperative retraction of the inner and outer pharyngeal muscular layers.

Pang and Woodson modified Cahali's technique and developed the expansion sphincter pharyngoplasty (ESP) for a selected group of OSA patients with small tonsils, Friedman [220] stage II or III, and lateral pharyngeal wall collapse noted on endoscopic examination [540]. Their principle is to isolate the palatopharyngeus muscle as the main part of the lateral pharyngeal wall bulk and rotate this muscle superoanterolaterally, to create the lateral wall tension and remove the bulk of the lateral pharyngeal walls. After bilateral tonsillectomy, the inferior end of the palatopharyngeal muscle is transected horizontally and rotated superolaterally with a figure 8 suture, through the muscle bulk itself, with a 3-0 resorbable suture with round body needle. The muscle is sufficiently isolated and left with its posterior surface partially attached to the posterior horizontal superior pharyngeal constrictor muscles. A superolateral incision is made on the anterior pillar arch bilaterally, identifying the arching fibers of the palatoglossus muscle. The palatopharyngeus muscle is then attached to the arching fibers of the soft palate anteriorly with a figure 8 suture, through the muscle bulk itself, with 3-0 resorbable sutures. After a partial uvulectomy, the anterior and posterior tonsillar pillars are approximated with resorbable sutures.

6.3.2
Effectiveness for SDB

Concerning the effectiveness of the UPPP modifications for treatment of sleep-related breathing disorders only few data have been published. Only one publication addresses the therapy of primary snoring [502]. Sixty-five patients received as sole surgical procedure an uvulopalatal flap. At follow-up 14 months postoperatively, both a significant subjective and objective reduction of the snoring sounds could be demonstrated. The polysomnography showed an unchanged RDI (preoperatively 3.2 ± 1.2 vs. 3.0 ± 1.8 postoperatively).

More data exist concerning the efficacy of the recent UPPP modifications for the treatment of OSA (Table 6.3.1). In an initial publication, 80 patients were diagnosed prospectively (EBM 3b) [573]; 59 of them received an uvulopalatal flap; the remaining 21 underwent a conventional UPPP. The results in regard to the polysomnographic and subjective findings were comparable in both groups. But it must be said that in 84% of the cases additional surgery on the hypopharynx was performed in the same session. Therefore, this study does not allow for inferences regarding the isolated effect of the uvulopalatal flap.

Our initial evaluation of 30 patients [293] who received an isolated uvulopalatal flap according to the technique described above resulted in a statistically significant reduction of the AHI (Table 6.3.1). Further significant improvements were found in the objectively determined snoring index (45.3 vs. 21.0) and in the minimal oxygen saturation (79.2% vs. 87.5%).

Table 6.3.1   Effectiveness of uvulopalatal flap and other recent modifications of UPPP for OSA

Author	N	Technique	Add. proc.	Follow-up (months)	AHI pre	AHI post	Success (%)	ESS pre	ESS post	EBM
Hörmann et al. [292]	30	Flap	None	1.5	19.2	8.2	46.7	5.5	3.0	4
Neruntarat [497]	31	Flap	GA HS	8.0	48.2	14.5	73.7	14.9	8.2	4
Neruntarat [499]	32	Flap	HS	8.1	44.5	15.2	78.0	14.1	8.2	4
Neruntarat [498]	49	Flap	GA HS	39.4	47.9	18.6	65.2	15.9	6.2	4
Li et al. [399]	33	EUPF	None	6.0	41.6	12.5	81.8	No data	No data	4
Cahali [88]	10	LP	None	6.0	41.6	15.5	53.3	14.0	4.0	4
Friedman et al. [212]	25	ZPP	RFT TB	6.0	41.8	20.9	68.0	12.5	8.3	2b
Cahali et al. [87]	15	LP	Nasal surgery	7.9	41.6	15.5	53.3	14.0	4.0	2b
Li et al. [395]	105	EUPF	None	12.0	43.8	15.0	80.0	No data	No data	4
Li et al. [396]	55	EUPF	None	6.0	43.6	21.1	82.0	11.8	7.5	4
Li et al. [397]	84	EUPF	None	6.0	46.5	14.6	No data	11.0	7.2	4
Li et al. [400]	12	EUPF	LLT/ MLG	6.0	53.5	30.4	41.7	No data	No data	3b
Li et al. [398]	50	EUPF	None	6.0	44.5	13.4	84.0	No data	No data	4
Hsieh et al. [297]	6	EUPF	MLG	6.0	50.7	11.6	No data	No data	No data	4
Lin et al. [417]	55	EUPF	None	6.0	43.6	12.1	No data	11.8	7.2	3b
Baisch et al. [35]	83	Flap	RFT TB, HS	1.0	36.4	19.4	59.7	9.7	6.4	4
Verse et al. [762]	45	Flap	RFT TB, HS	4.3	38.9	20.7	51.1	9.4	7.2	3b
Verse et al. [762]	15	Flap	RFT TB	5.9	27.8	22.9	40.0	9.1	4.1	3b
Pang and Woodson [540]	23	ESP	None	6.5	44.2	12.0	82.6	No data	No data	2b
Huang and Cheng [301]	50	MEUP	None	6.0	37.9	6.1	80.0	9.8	5.2	4
All	839			8,24	41.92	15.61	70.10	11.55	6.68	B

Add. Proc additional procedure; *AHI* Apnea Hypopnea Index; *ESS* Epworth Sleepiness Scale; *EBM* level of evidence based medicine; *Flap* uvulopalatal flap; *EUPF* extended uvulopalatal flap; *ZPP* z-pharyngoplasty; *LP* lateral pharyngoplasty; *ESP* expansion sphincter pharyngoplasty; *MEUP* microdebrider-assisted extended uvulopalatoplasty; *GA* genioglossus advancement; *HS* hyoid suspension; *RFT* interstitial radiofrequency treatment; *TB* tongue base; *MLG* midline laser glossectomy

Better results have been recently reported by Li et al. (Table 6.3.1), who use an extended technique not comparable to our own [400]. These authors also report a significant improvement of the snoring index and the minimal oxygen saturation. Furthermore, a significant improvement of daytime sleepiness and of quality of life in 7 of 8 domains of the SF-36 was observed.

Friedman et al. [213] compared the outcomes of ZPP (N = 25, BMI 31.0 kg/m^2) with UPPP (N = 25, BMI 29.6 kg/m^2) in patients with OSA and with already absent tonsils after 6 months follow-up. All of them also received a radiofrequency treatment of the tongue base. Subjective improvement was good for both groups, but objective clinical improvement was significantly better for the ZPP group. The AHI in the ZPP group was reduced from 41.8 to 20.9 and respectively from 33.4 to 25.2 in the UPPP group (Table 6.3.1). The authors consider a very significant limitation of their procedure that there is no landmark to describe the size of the flaps, that the procedure is technically more difficult and takes longer time than the classic UPPP. Further, the ZPP results in the absence of a uvula and many patients complain of a "foreign-body" sensation in the throat. We consider an essential limitation of this study that the efficacy of ZPP or UPPP cannot really be estimated because of the concomitant treatments of the tongue base with radiofrequency. In a more recent paper, the authors recommended ZPP as an effective and safe second-line treatment after unsuccessful UPPP [211].

In a randomized controlled trial, Cahali et al. [87] compared the clinical and polysomnographic outcomes of the LP procedure (N = 15) with UPPP (N = 12) according to the technique of Fairbanks [184] in adults with OSA incompliant of nCPAP. Concomitant nasal surgery was performed in 5/15 LP patients and in 8/12 UPPP patients. Comparing the preoperative data with those after a mean follow-up of 8 months, in the LP group a statistically greater reduction of body weight (mean BMI: 29.3 vs. 27.7 kg/m^2), excessive daytime sleepiness (ESS: 14 vs. 4), and AHI (mean AHI: 41.6 vs. 15.5) was found. There also was a statistical increase in the amount of deep sleep and a reduction of morning headache. In the UPPP group, there were no significant changes in the polysomnographic parameters (mean AHI: 34.6 vs. 30.0), while mean excessive daytime sleepiness also was significantly reduced (ESS: 14 vs. 5). Interestingly, there were similar cross-sectional measurements of computed tomography of the pharyngeal airways while awake in both groups preoperatively and at follow-up.

In a prospective, randomized controlled trial, Pang and Woodson [540] compared the outcomes of expansion sphincter palatoplasty (ESP) (N = 23) with UPPP (N = 22) in selected patients with OSA with a mean BMI of 28.7 kg/m^2 after a mean follow-up of 6.5 months. The AHI decreased from 44.2 to 12 (p < 0.005) following EPS and from 38.1 to 19.6 (p < 0.005) in the UPPP group. Using Sher's criteria, success was 82.6% in ESP compared with 68.1% in UPPP (p < 0.05). When selecting an arbitrary threshold of a 50% reduction in AHI and AHI less than 15, the ESP success rate was 78.2%, compared with that of the UPPP group at only 45.5% (p < 0.005). Postoperative endoscopic findings also demonstrated significant reduction of lateral pharyngeal wall collapse in the EPS group. This was not the case in the UPPP group, with some patients still having significant lateral pharyngeal wall collapse noted on Müller's maneuver, postoperatively.

6.3.3
Postoperative Care and Complications

The immediate healing phase after uvulopalatal flap proceeds as after conventional UPPP. This of course also especially holds of the healing phase after the additionally performed tonsillectomy. Therefore, we implement the same postoperative management as after UPPP, and refer the reader to our discussion in Chap. 6.2.

Several studies [87, 213, 293, 397, 498, 540, 573] also furnish information concerning the potential complications after uvulopalatal flap or LP.

6.3.3.1
Uvulopalatal Flap

Focusing on the uvulopalatal flap, it has to be said that orginally the uvulopalatal flap was regarded as a potentially reversible surgical technique. We want to challenge this evaluation; we do not consider the uvulopalatal flap as in principle reversible. Our experience has shown that the scarrings after completed healing of the wound cannot easily be opened up again.

The dreaded velopharyngeal incompetence has clinically neither been observed by the Stanford or our study group. Neruntarat described transient nasal regurgitation in two of his patients (4%). In the Finkelstein test [199], a flow of liquid into the nose was demonstrated endoscopically in 3 of our 30 patients, without it becoming clinically relevant. In the longer run, a nasopharyngeal reflux could no longer be demonstrated.

Although a few patients complained of the sensation of having a lump in the throat (7%; 4/55) and mild nasal regurgitation (6%, 3/55) after EUPF, none of them complained about any physical limitation in their daily activities [397].

A nasopharyneal stenosis, as it has been described after other, especially aggressive soft palate techniques, has not been observed either after uvulopalatal flap or after LP.

In the first weeks postoperatively, irritations and foreign-body sensations are to be expected. This is due to the principle of the surgery, which transports mucous membrane segments which originally have been in the posterior side of the velum to the anterior side. As a result, some patients initially experience an irritation in the nasopharynx when it comes to a contact with the flap. These sensations disappear after several weeks.

Permanent foreign-body sensations develop, especially in cases where not merely an incision of the posterior palatine arch is performed, but a cut is also performed in the anterior palatine arch. This is necessary in rare cases, in order to achieve a sufficient opening of the velopharyngeal segment; but this should always be performed as cautiously as possible, in order to not endanger the sensible innervation of the flap and the uvula, which pulls from laterocranial toward mediocaudal. If one abides by this principle, then such permanent foreign-body sensations, which severely burden the patient, can be avoided.

Our own investigations concerning language and articulation have not brought to light any disturbances in this respect.

As a further complication, a hematoma in the area of the uvula tip with secondary inflammation, which led to a revision of the flap, and a suture insufficiency with partial flap insufficiency, has been described [573]. We also have observed suture insufficiencies with partial or complete dislodgement of the flap from its bed. These suture insufficiencies can be reliably avoided with the help of an adequate suture technique with deep-reaching double sutures and atraumatic suture material. In order to prevent unnecessary postoperative wound pain, it must be ensured that the knots are tightly bound, but that the tissue is not squashed. A slack adaptation of the wound edges is aimed at. Some surgeons consider the use of knot slides as very helpful in this context.

These data are comparable with those of gentle UPPP, and they corroborate the assumption by Finkelstein, according to which the proof of a subclinical nasopharyngeal reflux in the first weeks after soft palate surgery depends on the intensity, with which the surgeon hunts it out.

6.3.3.2
Other Techniques

Pang and Woodson [540] reported of no significant complications in either group following ESP or UPPP. All patients started soft diet consumption on the first postoperative day. There was no significant difference in the use of narcotics or pain relief in the two groups, and there was no long-term dysphagia or voice change.

Friedman et al. [213] found that patients undergoing ZPP used narcotic pain medication for 6.4 days and required 6.4 days to return to a normal diet as compared with 9.4 days and 10.3 days, respectively in UPPP patients ($p < 0.005$ resp. $p < 0.002$). Tongue base infections, secondary to radiofrequency treatments, were found in 1 ZPP patient and 2 UPPP patients. Temporary velopharyngeal insufficiency (VPI) between 2 and 60 days was reported in 12/25 ZPP and 7/25 UPPP patients. The majority of postoperative complications were related to throat discomfort, including foreign-body sensation (11 of ZPP vs. 17 of UPPP), dysphagia (1 ZPP vs. 11 UPPP), postnasal drip (3 ZPP vs. 4 UPPP), and dry throat.

As to complications there was no bleeding, nasopharyngeal stenosis, or permanent palatal incompetence [87]. In the first 10 patients of the LP group, there were significant swallowing problems with dysphagia over a mean of 20.4 days (range 8–70 days). Four patients in each group reported mild episodes of oronasal reflux of liquids which disappeared within 2–6 months.

6.3.4
Indications and Contraindications

The uvulopalatal flap is a comparatively modern procedure. We see the indication for the most part in the area of OSA. For primary snoring, there exist techniques such as radiofrequency surgery, soft tissue implants, and other procedures, which can be used on an outpatient basis and under local anesthesia. Given the comparable efficacy, these procedures are to be preferred also in respect to the costs involved.

UPPP and uvulopalatal flap are similar in regards to their basic principle and their effects upon the upper airways; therefore, we assume the same indication areas for both surgical techniques, when they are employed in a muscle-preserving manner. For the isolated soft palate surgery (uvulopalatal flap with tonsillectomy) we perform either UPPP or the uvulopalatal flap as the first-line procedure in moderate to moderately severe OSA. In combination with surgery on the hypopharyngeal segment we also use the uvulopalatal flap for severe OSA.

On the whole, we see few advantages for the uvulopalatal flap, especially if a tonsillectomy had been performed prior to surgery; but in the end it appears that every surgeon will have to choose for themselves the technique with which they achieve better surgical results.

6.3.4.1
Extended Techniques

For treating OSA using EUPF, Li et al. [397] selected patients with a normal weight and a narrowed retropalatal space judged by nasofibroscopy with Müller maneuver and 3-dimensional computed tomography.

Friedman et al. [213] published a longer list of selection criteria, among them are the failure of CPAP or dental appliances, patients without tonsils or those who underwent prior tonsillectomy, Friedman OSA stages II or III, and the appearance of obstruction at the level of the soft palate (diagnosed by fiberoptic hypolaryngoscopy and Müller maneuver).

Velum surgery including the lateral pharynpgoplasty (LP and ESP) is indicated to splint the lateral pharyngeal muscular walls and to remove or reduce the bulk of the lateral pharyngeal walls. Therefore, Pang and Woodson [540] selected patients with small tonsils (tonsil size 1 and 2), BMI < 30 kg/m^2, Friedman clinical stage II and III [220], and lateral pharyngeal wall collapse noted on endoscopic examination who cannot tolerate CPAP. They excluded patients with large tonsils for whom they recommended the traditional UPPP.

Cahali et al. [87, 88] selected as inclusing criteria the presence of a low-lying soft palate (most of the patients were Malampatti type 3 with few type 4) associated with a fiberoptic pharyngoscopy finding of narrowing or collapse in the retropalatal region without narrowing in the hypopharynx (Fujita type 1), both at rest and during the Muller maneuver. All their patients had bulky lateral oropharyngeal tissues (either the tonsil or the posterior tonsillar pillar). They excluded patients with weight over 130 kg, morbid obesity, the presence of uncontrolled hypothyroidism, and gross maxillary or mandible deformities.

Summing up the results of the cited studies on uvulopalatal flaps and other recent modifications of UPPP we find some positive developments and also some limitations. All described modifications try to improve shortcomings of the conventional UPPP, and especially the LP attacks the problems of the lateral pharyngeal walls [87, 88, 540]. Most studies report on more reduction of sleep parameters than achieved with conventional UPPP. Clear criteria for patient selection are only given by some authors [87, 213, 540], especially for patients after prior tonsillectomy. Quality-of-life evaluation helps to improve the subjective outcomes of velum surgery [213, 397, 400].

Some surgical procedures are rather invasive and temporarily disturb the coordination of the velar muscles which results in postoperative problems with swallowing. Also the velar sensory innervation is disturbed by large incisions, thus enhancing the preexisting polyneuropathy of the patients with OSA. Another disadvantage is the uvulectomy performed by several working groups [88, 213, 397, 540, 573]. Most authors use nasopharyngeal endoscopy and Müller maneuver while awake to diagnose the level of pharyngeal obstruction, methods of questionable diagnostic value. No study described the use of sleep endoscopy. The numbers of operated patients are mostly small, especially when compared with conventional UPPP. The follow-up is very short, between 1.5 and 8 months. Most publications [87, 213, 397, 573] present outcomes of a two-level surgery instead of isolated velum surgery. Therefore, no long-term conclusions on the definite value of these new modifications are possible.

Take Home Pearls

> The uvulopalatal flap is an alternative to conventional UPPP, especially in patients after prior tonsillectomy.
> As in conventional UPPP complications frequently occur after aggressive surgery. The muscles of the soft palate should be handled with care. There is no need for broad resections.
> Techniques addressing the lateral pharynx should be reserved to patients with still narrow velopharyngeal segments after unsuccessful UPPP.

Laser-Assisted Uvulopalatoplasty (LAUP) 6.4

Thomas Verse and Wolfgang Pirsig

Core Features

> There are two kinds of laser-assisted soft palate surgeries. The so-called laser uvulopalatoplasty (LUPP) is similar to conventional UPPP, requires general anesthesia, and should be regarded as a modification of UPPP.

> The so-called laser-assisted uvulopalatoplasty (LAUP) comprises a resection of redundant mucosa of the posterior tonsillar pillar and the uvula. Some authors perform a parauvular incision into the muscles of the soft palate in order to achieve additional stiffening. Instead of lasers, various other technical aids can be used as well (LAUP related procedures).

> LAUP and related procedures are easy and quick to perform. They only require local anesthesia without sedation in an outpatient setting.

> LAUP and related procedures can be combined with other surgeries for SDB.

> Because of substantial postoperative pain, LAUP induces significant postoperative morbidity.

> Potential complications are numerous. Most of them can be avoided, be a gentle resection of only mucosa.

> LAUP and related procedures are only indicated to treat simple snoring. They are not sufficiently effective in treating OSA.

Since 1981, uvulopalatopharyngoplasty (UPPP) has gained acceptance as routine therapy in the surgical treatment of sleep-disordered breathing [224]. As an essential modification of the conventional UPPP technique, a laser-assisted velum surgery was developed, which was introduced by Carenfelt [91] in 1986, and which he called "laser uvulopalatoplasty" (LUPP). While Carenfelt performed the LUPP under general anesthesia and with sutures similar to those used with the UPPP, at the end of the 1980s, Kamami [339] introduced a further modification, which was carried out under local anesthesia in several sessions on an outpatient basis. This modification was called "laser-assisted uvulopalatoplasty" (LAUP); it has spread rapidly in Europe and since 1992 has also become increasingly popular in the United States [118].

K. Hörmann, T. Verse, *Surgery for Sleep Disordered Breathing*,
DOI: 10.1007/978-3-540-77786-1_6.4, © Springer Verlag Berlin Heidelberg 2010

Up to March 2008, more than 120 articles on LAUP have been published worldwide; however, only some of these articles are clinically relevant. Therefore, the present outline intends to structure the literature on the basis of clinical criteria in order to highlight the significance of LAUP/LUPP for the everyday routine work. In particular, the indication for LAUP/LUPP, their surgical prospects of success, and the complications associated with the procedure will be illuminated.

6.4.1
Surgical Techniques

We found 24 different descriptions of laser surgical techniques of the soft palate, explaining in detail which anatomical structures of the soft palate are involved in the surgery. Most of these publications are illustrated with explanatory drawings or photographs. Although the variability of the techniques described is very high, three basic techniques can be identified.

The oldest technique, applied by Carenfelt already in 1986 [91], is the LUPP, which some working groups [91, 809] reported to be more gentle to muscles, while others regarded it as being substantially more radical [197, 371]. The procedure performed with the LUPP is similar to that carried out with the UPPP, which means the preparation also extends to the pharyngeal walls and partly to the tonsils (Fig. 6.4.1). The Carenfelt and Haraldsson working group uses suture techniques for the adaptation of the posterior tonsillar pillar to the anterior tonsillar pillar in order to prevent uncontrolled scarring.

Most authors apply the LAUP technique introduced by Kamami [339]. The uvula is partly or totally removed. Then, two paramedian full-thickness, through-and-through trenches are made over the soft palate, on either side of the uvula, to a height of 1–2 cm. With few exceptions, the LAUP is performed under local anesthesia in an outpatient setting. There exists a more gentle procedure performed in several (up to five) sessions (Fig. 6.4.2) and a radical "one-stage-technique" (Fig. 6.4.3).

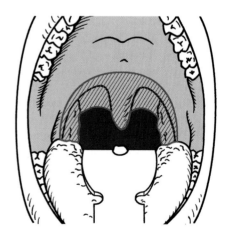

Fig. 6.4.1   Scheme of LUPP according to Wennmo et al. [809]

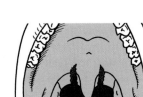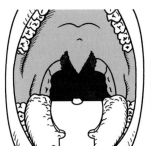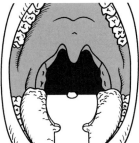

Fig. 6.4.2   Scheme of LAUP in multiple stages modified after Kamami [340]

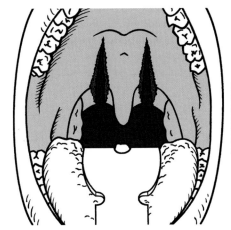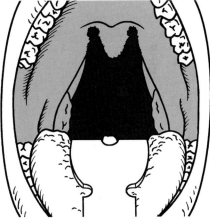

Fig. 6.4.3   Scheme of "One-Stage"-LAUP modified after Kamami [340]

In most cases, the CO_2-laser is used, sometimes the Nd:YAG [798] or the KTP laser [338]. No comparative information pointing to differences between various laser types has been found in the literature yet. However, Ducic et al. [164] were able to show in an animal test performed on six dogs that the CO_2-laser caused deeper thermal tissue damage and more intensive scarring than the conventional UPPP technique using bipolar coagulation.

According to our experience, we see the most advantages in a cautiously performed modified Kamami technique [775]. We strongly advise against radical incisions into the palatopharyngeal and the palatoglossal muscles. As we know from our extensive experience from the UPPP surgery, there is no rationale for an aggressive surgical technique. The surgical outcome will not improve after a more radical procedure, but the incidence of severe complications will increase. We do not believe that there are no or only little complications after procedures like the one-stage LAUP (Fig. 6.4.3) as reported by Kamami [340].

Based on our experiences we developed a modification of the multiple-stage Kamami technique. We operate on the sitting awake patient. In general, there is no need for sedation. We perform a local anesthesia using 5–6 mL prilocaine (2%) with adrenaline (0.01%).

Topical anesthesia is not advantageous because it often causes hypersalivation forcing the patient to swallow frequently. When we started to do LAUP surgery we used the CO_2 laser (8 W, continuous wave, superpulsed mode) in the majority of the cases. Important is the use of a backstop protecting the posterior pharyngeal wall from the laser beam. Comfortable to use in contact mode is the KTP laser. Today, we predominately use mono- or bipolar high-frequency cutting instruments mostly in argon atmosphere, the latter being used to reduce thermal penetration into the tissue. As no lasers are used, all these technique are subsumed using the term RAUP (radiofrequency-assisted uvulopalatoplasty). Depending on the devices used, there is little smoke formation. The staff does not need to use glasses to protect his or her eyes from the laser beam. To sum it up, we do not see any need for lasers for this kind of surgery. In our experience, it is much less important which surgical tool is used than to use an appropriate surgical technique.

While the tongue is held down with a blade, an inverse V-shaped incision is made bilaterally to the uvula, only cutting about 5 mm into the anterior pillar of the soft palate (Fig. 6.4.4).

If bleeding occurs it has to be coagulated carefully. To complete the procedure the tip of the uvula is pulled downwards with a forceps. Thereby the uvula muscle becomes apparent. Preserving muscular tissue the redundant mucosa is taken away (Fig. 6.4.5).

Figure 6.4.6 shows peri- and postoperative photographs of our technique taken in general anesthesia during one of our surgical courses.

6.4.2
Effectiveness for Simple Snoring

Up to now, there are no generally accepted techniques to quantify snoring. In the literature, either visual analogue scales (VAS) usually filled out by the patient's bed partner or the so-called snoring indices (SI) based on different algorithms analyzing the recorded snoring

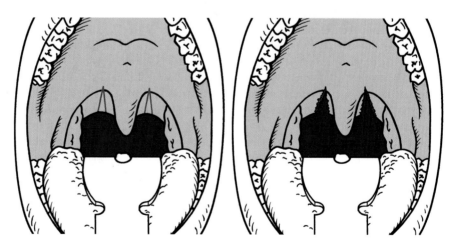

Fig. 6.4.4 (*Left*) palatal incision lines. (*Right*) incisions done

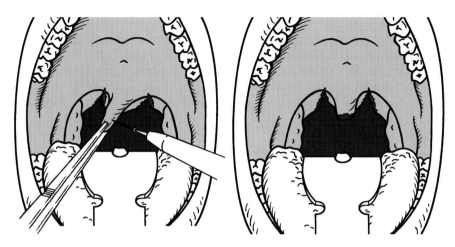

Fig. 6.4.5 (*Left*) uvula pulled downwards with forceps. (*Right*) uvula shortened

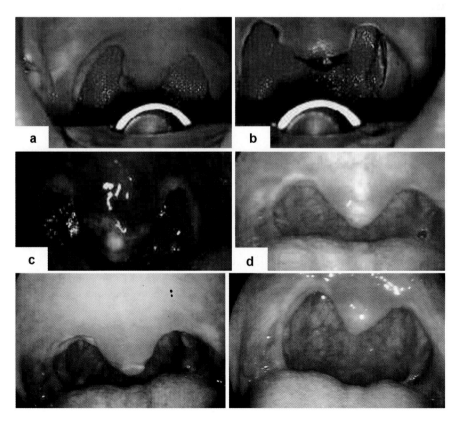

Fig. 6.4.6 Two cases of the Mannheim/Ulm/Hamburg Technique of LAUP. First case (a–d): (a) Preop. (b) immediately after surgery. (c) Six days postop. (d) 2 months postop. Second case (*bottom*). (*Left*) 2 weeks after surgery. (*Right*) three months after surgery.

sounds during sleep studies are used to describe the effectiveness of LAUP for simple snoring. Others use simple questionnaires with items such as "Do you still snore?" to verify treatment success.

Relevant data from prospective studies using VAS to evaluate the subjective improvements of either LUPP or LAUP for simple snoring are given in Tables 6.4.1 and 6.4.2. Extremely varying definitions of success complicate the interpretation of the results.

6.4.2.1
LUPP

Data concerning LUPP are taken from somewhat dated publications. More recent data including information about daytime sleepiness are not available.

LUPP seems to have a positive short-term impact if used in simple snorers. Long-term results are reported by Lysdahl and Haraldsson [430]. The authors prospectively performed LUPP in 60 patients. A control group of 61 snorers received a conventionally performed UPPP. Both techniques showed significant improvement of subjective parameters such as snoring, awakenings, apneas, daytime sleepiness, and sleep spells while driving, at short-term follow-up (3 months). UPPP was superior to LUPP in all mentioned effect parameters. Five to eight years after surgery, all subjective parameters except sleep spells while driving had worsened over time, with UPPP again showing better long-term results.

6.4.2.2
LAUP

All but one working group listed in Table 6.4.2 used the CO_2-Laser. Only Hanada and colleagues [263] used the Nd:YAG laser for LAUP.

Although every working group uses its own criteria of success, there is evidence that LAUP is effective in the treatment of simple snoring. Looking through the literature, there are many more studies on the effectiveness of LAUP on simple snoring, using other measurement tools than VAS. We recently summarized this information [775]. LAUP results in an at least short-term reduction of socially disturbing snoring. Some long-term subjective recurrence of snoring does occur [501, 661].

Similar to the findings in patients suffering from OSA, Berger et al. [48] describe a decrease of subjective snoring improvement after LAUP for simple snoring over time in a

Table 6.4.1 Effectiveness of LUPP for simple snoring

Author	N	Follow-up (months)	VAS	VAS pre	VAS post	Success rate (%)	Def. of success	Laser	EBM
Carenfelt [91]	60	3–4	1–4	No data	No data	85	Red >1	CO_2	3b
Wennmo et al. [809]	10	2–36	0–3	3	0.15	80	VAS ≤1	CO_2	4
Albu et al. [7]	90	No data	0–10	No data	No data	80	VAS <4	Nd:YAG	4
All	160	2–36				81.9			C

VAS visual analogue scale; *Red* reduction; *EBM* grade of evidence-based medicine

Table 6.4.2 Effectiveness of LAUP for simple snoring

Author	N	Follow-up (months)	VAS	VAS pre	VAS post	ESS pre	ESS post	Success rate (%)	Def. of success	EBM
Walker et al. [791]	105	1.5	0–100	66.7	No data	No data	No data	60.0	Red >70%	4
Hanada et al. [263]	35	1	1–10	No data	5.3	No data	No data	51.4	Red >50%	4
Vukovic and Hutchings [787]	25	6	0–12	No data	No data	No data	No data	84.0	VAS ≤6	4
Astor et al. [26]	38	No data	0–7	No data	No data	No data	No data	76.3	VAS <4 and Red >2	4
Schlieper et al. [649]	152	12	1–6	No data	No data	No data	No data	88.0	VAS ≤3	4
Uppal et al. [757]	31	19	1–6	4.0	2.7	10.0	No data	67.8	VAS ≤3	1b
Larrosa et al. [384]	13	3	1–10	6.6	5.5	10.4	9.6	0	No data	1b
Cincik et al. [112]	18	1.5	0–4	3.3	0.3	6.6	2.6	88.8	VAS ≤1	1b
Belloso et al. [44]	13	12	1–10	8.5	2.8	No data	No data	No data	No data	2b
Lim et al. [414]	17	6	1–10	8.0	3.4	12.1	5.4	85.0	Improvement	2b
All LAUP	447	1–19		5.6	2.8	9.6	5.5	75.1		B

VAS visual analogue scale; *ESS* Epworth sleepiness scale; *Red* reduction; *EBM* grade of evidence based medicine

group of 14 patients. Subjective improvement was stated in 79% 1 month after surgery and dropped down to 57% after 10.1 months. Increase of subjective snoring occurred in one patient after 1 month but in three patients after 10 months. Three of those patients (21%) who initially all were simple snorers developed mild OSA as a result of laser treatment. Similar findings of a decrease of success rates over time are reported by Kyrmizakis et al. [380].

On the other hand, Osman et al. performed objective analysis of snoring sounds using their Gal Clxyd Snore Box [532]; 22 patients underwent a single stage LAUP with the KTP laser, and another 16 patients received UPPP. At short-term follow-up (2–11 months), subjective snoring improvement was reported in 83% of LAUP patients and in 89% of the UPPP group. The objectively measured snoring index (SI) decreased statistically significantly in both groups [531]. Twenty-four patients (12 LAUP and 12 UPPP) out of the same pool of patients were reevaluated 29–56 months after surgery. The SI was still statistically significantly lower than before treatment. There was no statistical difference between short- and long-term follow-up in the SI [530]. There was still no difference between the UPPP and the LAUP patients.

Walker et al. [790] performed objective measurements of snoring sounds using the SNAP system in a series of 27 patients undergoing LAUP. The SI decreased with every new treatment session. The mean frequency of the snoring sounds increased, while the loudness of the low-frequent part of the sound spectrum which is thought to have its origin in the soft palate level decreased. A decrease of the relative loudness of snoring sounds below 180 Hz correlates well with the patients' subjective satisfaction.

6.4.2.3
Raup

The following Table 6.4.3 summarizes four other studies performing comparable surgeries but using other devices instead of lasers. Each one working group used a different device for monopolar electrocautery. Belloso at al. [44] used the Coblation technique. The basic surgical concept was in all cases identical with LAUP.

More important than the figures in Table 6.4.3 is the fact that all but one study are controlled trials comparing RAUP with LAUP. All the three studies achieved comparable results. This is why we think that RAUP and LAUP can be regarded as the same kind of surgery for SDB. It does not seem to be important which technical instrument is used to perform the surgery.

6.4.3
Effectiveness for OSA

In 2000, we conducted a meta-analysis on the efficacy of laser surgery to the soft palate for OSA [776]. At the time, we did not find any long-term results. Short-term results were given only in eight publications with altogether 232 patients providing pre- and postoperative polysomnographic information. The AHI decreased, not statistically significantly, from 29.1 to 23.4 after LAUP. The authors used diverse criteria of success, a fact that complicates sufficient comparison of the results. Mickelson and Ahuja [463] for example show a variation in the surgery success rate between 33 and 67% in the same patients merely by applying different criteria. This fact has already been criticized by the American Sleep Disorders Association [18] and by Hoffstein [288].

Today more substantial information exists. Therefore, we always used the criteria recommended by Sher et al. [665] (AHI reduction of at least 50% and AHI reduction to values below 20) to compare the literature results. Table 6.4.4 summarizes those studies presenting success rates according to Sher.

Table 6.4.3   Effectiveness of RAUP for simple snoring

Author	N	Follow-up (months)	VAS	VAS pre	VAS post	ESS pre	ESS post	Success rate (%)	Def. of success	EBM
Wedman et al. [803]	40	3	0–10	8.4	2.3	No data	No data	93	Will undergo RAUP again	4
Cincik et al. [112]	18	1.5	0–4	3.1	0.4	6.4	2.6	83.3	VAS ≤1	1b
Belloso et al. [44]	17	12	1–10	7.1	4.0	No data	No data	No data	No data	2b
Lim et al. [414]	24	6	1–10	7.9	3.3	12.2	5.1	83.0	Improvement	2b
All	99	1.5–12		7.1	2.5	9.7	4.0	87.9		B

VAS visual analogue scale; *ESS* Epworth sleepiness scale; *Red* reduction; *EBM*: grade of evidence based medicine

The working group of Walker et al. and Mickelson reported in earlier publications about their results with LAUP in patients with OSA [466, 791, 793]. Since the investigation periods are identical, only the more recent publications were considered in order to prevent patients being included twice in the evaluation.

Looking at the data of the 13 studies listed in Table 6.4.4, one finds polysomnographic data about 392 patients. The overall success rate is 31.2% using Sher's criteria. Medium-term results (>8 months of follow-up) are substantially worse than short-term results. Table 6.4.4 strongly corroborates the findings of the working group of Finkelstein et al. [49, 198] that promising short-term results after LAUP deteriorate over time.

The controlled studies imply that LAUP is more effective than doing nothing [192, 384] but much less effective as conventional UPPP [49] for OSA. The study of Kern [350] does not really add much new information, as there is a substantial bias in this trial. Patients undergoing LAUP combined with tonsillectomy were more severely affected than patients selected for LAUP. Therefore, we cannot agree with the authors' conclusion that LAUP with and without tonsillectomy shows comparable efficiency in the treatment of OSA.

Apart from their objective results stated in Table 6.4.4, Ryan and Love [633] were able to show that the quality of life significantly improved in all domains and daytime sleepiness decreased after LAUP.

The working group of Finkelstein at al. [49, 198] found out twice that their favorable subjective short-term results of LAUP for OSA deteriorated over time (mean follow-up 12.3 months). Postoperative polysomnography revealed that LAUP might lead to deterioration of existing apneas. The authors conclude that these findings are probably related to velo-pharyngeal narrowing and progressive fibrosis inflicted by the laser beam as found in human specimen after LAUP [47].

Fifteen working groups have searched for criteria to predict the operation's success. The following criteria are stated: lower BMI, lower severity of OSA, site of obstruction in the velopharynx, female gender, velo-pharyngeal obstruction pattern, lack of loud snoring and apneas, exclusion of cranio-facial malformations, and lower age [775]. A clear trend cannot be recognized, which is mainly explained by the fact that the definitions for success are too divergent.

Bassiouny et al. [41] conducted the only trial so far investigating the effect of RAUP on OSA. Twenty patients were included. Using the Coblation system, the mean AHI dropped from 17.2 at baseline to 8.1 four months after surgery. The surgical success rate according to Sher's criteria is given as 50%. A control group received interstitial radiofrequency treatment of the soft palate. RAUP turned out to be more effective but to cause significantly more postoperative pain.

There is a single study providing polysomnographic data on the efficiency of LUPP [559]. In this study, the Apnea Index (AI) of 30 patients decreased from 26 before to 7 five months after LUPP. The success rate according to Sher's criteria was calculated as 63.3%. It is important to keep in mind that this technique includes the removal of the tonsils. This fact makes the higher success rate understandable. In any case, this technique is very similar to the conventional UPPP technique and should be interpreted in this context.

Table 6.4.4 Effectiveness of LAUP for treatment of OSA

Author	N	Follow-up (months)	AHI pre	AHI post	Success (%)	Sessions	EBM	Control group
Lauretano et al. [386]	17	2	27.9	29.1	No data	2.6	4	None
Utley et al. [760]	12	4	8.9	10.3	33	2.4	4	None
Mickelson and Ahuja [463]	36	4	28.1	17.9	33.3	2.7	4	None
Pribitkin et al. [580]	29	2	15.8	41.3	24.1	1.9	4	None
Walker et al. [792]	38	3	30.3	22.2	44.8	4	4	None
Ryan and Love 2000 [633]	44	3	29	19	34.1	1	4	None
Seemann et al. [655]	43	2	No data	7.4	32.2	1	4	None
Finkelstein et al. [198]	26	12.3	29.6	25	19.2	1.5	4	None
Ferguson et al. [192]	21	8.2	18.6	14.7	19.1	2.4	3b	N = 24 No treatment
Berger et al. [49]	25	12.2	25.3	33.1	16	1	2b	N = 24 UPPP
Kern et al. [350]	33	3	35.6	24.1	42.4	3.2	3b	N = 31 LAUP+TE
Larrosa et al. [384]	13	3	13.6	15.1	No data	1	2b	N = 12 Sham surgery
MacDonald et al. [431]	55	6	9.6	10.1	No data	1	4	None
All	392	2–12.3	18.2	16.6	31.21	1–4	B	

BMI body mass index; *AHI* Apnea Hypopnea Index; *EBM* Evidence-based medicine

6.4.4
Postoperative Care and Complications

In a survey about complications that occurred in Sweden with soft palate surgery for SRBD [90], three deaths were reported with 9,000 UPPPs and one death with 2,900 LAUPs. The latter patient died from a sepsis on the fourth postoperative day, since a perioperative prophylaxis with antibiotics had not been carried out.

Generally any kind of soft palate surgery, in particular radical procedures, bears the danger of a limited acceptance of a later nasal CPAP therapy due to an occurring oro-nasal airflow leakage [789]. Moreover, in 25 publications, further complications with LAUP are mentioned,

Table 6.4.5 Complications of laser-assisted surgery on the soft palate according to frequency

Complication	Incidence (%)
Nasal regurgitation (short-term)	80
Sore throat	46
Scar fibrosis	27
Velopharyngeal incompetence	1.5–26.7
Dysphagia	6–26.6
Foreign body sensation	9–25
Paresthesia	22
Aspiration	21.5
Occurrence of other disturbing breathing sounds	20.5
Voice problems	1.3–20
Irritation of taste	0.7–18
Xerostomia	16
Wound infection	1.5–14
Odynophagia	1.4–12
Vomiting	10
Nasal regurgitation (long-term)	4.8–10
Postoperative bleeding	0.7–10
Hypersalivation	5
Nasopharyngeal stenosis	0.1–3.3

which are summarized in Table 6.4.5 together with the frequency, in cases wherein it was stated. The post-surgical observation period reached from 48 h [739] to 8 years [259].

Long-term complications are particularly strenuous for the patients. Hardly any data can be found regarding this problem. Petri et al. [559] describe a permanent reflux in the nasopharynx (Fig. 6.4.7) for 3 of 30 of their patients. Grontved et al. [243] report about a permanent reflux in the nasopharynx for 1 of 21 patients. In 2 of 60 patients Pinzcower et al. [564] described a foreign body sensation (Fig. 6.4.8) 6 months after surgery. The authors deal with this problem in more detail in their publication. They were able to prove that the parauvular incisions caused damage to the sensitive supply of the neo-uvula area, which is medial of the incisions. This in turn causes the sensation of a foreign body being there, which may sometimes lead to vomiting [366], but which apparently recedes in most cases. Nasopharyngeal stenosis (Fig. 6.4.9) was reported in 0.1–3.3% of all cases and must be considered as a permanent complication. This complication is difficult to correct. Basic surgical principles are stated in Chap. 6.2.

Particularly valuable for the assessment of complications occurring with the LAUP is the comparison with the UPPP when the same author uses both surgical techniques. Such a comparison can be found in five publications. Carenfelt [91] describes a significantly higher rate ($p > 0.05$) of scarred nasopharyngeal stenosis after LUPP when compared with the status after UPPP. Chabolle [97] found fewer cases of velo-pharyngeal incompetence after LAUP (5% vs. 10%) and fewer dysphagia (15% vs. 23%), but more often pharyngeal dysphagia (22% vs. 18%), wound infections (10% vs. 5%), and general painfulness (44% vs. 41%).

Fig. 6.4.7 Nasopharyngeal
incompetence after LAUP

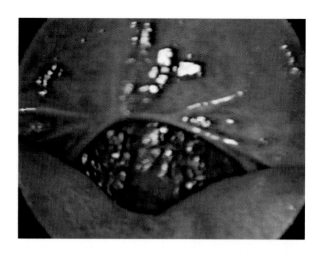

Fig. 6.4.8 Anesthesia (no
sensation with needle test)
with foreign body sensation
after LAUP. *Broken line*:
oral side. *Drawn line*: nasal
side

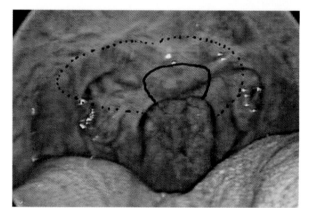

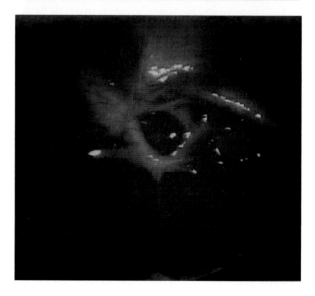

Fig. 6.4.9 Nasopharyngeal
stenosis after LAUP

On the other hand, in a radiocephalometric examination with contrast agent, Finkelstein et al. [197] proved an obstruction of the nasopharynx by LAUP and a dilation of the nasopharynx by UPPP. In an investigation carried out by Shehab et al. [662], the patients reported significantly more pain ($p = 0.0027$) on the seventh day postsurgery after LAUP than after UPPP. On the first postoperative day, no significant difference was found. For a collective consisting of 110 patients with OSA and 254 simple snorers Hagert et al. [259] reported about postoperative occurrence of other disturbing noises during sleep. Those other noises (smacking, grunting, whistling) were observed in 20.5% after LUPP, but only in 15.1% after UPPP.

6.4.4.1
Pain

Laser surgery of the soft palate is a painful procedure with a maximum of pain during the third to fifth day after surgery. If done as a multiple-stage procedure almost 20% of the patients were reported to be not willing to undergo a next session because of pain [26]. Even 2 years after surgery some patients stated that they would not undergo a LAUP again because of the painfulness of their procedures.

The mean duration of pain requiring pain killers is cited as between 5.3 days [118] and 15 days [380] after multiple-stage LAUP under local anesthesia. In individual cases pain killers were taken up to 3 weeks postoperatively. Soreness seems to decrease with the number of repeated sessions [26].

In comparison to conventional UPPP the LAUP procedure turned out to be slightly more painful during the first days after surgery but required pain killers for a shorter period of time [97, 623, 662, 748, 809]. This is in accord with our own experience. In the area of the soft palate, laser surgery is significantly more painful than RFQ treatments [56, 623, 748, 757].

Up to now, there is little information about specific postoperative pain management after LAUP. We treat our patients successfully with Cox-II antagonists and tramadol. Sometimes oral antibiotics are very helpful to control postoperative pain. Sucralfate was found to alleviate post-LAUP pain in a randomized clinical trial [381]. Sucralfate is known to adhere to proteins that promote healing by forming a protective coating against gastric acid, pepsin, and bile salts. Another future perspective may consist in the use of long-lasting local anesthetics.

6.4.5
Indications and Contraindications

In 2001 the Standards of Practice Committee of the American Academy of Sleep Medicine (AASM) issued a declaration with six statements regarding laser-assisted surgery of the soft palate [419]:

1. LAUP is not recommended for the treatment of the sleep-related breathing disorders including obstructive sleep apnea (guideline).
2. LAUP is not recommended as a substitute for UPPP in the treatment of sleep-related breathing disorders including OSA (guideline).
3. LAUP appears comparable to UPPP in relieving subjective snoring (guideline).
4. Surgical candidates for LAUP as a treatment for snoring should undergo a preoperative clinical evaluation and a polysomnographic or a cardiorespiratory study to determine if the candidate has a sleep-related breathing disorder including OSA (standard). Since snoring is a primary diagnostic symptom, patients who undergo LAUP should be informed of the need for periodic evaluation for subsequent development of OSA even if the procedure reduces or eliminates snoring (standard).
5. The need for medications that affect respiration during the perioperative period should be assessed during the preoperative clinical evaluation (standard).
6. Patients should be informed of the risks and complications of LAUP (standard).

We fully agree with this statement and do not perform any laser-assisted surgery of the soft palate in patients with OSA. The new guideline "obstructive sleep apnea in adults" of the German Society of Otorhinolaryngology, Head and Neck Surgery [768] is consistent with the statement of the AASM.

There are six publications dealing with the former "upper-airway-resistance-syndrome" (UARS). Five of these six groups of authors perform LAUP in patients with UARS. We do not as it has been documented that LAUP may narrow the nasopharyngeal valve while UPPP has been proven to widen it [49, 197, 633]. For this reason we only perform UPPP or a modified uvulopalatal flap, always in combination with a tonsillectomy, if tonsils are still present, in our patients with confirmed UARS, for the case that a CPAP therapy is not accepted.

Nevertheless, LAUP seems to be an adequate treatment modality for simple snoring. For this indication, LAUP competes with radiofrequency of the soft palate. While patients with long uvula and redundant mucosa at the posterior pillar (so-called web-bing) are good candidates for laser-assisted procedures, radiofrequency treatment is reserved for candidates with no or minimal redundant mucosa because radiofrequency does not remove any excessive tissue but stiffens the soft palate by intramuscular scarrification.

The following associated conditions are mentioned as contraindications for LAUP: overweight, arterial hypertension, and mental irregularities or lacking cooperation [775]. Being a professional speaker or singer was also seen as relative contraindication [371].

The following illnesses are named as local factors: tonsillar hypertrophy, trismus, cranio-facial malformation and cleft palate, macroglossia, prominent plication of the rear oropharyngeal wall, heavy retching, previously existing velo-pharyngeal incompetence, floppy epiglottis, and neuromuscular diseases of the pharynx [775]. A solely retro-lingual site of formation of snoring sounds is naturally also seen as contraindication.

Take Home Pearls

> We do not see any indication for LUPP.
> LAUP and related procedures (RAUP, etc.) are not adequate treatments for OSA.
> Outcome of LAUP or RAUP does not depend on the technical equipment used.
> LAUP and related procedures do not fulfill the criteria of minimally invasive surgery, because of substantial postoperative pain. Patients need to know that they cannot return to work for a couple of days.
> There is no need for aggressive LAUP or any other resections within the soft palate.

Radiofrequency Surgery

6.5

6.5.1
Interstitial Radiofrequency Treatment (RFT)

Boris A. Stuck and Thomas Verse

> ### Core Features
>
> > Radiofrequency surgery of the soft palate is a minimally invasive treatment for primary snoring and mild obstructive sleep apnea.
> > Radiofrequency surgery of the soft palate can be performed on an outpatient basis under simple local anesthesia, but usually requires multiple treatment sessions.

Already in 1995, Whinney and colleagues suggested a procedure that can be considered as a precursor of radiofrequency surgery on the soft palate [813]. The authors performed 10–15 punctate penetrations of the mucosa and diathermized the palatal muscles on each puncture to achieve a stiffening of the soft palate, palpable to the surgeon (Fig. 6.5.1.1).

Today, radiofrequency systems, which need fewer thermic lesions to achieve a treatment effect, have been established. In terms of the soft palate, this interstitial radiofrequency surgery competes more with the LAUP than with the classical UPPP. The fundamental aspects of radiofrequency surgery have already been discussed in Sect. 6.1.2 in the context of the tonsil treatment. But in contrast to tonsillar surgery, a plethora of data from clinical studies is available for the soft palate.

6.5.1.1
Surgical Technique

Surgery is usually performed under local anesthesia as an outpatient procedure on the sitting patient. In the case of an isolated soft palate treatment, sedation is usually not necessary.

K. Hörmann, T. Verse, *Surgery for Sleep Disordered Breathing*,
DOI: 10.1007/978-3-540-77786-1_6.5, © Springer Verlag Berlin Heidelberg 2010

Fig. 6.5.1.1 Punctate diathermy of the soft palate according to Whinney et al. [813]

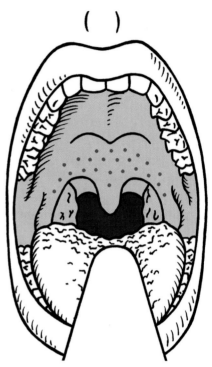

Monitoring by way of a pulse oximetry and an ECG is recommended for sedated patients, but otherwise not mandatory.

In the area of the soft palate, we also perform surgery without a mucosal disinfection. For the local anesthesia, we use prilocaine 2% with epinephrine (1:200,000). In many patients, surface anesthetics cause a bothersome hypersalivation; therefore, we do not regularly take recourse to this option. In order to achieve an adequate analgesia, the pathway of the sensible innervation needs to be taken into account. The nerve fibers run from lateral toward the uvula. It is important to begin the local anesthesia sufficiently close to the hard palate, due to the fact that the radiofrequency applicators need to be inserted approximately 2 cm further cranially than the expected lesion. As a rule, 5–8 mL local anesthetic is sufficient for the local anesthesia (Fig. 6.5.1.2).

It may be beneficial to lay the needle on the soft palate in order to determine the correct position for lesion and puncture before penetrating the mucosa with the radiofrequency applicator. It is crucial to check the position of the active probe in the tissue before applying energy. This can be done either by palpation or by back-and-forth moving of the probe. If the active electrode is situated too superficially, an ulcer may develop as a result of the thermic damage, causing an extended time of healing.

Currently, using the Somnus system (Somnus, Gyrus ENT, Bartlett, USA), we prefer 4–6 lesion at 85°C target temperature and 400–500 J for the initial treatment. In this respect, our concept differs from that of others, which either favor a single lesion [194, 664] or also several lesions with total energy amounts between 1,099 [738] and 2,100

Fig. 6.5.1.2 Local anesthesia.
(*Left*) Area of infiltration.
(*Right*) Application of local
anesthesia

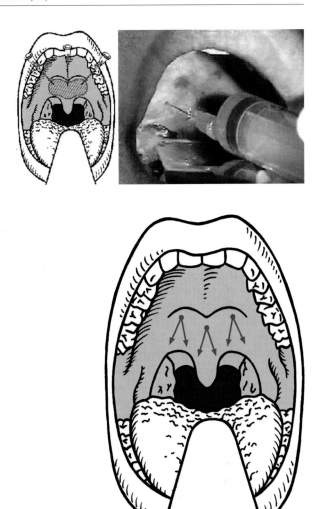

Fig. 6.5.1.3 Soft palate procedure. Six lesions

[749]. Either 80 or 85°C is used as target temperature. In the case of the Celon system (Celon AG medical instruments, Teltow, Germany) we use, depending on the thickness of the soft palate, 10–12 W, and also apply six lesions (Fig. 6.5.1.3). It is efficient to limit the amount of punctures of the mucosa by not pulling the needle completely out of the soft palate after the first lesion, but pushing forward again under slightly changed target direction. In this way the bleeding, which is minor in any case, can be even further minimized. Other potential treatment devices are the reusable bipolar probes of Sutter Medizintechnik (Sutter Medizintechnik, Freiburg, Germany).

In the case of soft palate therapy, two to three sessions are necessary until a satisfactory reduction of the snoring sound to a socially acceptable level is achieved. The follow-up sessions are basically performed in the same way as the first; but in the case of smaller soft palates we reduce the number of lesions to four.

Other authors proceed more aggressively, and apply up to nine lesions to the soft palate. Yet we have not found an increase in efficacy by applying larger or more frequent lesions. But the development in this field is still in flow.

6.5.1.2
Effectiveness for Simple Snoring

In 1998 Powell et al. [577] first reported the use of interstitial radiofrequency surgery for the human soft palate in the treatment of simple snoring. In the following 5 years, various study groups attempted to repeat or modify this study in order to assess the value of this new procedure.

Stuck and colleagues summarized the results in a meta-analysis in 2004 [718]. The survey of the literature at that time generated 22 original articles dealing with interstitial radiofrequency surgery of the soft palate in the treatment of snoring. 18 studies were prospective clinical trials, 15 of these focused on treatment efficacy, 3 of which included a comparison with other treatment modalities such as intraoral devices, LAUP or UPPP. One study was a medium-term follow-up of previously published material.

Nineteen of the 22 studies used temperature-controlled radiofrequency tissue ablation (Somnoplasty®). The remaining three studies used the Ellman (monopolar), VidaMed, or Coblation (bipolar) system. Between 1 and 4 application sites per treatment session were selected. Obstructive sleep apnea was ruled out with polysomnography in 19 of these studies, with a maximum RDI of 10 or 15 respectively. Furthermore, obese patients were excluded in most of the trials (16 out of 22), although the maximum BMI varied between studies (between 27 and 40 kg/m^2). Follow-up periods were usually 6–8 weeks, but especially retrospective trials had a significantly longer follow-up (2–18 months). Treatment efficacy was assessed with the help of visual analogue scales or snoring scores filled out by the bed-partner in 16 of the 18 studies addressing treatment efficacy.

The studies providing results of subjective snoring (visual analogue scales or snoring index) were summarized in terms of two meta-analyses. In the studies using the visual analogue scales a total number of 505 patients were treated. The weighted mean score of these studies was reduced from 8.2 to 3.7. The mean weighted treatment effect was 4.5. In the studies using the snoring index a total number of 167 patients were treated. The weighted mean ± SD was reduced from 8.1 to 3.3 and the weighted mean treatment effect was 4.8. The changes in mean snoring scores of the studies involved were significant at a level of $p < 0.01$.

In three trials, different treatment protocols concerning the number of applications sites per treatment session were compared (i.e., 3–4 vs. 1) [173, 194, 664]. One study was based on snoring scores [173] and compared a group of 19 patients receiving 698 J (mean value) at the midline as a single treatment to a group of 24 patients receiving three lesions with a mean total of 1,254 J per treatment session. The group receiving multiple lesions (total amount of energy per patient: 2,165 J) showed a slightly more pronounced reduction of mean snoring scores (7.8–2.3) compared to the group receiving single lesions (total amount of energy per patient: 2,196 J; 8.9–2.5).

The two studies comparing the effects of single vs. multiple lesion treatments based on visual analogue scales showed comparable effects for these two treatment protocols [194,

664], with a higher total amount of energy delivered per patient for the multiple lesion group (1,676 vs. 3,418 J, and 1,898 vs. 2,001 J). The main advantage of multiple lesion treatments seems to be the reduced number of treatment sessions necessary (3.3 vs. 1.75 [173], 2.38 vs. 1.94 [194], and 2.9 vs. 1.6 [664]) rather than a higher efficacy in respect to the final outcome.

Kania et al. [341] analyzed the influence of energy delivered on snoring outcome in 43 patients. One group received 1,250 J and the other group 1,500 J per treatment at three sites. The 1,500 J delivery led to a better snoring reduction with a significant difference after two treatment sessions.

In two studies with a longer follow-up a relapse over time was seen in 11–41% of the patients [407, 637]. The results for the VAS in this study increased from 2.1 to 5.7 after 14 months. Eight of the 9 patients showing a significant relapse were again treated with radiofrequency surgery. Their mean snoring score could again be reduced from 5.8 to 3.3. Two studies reevaluated initial success rates (3 months) after 12 and 9.5 months respectively. Mean postoperative snoring index increased from 4 to 5 in the first study (12 months) [31] and the success rate decreased from 33 to 28% in the second (9.5 months) [32].

Terris et al. [740] compared interstitial radiofrequency surgery of the soft palate with LAUP in a prospective, randomized manner. LAUP revealed a slight advantage over radiofrequency but resulted in a greater degree of postoperative discomfort.

In 2005 a placebo-controlled, prospective trial on radiofrequency surgery of the soft palate was published by our working group. An overall number of 26 patients with primary snoring were randomized to either two sessions of temperature-controlled radiofrequency surgery or placebo, the latter consisting of an insertion of the device needle under local anesthesia without energy application [722]. While no relevant changes were documented in the placebo group (snoring before treatment 8.4 and after treatment 8.0) snoring score were reduced from 8.1 to 5.2 in the radiofrequency group. This result demonstrates statistically significant differences between the two groups. Although the overall success was inferior to the results of the meta-analysis, this is the first study demonstrating the superiority of radiofrequency surgery of the soft palate over placebo in terms of a level I trial.

In 2006, Hofmann et al. compared radiofrequency surgery of the soft palate with tonsillectomy and UPPP (the surgical intervention was based on the individual anatomy) and came to the conclusion that UPPP was more effective in reducing snoring compared to interstitial radiofrequency surgery but associated with higher morbidity [289]. Our personal opinion, however, is that a relatively invasive treatment such as tonsillectomy and UPPP should only be used in highly selected cases and with particular caution to treat patients with primary snoring only, as other minimally invasive alternatives exist (e.g., RF-UPP combined with RFT of the tonsils).

6.5.1.3
Effectiveness for OSA

There is only a limited number of studies available dealing with isolated interstitial radiofrequency at the soft palate for OSA. A literature search in Pubmed (National Library of Medicine) was performed for the terms "radiofrequency," "palate," and "sleep apnea". Original studies published in English up to March 2008 were included if they addressed

Table 6.5.1.1 Interstitial radiofrequency treatment of the soft palate for OSA

Author	N	Device	Follow-up (months)	AHI pre	AHI post	Success (%)	EBM
Brown et al. [78]	12	Somnus	1.5	31.2	25.3	16.7	4
Blumen et al. [55]	29	Somnus	8.5	19.0	9.8	65.5	4
Bassiouny et al. [41]	20	Arthrocare	4.0	15.3	9.8	40	2b
All	61		5.6	20.2	12.8	47.5	C

AHI Apnea Hypopnea Index

radiofrequency surgery of the soft palate in the treatment of sleep-disordered breathing. For the analysis of clinical outcome, only studies using radiofrequency surgery as an isolated approach were analyzed; studies using combined approaches or studies with patients with primary snoring were only selected with regard to morbidity and complications. In addition, a recent review was evaluated regarding potential additional publications [189]. Several trials were not included, although they claimed to investigate the effects of radiofrequency surgery of the soft palate in sleep-disordered breathing. Those excluded trials either did not provide sufficient objective outcome measures [31, 738, 753] or the baseline AHI was below 5 [305, 577] or 10 [119, 734, 753] and the primary intention was to treat snoring.

Using the Somnus unit, Blumen et al. [55] treated 29 patients with an AHI of 10–30 and a body mass index of less than 30 kg/m². For the entire group the AHI significantly decreased 8.5 months after surgery. The cure rate (defined as an AHI below 10 after surgery) was estimated as 65.5%. Daytime sleepiness as measured with the Epworth Sleepiness Scale improved in 62.1% of the patients.

Brown et al. [78] performed interstitial radiofrequency at the soft palate in more severely affected patients with an AHI up to 78. Although the reduction in mean AHI was statistically significant in this sample too, no clinically significant differences were found between pre- and posttreatment groups with respect to any other sleep parameters.

Bassiouny et al. compared RFT of the soft palate with radiofrequency-assisted uvulopalatoplasty (RF-UPP) (see Sect. 6.5.2 in this book) [41]. In this trial, RF-UPP was superior to "standard" radiofrequency surgery (RFT), but associated with higher postoperative morbidity.

Detailed information using Sher's criteria of success is given in Table 6.5.1.1.

In summary, there is little information that interstitial radiofrequency treatment of the soft palate might be effective for mild OSA. In our personal opinion, radiofrequency surgery of the soft palate may be helpful for patients with mild OSA not requiring nasal ventilation therapy but seeking treatment of snoring as long as the individual anatomy appears suitable.

6.5.1.4
Postoperative Care and Complications

Concerning postoperative complications no serious adverse events were reported, though it should be mentioned that there was a significant variation in the overall complication rates provided, which ranged from 0 to 50% [551, 724]. The most frequently reported complication was a mucosal erosion/ulceration. Mucosal blanching was also reported as accompanying the treatment and to be related to the intensity of postoperative pain [31], but was not assessed by us as a complication. In general, the comparison between different studies concerning postoperative complications poses difficulties. Especially "mucosal erosion" seems to a certain extent be inevitable at the site of the intrusion of the needle (and is not regarded as a complication). It has to be distinguished from secondary erosions or ulcerations due to the energy delivered. Nevertheless, "mucosal erosion" is often listed as a complication without further description.

Four studies reported moderate complications in terms of palatal damage (palatal fistula, uvula loss/sloughing) [63, 173, 194, 551]. One of these studies reported the highest rate of overall postoperative complications with 50%, all being moderate complications such as major mucosal breakdown and uvula sloughing [551]. In this study, technical parameters and the intraoperative setting were comparable to the other studies using temperature-controlled radiofrequency surgery. One significant difference was the regular use of oral corticosteroids before and after treatment in every patient. This is the reason why we do not give any corticosteroids routinely. Series with a larger number of patients showed complication rates of about 1–5% [63, 664, 724].

In those studies where postoperative morbidity was compared with other surgical approaches (UPPP or LAUP), interstitial radiofrequency surgery was associated with the least amount of postoperative pain [56, 92, 623, 748, 757]. For example, mean postoperative pain duration was 2.6 days for radiofrequency surgery compared to 13.8 for LAUP and 14.3 for UPPP in the study of Troell et al. [748].

In a very recent publication of Birkent et al. the effects of radiofrequency surgery of the soft palate on voice was assessed [53]. The authors could demonstrate that there was no significant impact on fundamental frequency and formant frequency of vowels which appears particularly important in professional voice users. If a professional voice user asks for surgical treatment of snoring, radiofrequency surgery appears to be the favorable treatment alternative.

6.5.1.5
Indications and Contraindications

On the basis of the presented data, we currently see an indication for radiofrequency surgery of the soft palate mainly in case of primary snoring. In those cases wherein a mild OSA has been diagnosed but does not require ventilation therapy (for instance, in cases of an AHI below 15 or 20 without daytime symptoms in otherwise healthy subjects), radiofrequency surgery may be applied if the primary complaint is snoring and the anatomy appears suitable. As an alternative, a combined radiofrequency surgery of tongue base, tonsils, and soft palate may be performed. In the case of moderate-to-severe OSA a radiofrequency therapy is usually not sufficient.

For the indication of primary snoring radiofrequency surgery of the soft palate competes with LAUP, palatal implants, and RF-UPP. In this context, the individual anatomy is (again) of particular importance. In the case of pronounced webbing and particularly excessive mucous membrane at the soft palate an ablative procedure is needed which removes the redundant mucosa (LAUP or RF-UPP, see corresponding Sects. 6.4 and 6.5.2).

Soft palate implants (Sect. 6.6) compete directly with radiofrequency surgery of the soft palate due to the fact that indication and anatomical requirements are identical for both techniques. The soft palate implants also produce only a low postoperative morbidity and level I trials are available for both techniques. It is assumed that soft palate implants may have a better long-term efficacy; nevertheless, currently no comparative trials exist for the two techniques.

Take Home Pearls

> Radiofrequency surgery of the soft palate can successfully be applied in primary snoring. Its effects in obstructive sleep apnea are limited, but it may be used in mild cases where snoring is the major complaint.
> The morbidity of radiofrequency surgery of the soft palate is limited and it is associated with least postoperative pain compared to standard soft palate procedures (LAUP, UPPP).
> Level I data from placebo-controlled trials are available for radiofrequency surgery of the soft palate in primary snoring, demonstrating its superiority over placebo. The overall effect, however, is limited but can be further improved with a combination of soft tissue resection.

6.5.2
Radiofrequency-UPP

Boris A. Stuck

> **Core Features**
>
> › Radiofrequency surgery can also be used in a cutting mode to resect and excise excessive soft tissue at the soft palate. It has substantial advantages over laser-assisted resections in terms of morbidity and safety.
> › Combined approaches with interstitial radiofrequency surgery and radiofrequency-assisted surgical excision can be performed to increase clinical efficacy.
> › Radiofrequency-UPP alone or in combination with interstitial radiofrequency surgery can be performed in an outpatient setting under local anesthesia.

With regard to the significant morbidity associated with laser-assisted uvulopalatoplasty (LAUP) in terms of postoperative pain and with regard to the specific safety issues with laser systems, cutting devices based on radiofrequency energy were used instead of the laser to excise palatal tissue. According to the LAUP, this technique has often been labeled as "radiofrequency-assisted uvulopalatoplasty" RAUP [41, 414, 803]. Furthermore, various combinations have been proposed, the most interesting one being the combination of interstitial radiofrequency surgery (RFT) and RAUP, which we call RF-UPP [34]. This technique is particularly interesting as it overcomes the major limitations of interstitial radiofrequency surgery, being the fact that excessive soft tissue (webbing) cannot be successfully treated with interstitial radiofrequency surgery alone.

6.5.2.1
Surgical Technique

RAUP is usually performed analogous to standard LAUP under local anesthesia (see Sect. 6.4). We prefer the above-mentioned combination of interstitial radiofrequency surgery combined with cautious resection of excessive soft tissue at the posterior pillar and the uvula whenever present (RF-UPP). The procedure can be performed under local anesthesia. In upright position, the patient is comfortably seated either in the clinical chair or on a surgical table. Sedation is not generally recommended in this case but may be applied according to the patient's needs. If necessary, we administer sedation intravenously with Midazolam, by titrating the drug up to the desired level of sedation. A perioperative antibiotics prophylaxis is not required. First, the interstitial application of radiofrequency energy is undertaken (for RF-UPP, the bipolar Celon systems are used performing about 5–6 lesions at 10 W; Celon AG Medical Instruments, Teltow, Germany), as described in Sect. 6.1.3. In addition, careful resection of excessive mucosa is performed with a cutting device (Celon ProCut, Celon AG Medical Instruments). A triangular incision is done bilaterally of the uvula; hypertrophic mucosa at the posterior arch of soft palate is resected with the ProCut electrode with 20 W. With the same needle, uvular resection is done with transversal resection of mucosa (Fig. 6.5.2.1). Particular care is taken to resect only excessive soft tissue, leaving the palatal muscles intact. The session is usually repeated after 6–8 weeks.

6.5.2.2
Effectiveness for Simple Snoring

As presented in Table 6.5.2.1, both studies addressing RF-UPP in primary snoring demonstrated statistically significant improvement of snoring assessed with visual analogue scales (VAS) (0–10), with one study being a randomized controlled trial. In the study by Uppal et al., surgical outcome was compared between RF-UPP ($N = 30$) and LAUP ($N = 30$), and no differences were seen between the two groups [757]. The best outcome was reported by our own study group with RF-UPP, indicating that the additional soft tissue resection helps to improve overall outcome [34]. Nevertheless, data are sparse, and long-term data are not available to date.

6.5.2.3
Effectiveness for OSA

To date, only two studies from the same working group in Kairo are available with regard to RF-UPP and its use in obstructive sleep apnea. Both studies applied the Arthrocare system (Coblation, Arthrocare, Synnyvale, CA) as demonstrated in Table 6.5.2.2 [27, 41]. Bassiouny et al. compared interstitial radiofrequency treatment (RFT) of the soft palate with RF-UPP and demonstrated that RF-UPP was more effective in reducing respiratory parameters than RFT [41]. Atef et al. compared RF-UPP (they made three upward

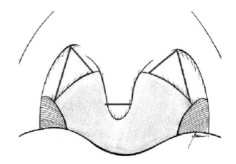

Fig. 6.5.2.1   Amount of soft tissue resection in RF-UPP

Table 6.5.2.1 RF-UPP for simple snoring

Author	N	Device	Follow-up (months)	Snore pre	Snore post	Success (%)	ESS pre	ESS post	EBM
Uppal et al. [757]	30	No data	19	4.0	2.9	70 (Improvement)	8.0	No data	2b
Baisch et al. [34]	21	Celon	2	8.5	2.0	86 (VAS < 3)	6.3	4.3	4
All	52		2–19						C

ESS Epworth sleepiness scale; *VAS* Visual Analogue Scale; *EBM* evidence-based medicine

Table 6.5.2.2 RF-UPP for OSA

Author	N	Procedure	Follow-up (months)	AHI pre	AHI short (3 months)	AHI post	Success 3 months (%)	Success 18 months (%)	EBM
Atef et al. [27]	64	RF-UPP vs. LAUP	18.0	26.3	14.4	16.6	73.1	41.2	2b
Bassiouny et al. [41]	20	RF-UPP vs. RFT SP	4.0	17.2		8.1		50	3b
All	84		4–18	24.1		14.6		43.3	B

AHI Apnea Hypopnea Index; *EBM* evidence-based medicine

interstitial channels through the incision made near the uvula) with LAUP [27]. A statistically significant reduction in Apnea Hypopnea Index (AHI) was achieved after RF-UPP after at least three treatment sessions while a statistically significant reduction was achieved in the LAUP group already after the first session. The overall outcome was comparable but a higher number of sessions was necessary in the RF-UPP group. Surgical success decreased over time. This is a result that is known from almost all other soft palatal surgeries for SDB.

More controlled trials with regard to a real control group are not available to date; the same is true for long-term follow-up studies.

6.5.2.4
Postoperative Care and Complications

As described above and in accordance with interstitial radiofrequency surgery and LAUP, the above-mentioned techniques can be performed on an outpatient basis. In general, postoperative pain after RAUP is significantly less pronounced and postoperative morbidity is significantly lower compared to LAUP [414]. Nevertheless, postoperative morbidity, especially in terms of postoperative pain, after RAUP is still higher compared to simple interstitial treatment with radiofrequency [41]. With regard to our own data and our increasing experiences with RF-UPP, significant postoperative pain after RF-UPP has to be expected in the first 2–3 days.

In the majority of the trails cited above, no relevant complications were described. Lim et al. reported foreign-body sensation and dry mouth in 2 of their 24 patients with RAUP (which was significantly less than in the LAUP group) [414].

6.5.2.5
Indications and Contraindications

According to the current literature and our own experiences, RAUP has substantial advantages compared to LAUP, especially with regard to postoperative morbidity and technical simplicity. RAUP can easily be combined with interstitial radiofrequency surgery (RF-UPP), which significantly improves the outcome compared to interstitial radiofrequency surgery only. We would recommend performing RAUP or better RF-UPP instead of interstitial radiofrequency surgery alone, especially in those cases where excessive soft tissue is found at the soft palate. To our understanding, there is little support for still using the Laser at the soft palate in patients with snoring (and no indication in obstructive sleep apnea according to current guidelines).

RAUP and RF-UPP significantly improve snoring, although to date no controlled trials are available. In terms of obstructive sleep apnea, we see an indication for these procedures in cases with mild obstructive sleep apnea not requiring ventilation therapy, as long as snoring is the major complaint and the individual anatomy appears suitable.

Take Home Pearls

> RF-UPP is the combination of interstitial RFT and the resection of redundant mucosa at the posterior palatal pillar and uvula, as for example in LAUP.
> In cases of excessive soft mucosa at the soft palate (webbing, uvula hypertrophy), radiofrequency-UPP can significantly reduce snoring. In our hands, RF-UPP is more effective than its isolated components.
> With regard to postoperative morbidity and safety, radiofrequency-UPP has significant advantages over LAUP and can also be used in cases of mild obstructive sleep apnea, where Laser resection is contraindicated.

Palatal Implants

6.6

Joachim T. Maurer and Thomas Verse

Core Features

> Three palatal implants are used to stiffen the soft palate.
> Palatal implants fulfill the criteria of minimally invasive surgery.
> Satisfaction rates for simple snoring vary between 22 and 75%.
> Palatal implants seem to be effective in mild OSA.

UPPP and LAUP are standard procedures for the treatment of simple snoring and the palatal site of obstruction in OSA or UARS. However, these treatments are invasive, destructive, painful, and, to a certain extent, irreversible. Furthermore, UPPP requires general anesthesia. Radiofrequency of the palate being the first minimally invasive palatal procedure is a multiple-step procedure. Furthermore, a considerable relapse of snoring has been reported 1 year after treatment [405]. Therefore, a new minimally invasive, single-step procedure that places cylindrical implants within the soft palate has been developed [442]. Shortly afterward, the technique (Pillar®) was used for OSA patients as well.

The Pillar® implant consists of polyethylenterephthalat (PET). This material has been used as a vascular endoprosthesis (since 1960), as mesh in stomach surgery (since 1970), and in heart valves (since the end of the 1970s). Three rod-shaped implants are inserted in the soft palate. The implants themselves and the surrounding scarring induce a stiffening of the soft palate, which shall reduce or eliminate snoring sounds and respiratory events.

6.6.1
Surgical Technique

As in the case of LAUP and interstitial radiofrequency surgery of the soft palate, this technique is performed on an outpatient basis in the sitting patient. A perioperative antibiotic prophylaxis is started (e.g., with 2 g Cefazolin intravenously) and will be continued per os for 5 days (e.g., with 2 × 500 mg Cefuroxim per day). After mucosal disinfection with Hexetidine 0.1% and topical anesthesia with Lidocain spray or gel 2%, the palate is infiltrated with approximately 3 mL of Prilocain 2% with epinephrine 1:200,000. If required, sedation is induced (e.g., with Dormicum® = Midazolam, titrated according to effect), but in most cases,

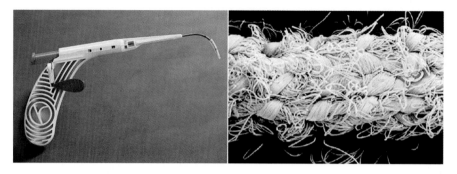

Fig. 6.6.1   Left side: delivery tool. Right side: magnification of implant

this is not necessary. Of course, the operation can also be done as an adjunct procedure under general anesthesia. Then, the patient has to be in the tonsillectomy position.

The implants are 18 mm long and have a diameter of 1.5 mm. They are delivered in a 14-gauge hollow needle (Fig. 6.6.1), which has three markings at the curved end of the needle. The complete hand piece is a disposable instrument with one preloaded implant per hand piece; therefore, three hand pieces have to be used for one patient. Before the procedure, the plastic sleeve must be stripped off the needle, and the implant can be seen inside the hollow needle. Then, the transport lock has to be removed.

The needle is inserted in the midline directly at the junction of soft and hard palate and then pushed forward toward the free margin of the soft palate to an extent that the most proximal, i.e., full insertion marking just remains visible. The implant is supposed to settle intramuscularly. It is crucial that the implant neither anteriorly nor posteriorly bulges through the mucosa. When the correct position is checked by gently moving the palate anterioly and posteriorly with the inserted needle, the lock beneath the slider is pushed downwards. The implant is deployed by advancing the slider halfway until a click is heard. Then, the needle is pulled out until the halfway marker becomes visible. Finally, the slider is advanced to the end, and the needle is withdrawn in a curved motion. The other two implants are placed in the same way 2 mm parallel to the first one on both sides. After implantation, a perforation of an implant at either surface of the palate is ruled out by inspection, palpation, and transnasal pharyngoscopy (Fig. 6.6.2).

After the surgical procedure, the implant can no longer be discerned. In Fig. 6.6.3, one can still distinguish the punctures, but not the implants themselves (Fig. 6.6.3).

6.6.2
Effectiveness for Simple Snoring

During the first 3 years after the inauguration of the method, prospective case series focused on simple snorers. Today there is data from 268 patients covering a follow-up of 3–12 months. Three month data in average is superior to 12 month data pointing at a possible decrease in efficacy during the first year after the procedure. Subjective snoring (bed-partner

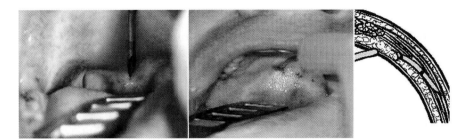

Fig. 6.6.2 (Left) Mimicking the final position of median implant. (Center) Insertion of right implant. (Right) Intramuscular position of implant within the soft palate

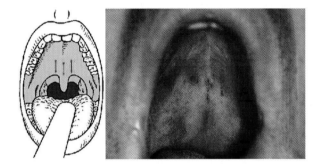

Fig. 6.6.3 Postoperative situation

evaluation by visual analogue scale) can be reduced by approximately 3 cm to a final value of 4 cm on the 10 cm scale (Table 6.6.1). A complete elimination of snoring is rare. As values below 3 cm are considered as nonbothersome snoring, one has to admit that a considerable number of patients may not be satisfied by this procedure. It has to be investigated whether additional implants can reduce snoring further. Similarl to other operations, subjective data do not necessarily match with objective data obtained in a few studies [449, 514] with the SNAP®-system. This may be due to the fact that the description of snoring is very subjective and strongly depends on the bed-partner. There is a lack of randomized data till date.

6.6.3
Effectiveness for OSA

After several case series presenting short-term data two randomized, placebo-controlled trials have been published in 2008 (Table 6.6.2). All patients had mild OSA. Unanimously, the case series show some reduction of AHI and a success in 20–40% of the cases. The study of Nordgard [511] has a higher success rate because 15 of 41 patients were lost to 1-year follow-up. Some had received additional treatment due to insufficient 3-month data, others rejected follow-up visits because they felt subjectively relieved, and the rest could not be contacted any more. In an intention-to-treat analysis the success rate of this

Table 6.6.1 Efficacy of Pillar® implants for simple snoring

Author	N	Follow-up (months)	Method	Snore pre	Snore post	Success (%)	ESS pre	ESS post	EBM
Ho et al. [283]	12	3	VAS	7.9	4.8	No data	8.9	5.7	4
Nordgard et al. [514]	35	3	VAS	7.3	3.6	53 (VAS <3)	9.3	4.6	4
Maurer et al. [449]	15	3	VAS	7.3	2.5	73 (VAS <3)	5.3	3.4	4
Maurer et al. [448]	40	12	VAS	7.1	4.8	22 (VAS <3)	6.1	4.9	4
Kühnel et al. [377]	106	6	VAS	7.6	3.9	<50 (quest)	8.0	5.1	4
Romanow et al. [622]	25	3	VAS	8.5	4.4	75 (quest)	8.3	7.3	4
Nordgard et al. [512]	35	12	VAS	7.1	4.8	23.5 (VAS <3)	9.3	5.6	4
All	268	6.7	VAS	7.5	4.1		8.0	5.2	C

Quest questionnaire; *ESS* Eporth Sleepiness Scale, *VAS* Visual Analogue Scale; *EBM* evidence-based medicine

Table 6.6.2 Effectiveness of Pillar® implants in OSA

Author	N	Follow-up (months)	AHI pre	AHI post	Success (%)	ESS pre	ESS post	p ESS	EBM
Friedman et al. [222]	29	7.5	12.7	11.5	24.1	No data	No data	No data	4
Walker et al. [794]	53	3.0	25.0	22.0	20.8	11.0	6.9	<0.001	4
Nordgard et al. [513]	25	3.0	16.2	12.1	36	9.7	5.5	<0.001	4
Nordgard et al. [511]	26	12.0	16.5	12.5	50	8.3	5.4	<0.001	4
Goessler et al. [233]	16	3.0	16.5	11.2	37.5	7.2	4.6	<0.05	4
Friedman et al. [217]	29	3.0	23.8	15.9	41.9	12.7	10.2	<0.001	2b
Steward et al. [705]	47	3.0	16.8	19.7	26	10.6	8.7	<0.01	2b
All	225	4.6	18.9	16.4	31.3	8.9	7.3		B

AHI Apnea Hypopnea Index; *ESS* Epworth Sleepiness Scale; *EBM* evidence-based medicine

study group drops to 32% which is in line with the other short-term data. This indicates that the results remain stable over 1 year.

A Chinese group also treated patients with an AHI >60 showing a reduction as well, but with success in only one of the six patients, whereas patients with mild OSA were successfully treated in 68% [105]. This indicates that the Pillar® system is more appropriate in mild OSA. Unfortunately this publication is in Chinese language only.

Both randomized, placebo-controlled studies show a superiority of implants over placebo. However, results are conflicting as Steward et al. had to recognize an increase of AHI [705] in contrast to Friedman et al. who reported a pronounced reduction of AHI [217]. Friedman also tried to put Pillar® implants after UPPP failure. He was successful in 21.7% of the patients with this adjunct minimally invasive treatment [216]. There is a lack of long-term data. Walker et al. reevaluated their short-term results (90 days) [794] again after 436 days [795]. Initial response or nonresponse to palatal implants remained stable over this extended period.

Palatal implants can also be used in multilevel treatment under general anesthesia [214].

6.6.4
Postoperative Care and Complications

The procedure can be performed on an outpatient basis. Perioperative antibiotic prophy-laxis with 2 g Cefazolin intravenously which will be continued orally for 5 days with Cefuroxim 2 × 500 mg per day may not be forgotten. Up to now, all implants have been placed without complications. Improvements of the delivery tool simplified the procedure and reduced the risk of malpositioning of the implants.

Only minor discomfort (minor sore throat) is reported in a few patients within the first 3 days postprocedure. Pain scores on the VAS are minimal (always below 3 at day 2, no more pain at day 90). In the majority of patients, Paracetamol at low dosage is sufficient. Narcotic analgesics or nonsteroidal anti-inflammatory drugs (NSAID) are not required. There is no significant speech disturbance after the procedure.

The patient has to be informed about the possibility of partial extrusion of an implant. Implants can extrude to both sides. Therefore, the surgeon has to check the oral as well as the pharyngeal surface of the soft palate. Implants never extrude com-pletely thus making an aspiration impossible. This complication may cause mild pain and a foreign-body sensation, but there is no need for analgesics in the majority of cases. A partial extrusion happens in 8.6% of the patients on average. There has been a marked decrease of extrusion rates over the years indicating that there is a certain learning curve the surgeon should be made aware of. The implants can be removed easily under local anesthesia. If a patient desires the removal of all three implants even though they are well-incorporated into the palatal tissue, it can be difficult because of relevant scarring. We have done that in two patients and general anesthesia was required. The trauma generated is far bigger than during implantation or removal in cases of partial extrusion. Nevertheless, the lesions heal without any further clinical sequelae. Despite a partial extrusion snoring may decrease further over time. No severe adverse events were observed in 390 patients with a mean follow-up of 237 days (Table 6.6.3).

6.6.5
Indications and Contraindications

The technique can be used for simple snorers as well as patients with mild OSA who have palatal obstruction without a long uvula or big tonsils. Its short-term results are compara-ble to interstitial radiofrequency surgery of the soft palate. Soft palate implants directly compete with this procedure. One-year follow-up seems to be slightly superior to RF of the soft palate. However, further studies have to show whether one of these two minimally invasive techniques will turn out to be preferable.

In comparison with the soft palate implants, interstitial radiofrequency surgery has the advantage that it can be additionally extended to the tongue base, the inferior turbinates, or

Table 6.6.3 Extrusions of Pillar® implants

Author	N	Follow-up (days)	Extrusions per implant	Per patient
Ho et al. [283]	11	90	3 (9.1%)	2 (18.2)
Nordgard et al. [512]	35	365	9 (8.6%)	6 (17.1)
Maurer et al. [448]	40	365	13 (10.8%)	10 (25%)
Romanow et al. [622]	25	90	2 (2.7%)	1 (4%)
Friedman et al. [222]	125	300	10 (2.7%)	10 (8%)
Friedman et al. [216]	23	180	0 (0%)	0 (0%)
Skjostad et al. [688]	10	180	0 (0%)	0 (0%)
Nordgard et al. [511]	26	365	3 (3.8%)	3 (11.5%)
Goessler et al. [233]	16	90	0 (0%)	0 (0%)
Friedman et al. [217]	29	96	2 (2.3%)	2 (6.9%)
Steward et al. [705]	50	90	2 (1.3%)	2 (4%)
All	390	237	44 (3.8%)	36 (8.6%)

the tonsils. This is especially of advantage in those cases where the surgeon is not certain whether he or she is dealing with an exclusive palatal snoring.

Candidates for palatal implants differ from candidates for LAUP or RF-UPP, respectively. The latter are ablative procedures in which the posterior palatine arch and the uvula are shortened. This is not the case for the soft palate implants. Therefore, patients with pronounced webbing and a long uvula should not receive implants; on the other hand, in cases wherein no excessive mucosa exists, the soft palate implants or interstitial radiofrequency surgery are to be preferred because of the significantly lower postoperative morbidity rate.

Take Home Pearls

> Palatal implants are minimally invasive.
> They are effective for simple snoring and (very) mild OSA.
> A complete elimination of snoring is rare.
> Good candidates for palatal implants differ from candidates for LAUP or RF-UPP respectively.

Other Soft Palate Procedures

6.7

Thomas Verse

Core Features

> There are various types of surgery addressing the soft palate to treat simple snoring and OSA.
> This chapter will compile the current knowledge about uvulectomy, palatal stiffening, injection snoreplasty, and transpalatal advancement pharyngoplasty.

Apart from the procedures previously described, there exists a plethora of surgical techniques for the soft palate which have been suggested for the treatment of SDB. Illustrating all these techniques or modifications would go beyond the scope of this book. But a few of these techniques have recently received more attention or are so fundamentally different in their approach that we consider a brief presentation of these techniques to be worthwhile.

6.7.1
Uvulectomy

A search of the literature generated more than 60 hits for this topic. Most of the hits refer to ritual indications and not to SDB. Only one publication recommends uvulectomy as a simple and complication-free method for the treatment of primary snoring [25]. The success rate is approximately 61%. However, it must be said that the majority of the respondents requested further treatment for the reduction of their snoring. Uvulectomy is described as a very painful treatment, comparable to a complete uvulopalatopharyngoplasty (UPPP).

Another publication recommends uvulectomy for the therapy of UARS [503]. Yet the study offers no success rates. In this context, we once again wish to draw attention to the study by Mortimore et al. [485]: the study was able to demonstrate that in the case of a CPAP therapy after an isolated uvulectomy already for low respiratory pressures oronasal air leaks occur. These can make an effective respiratory treatment impossible. In our opinion, uvulectomy is generally not to be recommended. It is crucial that the musculature of the soft palate be preserved during surgery. Solely excessive mucosal folds may be resected.

K. Hörmann, T. Verse, *Surgery for Sleep Disordered Breathing*,
DOI: 10.1007/978-3-540-77786-1_6.7, © Springer Verlag Berlin Heidelberg 2010

Today, there exist safer and more effective procedures in the treatment of obstructive sleep apnea (OSA) as well as for the therapy of primary snoring.

6.7.2
Palatal Stiffening Operation

6.7.2.1
Surgical Technique

Ellis et al. [168] investigated the mechanics of snoring in the laboratory as an aid for devising a more effective operation. These studies have shown that there are several methods by which snoring can be generated, but palatal flutter is probably the most important factor. The dominant parameters in the generation of flutter of the palate are its length and stiffness. Any removal of tissue to shorten the palate as in UPPP inevitably risks impairing its function. Therefore, the authors were the first to choose the stiffening alternative. Using a laser, a central longitudinal strip of mucosa – but not the muscles in the area of the anterior palatine arch (M. palatoglossus) – is removed from the surface of the soft palate, which heals by fibrosis, producing the required stiffening. Some authors additionally [481, 687] treated the uvula and the posterior palatine arch as in the case of laser-assisted uvulopalatoplasty (LAUP) and laser uvuloplatatoplasty (LUPP) and call this modification "mucosal strip technique" (MST) (Fig. 6.7.1). Other authors do not address the uvula and call their technique "palatal stiffening" [798].

A third group of surgeons adopted this idea of palatal stiffening using electrocautery to remove the anterior palatal mucosa. Mair and Day [433] removed a 2 cm central palatal mucosal flap under local and topical anesthesia. The resection starts 1 cm from the junction of the hard and soft palate, which is gently dissected down to the uvula. Finally, the redundant mucosa of the uvular tip is resected preserving the uvular muscle (Fig. 6.7.2 left side and middle).

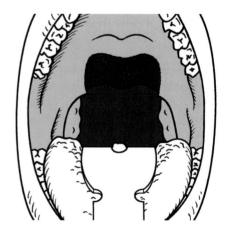

Fig. 6.7.1 Scheme of MST. Coagulation of the palatine mucosa combined with a shortening of the uvula according to Skatvedt [687]

Throughout the operation the palatal muscles remain intact. By week 2 or 3 the palate has stiffened (Fig. 6.7.2 right side). For further details on the precise surgical procedure, we refer the reader to the original publication [433].

Finally, a combination of both palatal stiffening and LAUP is recommended by Remacle et al. [595]. These authors perform three steps. First, they vaporize the palatal mucosa (Fig. 6.7.3 left side) in a method similar to the MST technique. Second, the palatal arches are trimmed very cautiously, completely protecting the anterior pillar (Fig. 6.7.3 middle). Finally, the uvula is either cut or vaporized (Fig. 6.7.3 right side). We do not have personal experience with this technique but is seems reasonable, because it is a very careful technique not disturbing the palatine arches and combines two established techniques. We ourselves combine the interstitial radiofrequency treatment (RFT) of the soft palate with a cautious resection of the redundant mucosa and call our technique radiofrequency-assisted uvulopalatoplasty (RF-UPP). For more details, please refer to Sect. 6.5.2.

As all the techniques mentioned here are very similar, and they will be discussed together in the following section.

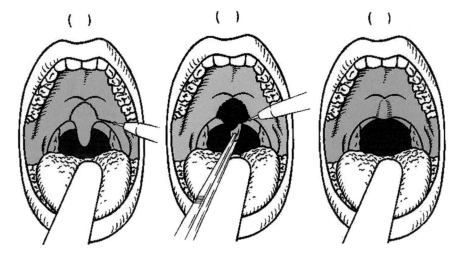

Fig. 6.7.2   Cautery-assisted palatal stiffening operation (CAPSO). *Left*: incision. *Middle*: resection of palatal mucosa and shortening of the uvula. *Right*: stiffening after secondary wound healing 3 weeks postoperatively

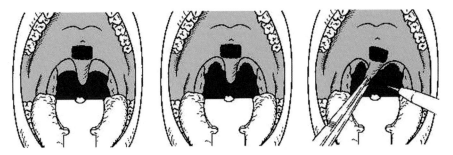

Fig. 6.7.3   Scheme of combined palatal stiffening with LAUP according to Remacle et al. [595]. *Left*: coagulation of the palatal mucosa. *Center*: resection of posterior pillars. *Right*: shortening of the uvula

Table 6.7.1 Palatal stiffening for simple snoring

Author	Device	N	Follow-up (months)	VAS	Success (%)	Definition of success	EBM
Ellis et al. [168]	Nd:YAG	16	3	1–10	87.5	VAS < 4	3b
Ellis [170]	Nd:YAG	16	15–18	1–10	68.8	VAS < 4	4
Shehab et Robin [662]	CO_2	24	3–52	1–10	79.2	Red. > 2	3b
Morar et al. [481]	CO_2	25	6	1–100	72.0	Red. ≥ 25%	4
Mair and Day [433]	electrocautery	206	12	No VAS	77.0	Telefone interview	4
All		287	3–52		76.88		B

VAS Visual Analogue Scale; *EBM* grade of evidence-based medicine; *Red.* reduction

6.7.2.2
Effectiveness for Simple Snoring

Palatal stiffening procedures show satisfying short-term results (Table 6.7.1). Again, patients' satisfaction decreases over time [170, 424, 757]. The two controlled trials showed comparable effectiveness of laser-assisted palatal stiffening and conventional UPPP [168, 662]. One fact in the latter trial is remarkable: there was no positive impact of an additionally performed tonsillectomy on the snoring outcome. Uppal et al. [757] compared laser-assisted palatal stiffening and a punctate diathermy both combined with uvulectomy in a single-blinded randomized controlled trial ($N = 62$). Results with regard to the subjective reduction of snoring were comparable with significantly more postoperative pain in the group after laser surgery.

Mair and Day investigated 206 patients who underwent isolated cautery-assisted palatal stiffening operations (CAPSO) for habitual snoring [433]. No sleep studies were performed. Four to six weeks after surgery, 190 patients (92%) reported successful reduction or elimination of snoring. Follow-up evaluation 6–36 months postoperatively (mean 12 months) revealed a 77% drop in the success rate (145 successes from 188 patients).

6.7.2.3
Effectiveness for OSA

Wassmuth et al. [800] evaluated the effect of CAPSO for OSA. As they are part of the same working group, the surgical technique used was identical to that of Mair and Day [433]. The authors included 25 sleep apneics with a baseline Apnea Hypopnea Index (AHI) of 25.1 ± 12.9. Three months postoperatively, the AHI had statistically significantly

Table 6.7.2 Palatal stiffening OSA

Palatal stiffening	Device	N	Follow-up (months)	AHI pre	AHI post	ESS pre	ESS post	Success (%)	EBM
Wassmuth et al. [800]	Electrocautery	25	3	25.1	16.6	12.7	8.8	40.0	4
Pang and Terris [539]	Electrocautery	8	3	12.3	5.2	12.2	8.9	75.0	4
All		33	3	22.0	13.8	12.6	8.8	48.5	C

EBM grade of evidence-based medicine; *AHI*: apnea hypopnea index; *ESS*: Epworth Sleepiness Scale.

dropped to 16.6 ± 15.0. Using Sher criteria, the success rate was estimated as 48%. Daytime sleepiness as measured with the Epworth Sleepiness Scale improved highly significantly from 12.7 at baseline to 8.8 after surgery (Table 6.7.2).

6.7.2.4
Indications, Complications, and Postoperative Care

Palatal stiffening operations are designed as an outpatient office procedure under local anesthesia. The surgical setting and postoperative care is the same as with LAUP. No sedation is required. No antibiotics or steroids are administered.

The use of lasers at the soft palate has proven to be safe in several animal models [127, 383, 798]. No perioperative complications have been reported so far. Postoperative complications include minor bleedings (1%), temporary velopharyngeal incompetence (<1%), prolonged throat pain (4%), and intermittent tiny vesicles at the scar site for up to 2 months after surgery [433]. Hoolsema [291] described subjective complaints in some patients such as an inability to articulate a rolling/r/, increased gag reflex, aspiration, and altered taste sensations at short-term follow-up.

CAPSO is a painful surgery. Pain has been rated at between 50 and 60 for the first 8 days on a Visual Analogue Scale (VAS) with its end-points 0 = no pain and 100 = maximum pain [800]. This means that CAPSO is as painful as our conventional UPPP technique (see Sect. 6.2).

In summary, CAPSO shows similar short-term results for simple snoring and for mild OSA as other soft palate procedures. We do not use it for simple snoring as we think there are less-invasive procedures available, producing less postoperative morbidity. In cases of redundant mucosa, we prefer the LAUP, which reshapes the free margin of the palate. In other cases, we prefer either interstitial radiofrequency surgery or palatal implants, as these techniques are much less painful. For OSA, we perform a conventional UPPP or an uvula-flap, always combined with a tonsillectomy if tonsils are still present, because for this procedure, there exists a reliable long-term data documenting superior efficiency.

6.7.3
Injection Snoreplasty

6.7.3.1
Surgical Technique

Injection snoreplasty was introduced in 2001 to treat palatal snoring [70]. The surgical concept consists of the injection of sclerosing agents into the soft palate. As a result, scarring ensues a stiffening of the soft palate. The authors initially used 3% sodium tetradecyl sulfate (STS) as an effective agent. In Europe, this substance has not been approved for this usage. Therefore, no European study reports exist, and for the same reason, we ourselves do not employ injection snoreplasty. In a recent publication, further agents were assessed with respect to their efficacy [71]. None of the tested substances produced better results than STS. Only 50% ethanol was found to produce equivalent subjective and objective snoring efficacy and equivalent pain and recovery time compared to STS. However, a higher rate of transient palatal fistula was found in the case of ethanol.

The patient is maintained in a sitting position in the surgical chair. The authors only perform topical anesthesia first using a spray followed by a local anesthetic gel. The latter is placed on the end of a tongue depressor and placed against the soft palate for up to 10 min. Injected local anesthesia is not thought to be necessary. During the first treatment, 2.0 mL of 1% STS (10 mg/mL Sotradecol, Elkins-Sinn, Cherry Hill, NJ) is injected with a single needle penetration into the midline soft palate. The desired anatomic plane of injection is the submucosal layer of the soft palate. After approximately 2 min, the injected midline palate turns into a purple, hemorrhagic color as the sclerotherapy agent begins to take effect. Over a period of weeks, the mucosa heals, and a midline scar remains. For patients undergoing a second treatment, the site of injection is modified (Fig. 6.7.4).

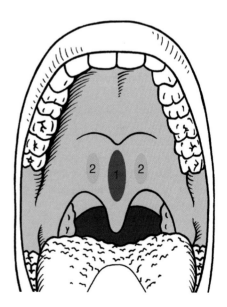

Fig. 6.7.4 Injection snoreplasty with 3% sodium tetradecyl sulfate. During the first treatment session the agent is applied in the midline. In case of a second treatment session, the agent is injected paramedially on both sides

Breitzke and Mair [70] used 3% Sotradecol for repeated treatment sessions in most cases. For more details see [70].

6.7.3.2
Effectiveness for Simple Snoring and OSA

Although the data is still limited, initial preliminary conclusions can be drawn from Table 6.7.3. All the authors used tetradycil sulfate (TDS) for treatment. In all studies, satisfaction was defined as the bedpartner`s satisfaction with regard to the decrease of snoring.

Two working groups [9, 69, 70] documented a decrease in the bedpartner`s satisfaction with injection snoreplasty over time. This finding is in accordance with all other palatal treatments for simple snoring. Iseri and Balcioglu [317] compared injection snoreplasty with interstitial RFT of the soft palate. Both the treatments were effective for simple snoring but tended to produce little benefit for RFT (87.5% satisfaction vs. 76.7%).

There is no information concerning the isolated use of injection snoreplasty for OSA. A recently published study describes the combined use of injection snoreplasty and bipolar radiofrequency uvulopalatoplasty as effective for both simple snoring and OSA [520].

6.7.3.3
Indications, Complications, and Postoperative Care

So far, intraoperative complications have not been reported. There is no specific postoperative care. The overall discomfort level created by the procedure was reported to be 3.5 on the VAS with its end-points 0 = no discomfort and 10 = maximum discomfort. To date, four patients have developed a transient, asymptomatic palatal fistula. One had received STS and the other three 50% ethanol. As with palatal tissue breakdown, treatment was entirely supportive without the use of antibiotics or steroids. All four patients healed spontaneously without complications and with good snoring results. In an animal model, injection snoreplasty produced more scarring within the palate as compared with interstitial RFT [579].

Table 6.7.3 Effectiveness of injection snoreplasty for simple snoring

Author	Agens	N	Follow-up short (weeks)	Success short (%)	Follow-up long (months)	Success long (%)	EBM
Breitzke et al. [69, 70]	TDS	27	6	92.6	19	74.1	4
Iseri et al. [317]	TDS	70	6	76.7	No data	No data	3b
Al-Jassim et al. [9]	TDS	60	6	66.7	12	48.3	4
All		157	6	75.61	12–19	56.31	C

EBM grade of evidence-based medicine; *TDS* tetradycil sulfate

The data are limited in their scope by the fact that they stem from merely one study group and only encompass a small number of patients. Having said this, the method does appear to produce comparable results in simple snorers as other minimally invasive surgeries of the soft palate.

6.7.4
Transpalatal Advancement Pharyngoplasty

Evaluations of pharyngeal properties before and after UPPP, using both computerized tomography and acoustic reflection, have demonstrated increases in oropharyngeal size and decreases in oropharyngeal collapsibility. Larger increases in these characteristics are associated with a successful clinical response to UPPP [663, 837]. However, UPPP failures are associated with smaller volume increases, compliance changes, and subsequently are observed to have a persistent palatal site of obstruction. Woodson and Toohill [829] concluded from these findings that in some patients technical failure may occur and introduced a new surgical alternative to UPPP, the so-called transpalatal advancement pharyngoplasty (TAP).

The surgical principle consists of not only altering the inferior edge as in a UPPP, but also in advancing the base of the soft palate at the hard palate. This entails a partial resection of the posterior edge of the hard palate. Surgery is performed under general anesthesia. The preparations and the surgical setting are analogous to the procedure in the case of a UPPP. All patients were administered perioperative antibiotics and dexametasone (10 mg). In the original publication [829], local infiltration with an adrenal local anesthetic and the superficial insertion of 4% cocaine solvent along the floor of the nose was recommended.

Initially, a conventional UPPP is performed. In the second phase, the advancement of the soft palate (Fig. 6.7.5) occurs. First, a reverse V-shaped mucous membrane soft tissue flap is prepared and the transition from the hard to the soft palate is exposed (Fig. 6.7.5 left side). Subsequently, soft and hard palate are separated exposing the nasopharynx (Fig. 6.7.5 half left). Now, the posterior edge of the hard palate is partially resected. For the reinsertion of the soft palate, drill holes are placed in the hard palate (Fig. 6.7.5 half right). Finally, the adaptation of the soft palate to the hard palate and the realignment of the soft tissue flap are performed (Fig. 6.7.5 right side). With regard to the exact surgical technique including potential pitfalls, we refer the reader to the original publication by Woodson and Toohill [829].

In a first series including 6 patients with severe OSA, the authors were able to achieve a reduction of the AHI from 52.8 to 12.3 after isolated TAP. Four of these 6 patients (67%) fulfilled the healing criteria according to Sher. In a second series, 6 more patients first underwent a UPPP and in second session a TAP [835]. Four patients received solely a TAP in the

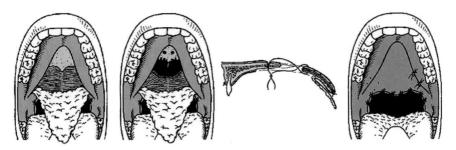

Fig. 6.7.5   Transpalatal advancement pharyngoplasty (TAP) according to [829]. Left) palatal incisions. Center left) separating hard and soft palate and resection of the dorsal edge of the hard palate. Center right) readaptation of soft palate to hard palate using drill holes. Right) situation after surgery

second session; three of them fulfilled the healing criteria according to Sher (AHI pre 74.5 vs. post 29.2). The maximal area behind the soft palate increased by 321% and the retropalatal closing pressure decreased significantly as compared with the situation after UPPP. In two other publications concerning the matter, Woodson describes an increase both in the anterioposterior and the lateral dimensions of the retropalatal airway after TAP [833, 834]. His most recent publication [827] compared TAP ($N = 30$) with UPPP ($N = 44$). Baseline AHI, age, and BMI did not differ between the two groups. In the TAP group, AHI decreased from 48.3 ± 25.6 at baseline to 19.8 ± 16.8 after surgery. In the UPPP group, AHI decreased from 47.9 ± 30.0 at baseline to 30.9 ± 28.5. The postoperative change was greater in the TAP group as compared with UPPP ($p = 0.02$). Especially in patients with preoperative Friedman III classification (mainly tongue base obstruction), TAP offered benefit over UPPP.

Postoperative care is similar to that after conventional UPPP. Antibiotic prophylaxis is recommended for 5 days. Additionally, 10 mg dexamethasone is given perioperatively.

As there are data only for a limited number of patients after TAP, it is not possible to determine the frequency of potential complications. In his publications, Woodson reports on transient palatal fistulas, mild intermittent oropharyngeal dysphagia, partial flap necrosis, and one case of severe otitis media. Oronasal fistulas may be avoided by a "propeller" incision as recommended by Shine and Lewis [670].

The TAP is a treatment modality for OSA, especially for those patients who still show a narrow retropalatal airway after a UPPP. Only very few reports exist documenting TAP as a primary technique. Woodson has employed the technique for the treatment of more severely affected sleep apneics. No data exists concerning the efficacy for mild OSA, especially in comparison with UPPP for a larger patient pool. The technique is more invasive than conventional UPPP and therefore it poses more potential risks. For this reason, we have not included TAP in our surgical repertoire but consider it as a solution for specific individual cases.

Take Home Pearls

> Uvulectomy is not recommended for either simple snoring or OSA. Resection of
> the uvula muscle may seriously affect the physiological functions of the soft
> palate.
> Palatal stiffening is achieved by partial removal of the oral mucosa of the soft
> palate. Various technical aids are used for surgery. Only short-term data exists.
> So far, palatal stiffening may be used to treat simple snoring and contingently
> mild OSA.
> Tetradycil sulfate is mainly used for injection snoreplasty (IS). This agent has no
> administration in Europe. Elsewhere, short-term results for simple snoring are
> promising but decrease over time. Data on the isolated use of IS for OSA does
> not currently exist.
> Transpalatal advancement pharyngoplasty (TAP) is recommended for moderate
> to severe OSA. In patients with preoperative Friedmann III staging, TAP seems
> to be superior to conventional UPPP.

7

Lower Pharyngeal Airway Procedures

Interstitial Radiofrequency Treatment (RFT)

7.1

Boris A. Stuck and Thomas Verse

Core Features

> Radiofrequency surgery of the tongue base is the only minimally invasive surgical treatment for retro-lingual obstruction in obstructive sleep apnea.
> Radiofrequency surgery may be performed as an insolate approach or in a multilevel surgical concept.

The feasibility of interstitial radiofrequency treatment (RFT) of the tongue base was first investigated in a porcine model [576] using the Somnus unit. The authors found a mild initial edematous response that tapered off 24 h after surgery. Ten days after RFT, a volume reduction was documented at the treatment site. The procedure turned out to be safe and was transferred to use in patients suffering from obstructive sleep apnea.

7.1.1
Surgical Technique

We prefer performing RFT of the tongue base under local anesthesia. In upright position, the patient is comfortably seated either in the clinical chair or on a surgical table. As perioperative monitoring, we initiate an ECG and a pulse oximetry. In contrast to the application at the nasal concha and the soft palate, sedation is recommended in this case. We administer sedation intravenously with Midazolam, by titrating the drug up to the desired level of sedation. Also, in contrast to the application of the RFT on the soft palate, we consider a perioperative antibiotics prophylaxis as essential in the application of RFT on the tongue base. We administer 2 g Cephazolin intraoperatively and perform a postoperative prophylaxis for 5 days with 500 mg Cefuroxim two times daily per os. In terms of cost-efficiency, a different antibiotic management, e.g., with

K. Hörmann, T. Verse, *Surgery for Sleep Disordered Breathing*,
DOI: 10.1007/978-3-540-77786-1_7.1, © Springer Verlag Berlin Heidelberg 2010

an oral penicillin, can certainly be envisioned. Yet, a general omission of an antibiotic prophylaxis is not recommended.

Following an optional surface disinfection with Hexetidine 0.1%, an infiltration anesthesia is performed. We use 2% Prilocain with adrenalin additive (1:200,000). We do not perform a surface anesthesia because some patients develop a discomforting hypersalivation, which can impede the patient's cooperation. Between 5 and 10 mL, local anesthetic is applied.

We employ different RFT systems. Among others, we use the Celon system (Celon AG Medical Instruments, Teltow, Germany) and the instruments provided by Sutter (Sutter Medizintechnik, Freiburg, Germany), both being bipolar-controlled systems (for more information, see Sect. 6.1.2). The vast majority of study was performed with the Somnus device (Somnus, Gyrus ENT, Bartlett, USA), a monopolar system which necessitates the attaching of a neutral electrode to the patient. Using this system, we were able to realize a series of in vitro and MRI-based in vivo studies regarding lesion sizes and optimal energy application. A setting of 600 J with a target temperature of 85°C creates optimal lesions [716, 717]. Therefore, we have substantial evidence to recommend this setting. Nevertheless, due to practical considerations, especially the time needed for energy application and the declining distribution of the system in Europe, we have discontinued its use. When using the Celon system, we set the generator to an output of 6–7 W (Fig. 7.1.1). With the Sutter system, 14 W in the autostop mode appears to be the optimal setting. In general, the lower the output is set, the larger the lesions in the tissue will become.

Given the high number of lesions, it is difficult to maintain a fixed application pattern for repeated treatment sessions. Nevertheless, one should attempt to avoid placing the application needle twice on the same location. The idea of multiple treatment session goes back to the initial publications using the Somnus unit, where lesion formation takes significant amount of time. Due to the limited experiences, only 2–4 lesions were applied in the beginning. With the more rapid bipolar systems, up to 10 or 12 lesions or more may be created in one session depending on the system used without increasing the associated morbidity in a relevant way. We now consider radiofrequency surgery of the tongue base as a single-step procedure.

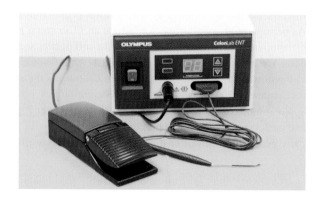

Fig. 7.1.1 Radiofrequency generator Celon with foot switch

It is much more difficult to penetrate the tongue surface than the surface of the soft palate. Therefore, special device needles are necessary for the application at the base of tongue. Together with Celon, we have developed a special faceted tongue base applicator, the so-called Celon Pro Sleep Plus (Fig. 7.1.2). The applicator is covered in a synthetic coat. Only the tip of the probe with the active electrode is exposed. The coat prevents the applicator from being inserted too far into the tissue. This reliably protects deeper lying structures, as for example the neurovascular bundle of the tongue. Substantial additional force would be needed in order to push the probe beyond the coat into the tongue. A radiofrequency energy application accidentally going too deep is made all but impossible. Comparable protection systems are realized with the majority of radiofrequency systems used to date. Nevertheless, special care for correct needle placement should be taken at any time. In Fig. 7.1.3, needle placement during surgery is demonstrated. The lesions should be as posterior as possible at the base of tongue in an area around or posterior to the wall papilla (see Fig. 7.1.4). The needle has to be inserted in an angle as close to 90° as possible to avoid superficial lesions with associated ulceration (see morbidity and complications).

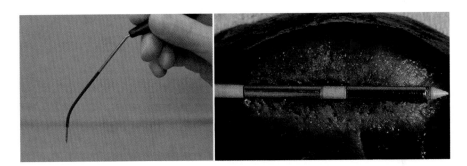

Fig. 7.1.2 (*Left*) Faceted radiofrequence probe Pro Sleep Plus with coat. (*Right*) Detailed view of the active electrodes

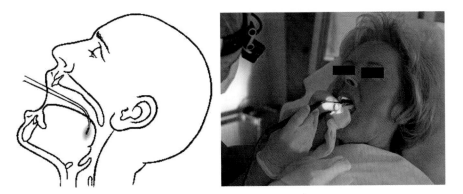

Fig. 7.1.3 (*Left*) Outline of the RFT of the tongue base. (*Right*) Intraoperative situation

Fig. 7.1.4 Correct area of treatment at the tongue base

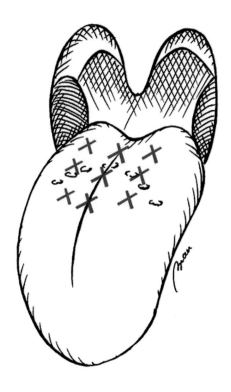

7.1.2
Effectiveness for Simple Snoring

A recently published trial by Welt and coworkers has investigated the effect of isolated tongue base RFT in the treatment of simple snoring [808]. While in obstructive sleep apnea RFT of the tongue base does indeed improve snoring [720]; this trial has clearly shown that RFT of the tongue base alone is not an effective treatment of primary snoring – not even in patients where palatal snoring was excluded and tongue base hypertrophy was the only clinical finding [808]. In another trial the effects of RFT on the tongue base was also assessed in cases of primary snoring [144]. Nevertheless, in this trial the study group ($n = 22$) consists of only a subgroup patients with simple snoring ($n = 9$) and a larger subgroup with obstructive sleep apnea. The results with regard to snoring reduction are not given for the different groups but only for the entire (mixed) group of patients. Therefore, the specific effect in snoring patients cannot be assessed in this trial.

No data exist with regard to a combined approach, but based on recent data we cannot recommend isolated RFT of the tongue base in the treatment of simple snoring (Table 7.1.1).

Table 7.1.1   Effectiveness of RFT of the tongue base for treatment of simple snoring

Author	N	Device	Les/treat	Method	Snore pre	Snore post	Success (%)	ESS pre	ESS post	EBM
Welt et al. [808]	20	Celon	12 (7 W)	VAS	7.5	6.1	15.0 (VAS <3)	6.0	6.1	4

Les/treat: lesions per treatment session; *Snore* score on the Visual Analogue Scale snoring; *ESS* Epworth Sleepiness Scale; *EBM* evidence-based medicine; *VAS* Visual Analogue Scale

7.1.3
Effectiveness for OSA

A literature search in Pubmed (National Library of Medicine) was performed for the terms "radiofrequency," "tongue," and "sleep apnea." Original studies published in English up to March 2008 were included if they addressed interstitial radiofrequency surgery of the tongue in patients with diagnosed obstructive sleep apnoea. In addition, a recent review was evaluated regarding potential additional publications [354]. For the analysis of clinical outcome, only studies using interstitial, transoral radiofrequency surgery as an isolated approach were analyzed. Studies using combined approaches in terms of multilevel surgery were only selected with regard to morbidity and complications. Data regarding a transcervical radiofrequency approach are limited to two pilot studies only with different techniques [54, 615]. In addition, it is regarded as a substantially different technique, so the data were not included in the analysis. One study was excluded due to the high number of dropouts and the inhomogeneous mixed patient sample (snoring and obstructive sleep apnea) [144]. The comparison of the cited studies is facilitated by the fact that all study groups but one worked with the same system. The total energy applied varies from 7,915 [575, 404] to 13,394 J [826]; yet no clear correlation between the energy applied and the surgery result can be deduced.

An analysis of the success rates given in Table 7.1.2 produces the following result: for altogether 118 patients (excluding the study of Li et al. [404], as the patient pool is partly identical with Powell et al. [575]) a surgical short-term success rate employing Sher's criteria of 33.2% for RFT of the tongue base was achieved for (on average) moderate OSA. This seems to indicate that the efficacy of this technique is almost equal to invasive tongue base resections (Sect. 7.3). Nevertheless, in our opinion the data from Table 7.1.2 need to be cautiously interpreted. This is due to the fact that the study design of the RFT studies is a very different one. In all of the other procedures, a sleep lab evaluation is performed before and after surgery. But in the case of the RFT surgery which is based on subsequent treatment sessions, therapy continues until the polysomnography produces a satisfactory result. This is the issue at stake: the polysomnography exhibits a high night-to-night variance, which in this case only becomes evident in a positive manner for the surgical result

Table 7.1.2   Effectiveness of RFT of the tongue base for treatment of OSA

Author	N	Device	Follow-up	AHI pre	AHI post	ESS pre	ESS post	Success (%)	EBM
Powell et al.[a] [575]	15	Somnus	4.0	47.0	20.7	10.4	4.1	46.7	4
Woodson et al. [826]	56	Somnus	1.5	40.5	32.8	11.1	7.4	20	2b
Stuck et al. [720]	18	Somnus	1.0	32.1	24.9	7.9	4.9	33	4
Li et al.[a] [404]	16	Somnus	28.0	39.5	28.7	10.4	4,5	No data	4
Riley et al. [611]	19	Somnus	3.0	35.1	15.1	12.4	7.3	63.2	4
den Herder et al. [144]	9	Celon	12.0	12.9	10.6	5.1	4.4	30	4
All	117		5.8	37.4	25.8	10.3	6.1	33.2	C

Follow-up in months; *AHI* Apnea Hypopnea Index; *ESS* Epworth Sleepiness Scale; *EBM* evidence-based medicine

[a]In part identical patients

[459, 462]. In other words: we doubt that the presented results would be corroborated by a therapy design delineated from the start by a defined number of sessions, lesions, and a defined amount of energy input. In addition to that, controlled studies are not available for tongue base RFT to date.

The best results are described by Riley and colleagues [611]. This study is distinguished from the other studies by the fact that besides two lesions at the tongue base it also applies a lesion on the anterior part of the tongue. Possibly this procedure contains a potential for an improvement of the objective results of RFT on the tongue base. Steward et al. performed an extended follow-up study [707] on a subgroup of patients published previously [708] and came to the conclusion that the improvements achieved with treatment remain stable over time (mean follow-up was 23 months).

A number of additional studies exist investigating the effects of RFT of the tongue base in the treatment of OSA. Nevertheless, these studies used this treatment as an adjunctive method together with, e.g., uvulopalatoplasty [212] or nasal surgery and palatal implants [214]. These studies basically document the feasibility of a combined approach; a reliable assessment of the specific effects of RFT of the tongue base cannot be performed with these studies. This is also true for those studies investigating the effects of combined RFT approaches at the tongue base and the soft palate [201, 708, 722]. Nevertheless, these data are specifically interesting, as a combination of the two RFT applications combines numerous advantages: the minimal invasiveness of both treatments and the fact that the application needles can often be used for both treatment sites without additional costs. The addition of a soft palate RFT, e.g., does not increase postoperative morbidity compared to tongue base RFT only. In this context, Steward et al. documented a significant symptomatic improvement of OSA after three RFT treatments at the tongue base with further improvement after additional two treatment sessions together with two soft palate treatments [706].

We are also of the basic opinion that the RFT therapy of the tongue base has been proven to have an effect in the treatment of OSA; but in terms of objective results it cannot compete primarily with the standard therapy CPAP. Yet the subjective results are absolutely equivalent with regard to daytime condition and quality of life [826]. Altogether, a careful reading of the raw data in the cited studies indicates that mainly mild forms of OSA are suitable for a therapy with RFT at the tongue base.

A series of trials has been published regarding combined radiofrequency surgery at the tongue base and the soft palate. This issue will be discussed in Chap. 10 multilevel surgery.

7.1.4
Postoperative Care and Complications

In the beginning of our RFTs at the base of tongue all patients were kept overnight for clinical monitoring after every treatment session. Over the last 100 treatments we have observed virtually no complications; therefore, this requirement can no longer be upheld as a general rule. Yet it is necessary to observe the patients until the sedation has sufficiently worn off. Due to the short half-life we solely use Midazolam. In our experience nothing is to be said against performing RFT at the tongue base on an outpatient basis.

The patient requires a perioperative and postoperative antibiotics prophylaxis [719]. We administer 2 g Cephazolin intraoperatively and 2 × 500 mg Cefuroxim per os postoperatively for 5 days. The administration of corticosteroids is not routinely necessary and we discourage its regular use.

In contrast to the application at the soft palate, postoperative pain is to be expected. In the case of our own patient pool, we have analyzed the level of pain with the help of a Visual Analogue Scale with the endpoints 0 = no pain and 10 = maximal pain [720]. The results, compared with the pain level after combined UPPP with tonsillectomy, are given in Fig. 7.1.5.

The patients require analgesics for approximately 4–5 days. We have achieved good results with retarded Dicflofenac (3 × 100 mg), if necessary in combination with also retarded Tramadol (2 × 200 mg). Nevertheless, an individualized pain management is necessary.

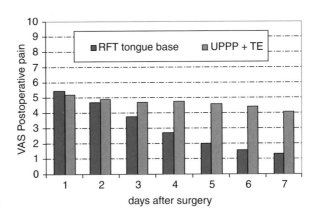

Fig. 7.1.5 Mean postoperative pain scores over 1 week after RFT of the tongue base

Apart from vasovagal reaction no intraoperative complications have been reported so far.

The postoperative complication rate is reported widely divergent, namely between 41 [551] and 0% [611]. But with its complication rate of 41%, the study by Pazos and Mair is an exception. All other studies report complication rates of below 5% [355, 720, 723, 724, 746]. We believe the most probable explanation for these divergent results lies in the perioperative management. In contrast to our own procedure, Pazos and Mair [551] recommend the general use of corticosteroids, whereas antibiotics were only administered in the case of inflammatory complications. The prophylactic administration of corticosteroids may predispose to infections. We therefore advise against their use.

A severe potential complication is the formation of an abscess of the tongue base, which has been reported by four study groups [551, 575, 724, 826]. We have taken our own case as an incentive to always perform a peri- and postoperative antibiotics prophylaxis. Since then, 6 years have passed, and we have not encountered a further abscess in over 1,000 treatments. A much more frequent complication is the occurrence of ulcerations at the tongue base (Fig. 7.1.6). They usually develop as a result of a too superficial positioning of the active electrode below the mucosa; in rare cases they are caused by a leak in the protective electrode sheath caused by excessive flexing of the electrode during treatment. These lesions at the tongue base cause a prolonged odynophagia of up to 3 weeks. Other complications are rare and consist in infection, edema, tongue pain well beyond 1 week, neuralgia up to 3 months, and thrush. A comparable safety profile has been documented for combined approaches with RFT at the tongue base and the soft palate [724]. Concerning functional parameters (swallowing, speech), no changes after RFT of the tongue base were observed in the majority of the trials [720, 723, 724, 826]. In a recent trial, high-energy single-session tongue base procedures were investigated by Nelson et al. [493]. The authors observed 2.8% superficial tongue ulcers and 1.7% persistent taste disturbances, but no serious complications. According to the statements made above regarding multiple and single treatment session, the authors came to the conclusion that high-energy single-session tongue base RFT is a safe procedure with low morbidity.

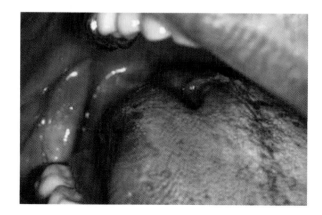

Fig. 7.1.6 Ulceration at the base of tongue after RFT treatment

Fig. 7.1.7 Complication rate
of RFT depending on the
surgical experience

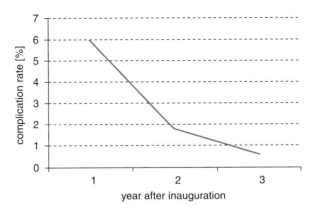

For our own patient pool we have analyzed the complication of altogether 711 treatments of 477 patients with the Somnus system and the Celon system. All in all, the complication rate lay by 2.4%, with a slight advantage for the Somnus system. At the tongue base, one abscess, five ulcers, and seven prolonged odynophagia for maximally 3 weeks were registered. It is interesting to note that the complications diminish with an increase of treatment experience (Fig. 7.1.7) [724].

Apparently, a surgical learning effect exists. Today we have reached complication rates of below 1%. By observing the recommended perioperative management RFT surgery at the tongue base has established itself as a safe procedure with a low postoperative morbidity.

7.1.5
Indications and Contraindications

With RFT, for the first time, a minimally invasive and effective procedure for the tongue base is at our disposal. The postoperative morbidity and complication rate is strikingly low. Therefore, we regard RFT at the tongue base as a significant broadening of the surgical therapy spectrum. Accordingly high is the number of operations performed in our centers.

With regard to the most recent literature, RFT of the tongue base cannot be recommended in the treatment of primary snoring unless it is performed as combined procedures, e.g., together with RFT of the soft palate. From the data presented in Table 7.1.2 we infer an indication for RFT at the tongue base for mild OSA although a precise threshold cannot be given. In the case of more severe OSA, RFT at the tongue base is additionally an essential element of our multilevel surgical concept (see Chap. 10).

Contraindications are very limited. RFT of the tongue base should not be performed in patients with preexisting unilateral hyoglossal paralysis, although persistent paralysis of the hypoglossal nerve has not been documented in our centers.

Take Home Pearls

> Radiofrequency surgery of the tongue base can successfully be applied in obstructive sleep apnea; as an isolated approach it is not recommended for primary snoring.
> Radiofrequency surgery of the tongue base is associated with limited postoperative morbidity and low complication rates as long as an antibiotic prophylaxis is ensured.
> The overall efficacy of the procedure is limited. When performed as an isolated approach, about one-third of well-selected patients may be treated successfully, although the underlying data are limited.

Hyoid Suspension

7.2

Nico de Vries and Thomas Verse

Core Features

> In OSA, due to retrolingual obstruction, it is an option to employ hyoid suspension (HS) as isolated procedure, not combining it with other procedures.

> Several modifications exist, with and without cutting of the strap muscles, with and without cutting of the tendon of the stylohyoid muscle, and with several forms of suture or steel wire.

> Overall, the results of HS as isolated procedure in OSA with retrolingual obstruction are slightly above 50%, in small series and without long-term follow-up.

> Success rates of HS in OSA due to retrolingual obstruction assessed by sleep endoscopy as only and as first procedure in a small series are above 70%.

> Results of HS in OSA with retrolingual obstruction as salvage surgery in patients after UPPP failure are around 35%.

> There is a trend to routinely combine HS with radiofrequency of the tongue base in OSA due to retrolingual obstruction.

> HS is an integral part of multilevel surgery in severe OSA, CPAP failure, and multilevel obstruction.

> Morbidity and complication rates of the procedure are acceptable.

7.2.1
Introduction: Hyoid Suspension Alone and As Part of Combined Treatment

While over the last 20 years gentle surgical procedures have been developed for the retropalatal obstruction site, much less techniques have been established for obstruction at retrolingual level. Series are small and long-term results are still lacking. Due to their invasive nature and their peri and postoperative morbidity, many of these procedures need to be critically evaluated.

K. Hörmann, T. Verse, *Surgery for Sleep Disordered Breathing*,
DOI: 10.1007/978-3-540-77786-1_7.2, © Springer Verlag Berlin Heidelberg 2010

As in all surgery, meticulous patient selection is crucial. In addition to polysomnography, topical diagnostic work-up is of paramount importance in this regard. We routinely perform sleep studies first. After this, in case surgery is considered, and in case of an AHI below 30, we schedule patients for sedated endoscopy ("sleep endoscopy"). In patients with an AHI >30, who refused nCPAP treatment upfront, or in patients who cannot accept nCPAP for whatever reason, sedated endoscopy is performed as well.

In case of retrolingual obstruction only, and simple snoring up to mild OSA (AHI <20), we either perform interstitial radiofrequency treatment of the tongue base (RFT TB) or we offer a mandibular advancement device if during sedated endoscopy the so-called chin lift (synonyms: mandible lift, chin thrust, Esmarch maneuvre) prevents tongue base collapse. Good candidates for a mandibular advancement device usually show a partial but not total tongue base collapse during sedated endoscopy.

In the period from March 2000 till June 2004 in case of retrolingual obstruction only, and moderate-to-severe OSA (AHI >20), we used to perform hyoidthyroidpexia (hyoid suspension, HS) as isolated procedure [145]. Usually in these patients the tongue base collapse during sedated endoscopy is more outspoken than in cases of mild OSA. Mandibular advancement devices have proven to be less effective in cases with a relatively higher AHI (moderate-to-severe OSA) and in cases that show total tongue base collapse and little effect of the chin lift within the sleep endoscopy.

Since 2005 till present, in case of retrolingual obstruction only, and moderate-to-severe OSA, we now more or less routinely combine hyoidthyroidpexia with RFT TB.

In case of combined retropalatal and retrolingual obstruction, moderate-to-severe OSA, we perform a form of multilevel surgery [600] (see Chap. 10). This, at our institute, is usually a combination of hyoidthyroidpexia, RFT TB, and UPPP with tonsillectomy. We have added genioglossal advancement (GA) to these three procedures in this period, but since we found that adding GA to the other three procedures did not lead to further improvement, we later abandoned this again.

7.2.2
Surgical Technique

7.2.2.1
Original Surgical Technique (1986), Historical Perspectives, and Nomenclature

The idea of preventing the collapse of the tongue musculature, which relaxes during sleep, toward dorsal into the upper airway with the help of a suspension of the hyoid bone is not new. Already at the beginning of the 1980s a widening of the upper airway after HS was demonstrated, first for the animal model [548, 762], and later for humans [348]. Initially it was attempted to fixate the hyoid on the chin.

Based on the findings from radiocephalometric studies, that in sleep apneics the hyoid is positioned lower than in healthy subjects, in 1986 a new therapy concept was presented for the treatment of hypopharyngeal obstruction: the inferior sagittal osteotomy of the

Fig. 7.2.1 Original technique of hyoid suspension (HS) with homologue fascia lata according to Riley et al. [606] here combined with genioglossus advancement

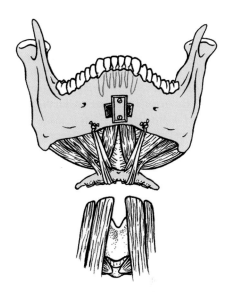

mandible with hyoid myotomy suspension [606]. The hyoid was moved upwards and forwards. This was achieved on the one hand with the help of a medial osteotomy at the chin with advancement of the origin of the M. genioglossus (see Sect. 8.1) and on the other hand with the help of a suspension of the hyoid at the chin with homologous fascia lata strands after myotomy of the intrahyoidal musculature (Fig. 7.2.1).

This original suspension technique of the hyoid to the chin with homologous fascia lata strands with myotomy of the intrahyoidal musculature has now more or less been abandoned by opinion leaders worldwide.

7.2.2.2
First Modification (1994)

Although this procedure was shown to be effective in improving OSA, it involved extensive surgical dissection of the submental region as well as the need of fascia lata harvest [413]. Other authors used, instead of the homologous fascia lata, other material, as for example nonresorbable suture material or special anchor systems [137, 368, 587, 641, 650]. In the meantime, the Stanford group modified its technique in reaction to these downsides. In this modification, originally presented by Riley and colleagues [608], the hyoid is no longer fixated on the mandible but on the upper edge of the thyroid cartilage. The resulting movement of the tongue base toward anterior and caudal increases and stiffens the upper airway.

Although in particular in the American literature the procedure is referred to as "Hyoid Suspension" this is in fact a misnomer and the correct term – albeit longer- is hyoidthyroidpexia. The reader has to make his own choice: the use of the short, easy term HS or the longer, more correct term hyoidthyroidpexia (HTP).

HTP involves stabilization of the hyoid bone inferiorly and anteriorly by attachment to the superior border of the thyroid cartilage. The underlying principle for altering the hyoid is that anatomically, the hyoid complex is an integral part of the hypopharynx. Anterior movement of the hyoid complex increases the posterior airway space (PAS) and neutralizes obstruction at the tongue base. In fact it is still not completely understood why it works. MRI studies have not shown an increase of PAS in wake, and possibly it is more a prevention of collapse during sleep only.

Under general anesthesia, with the head in slightly extended position, a horizontal incision of approximately 5 cm is made in a relaxed skin tension line at the level between hyoid and thyroid cartilage. Excessive fat tissue is excised, if useful for better visualization. Especially in case of a further posterior positioned hyoid, removal of fat is recommended as well, since otherwise the anterior placement of the hyoid will result in a somewhat turkey-like neck contour.

Secondly, the strap muscles are severed just below the attachment to the hyoid. Partial removal of the severed strap muscles at the level between hyoid and thyroid cartilage is sometimes also to be considered for the same cosmetic reasons while there is also little use to leave the nonfunctional cut strap muscles in situ.

The tendon of the stylohyoid muscle is cut only if after release of the strap muscles insufficient mobilization is gained. Otherwise the stylohyoid tendon is preserved. Gradually we ourselves have almost completely stopped cutting the stylohyoid tendon, as we feel that almost always the cutting of the strap muscles provides sufficient mobility.

By mobilizing the hyoid bone in an anterocaudal direction and fixing it to the thyroid with two permanent sutures per side (we use Mercilene 0) through the thyroid cartilage and around the hyoid bone, more space is created retrolingually. Although with increasing age ossification of the thyroid will take place, in more than 100 cases we have never needed to make drill holes. A sharp cutting needle has so far always been sufficient to pierce the thyroid cartilage.

Antibiotics are not routinely applied, in case HTP is the only procedure, but will be applied in case the procedure is combined with RFT TB. A surgical drain is placed and usually removed after 24–48 h postoperatively if drainage is less than 10 mL per 24 h. Nocturnal oximetry is monitored throughout the first postoperative night in the intensive care unit and nonopioid analgesics are used for pain relief, if necessary (Fig. 7.2.2).

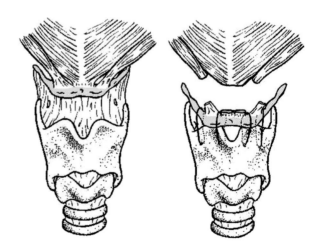

Fig. 7.2.2 Modified HS according to Riley et al. [608]

Usually intubation anesthesia is used. The procedure can also be performed under local anesthesia [500], but then intravenous sedation with Midazolam of Propofol is recommended.

7.2.2.3
Hörmann's Modification (2001)

In Mannheim, Hörmann and coworkers have modified the method rigorously [292, 294]. In order to be less invasive, the group does not cut the ligamenta stylohyoidea or the supra- and infrahyoidal musculature at all. Usually intubation anesthesia is used. The procedure can also be performed under local anesthesia [500], but then intravenous sedation with Midazolam of Propofol is recommended. The patient receives an intraoperative single shot with 2 g Cefazolin.

The patient is placed on the operating table with slightly reclined head. Initially it may be helpful to mark the position of the hyoid and the upper edge of the larynx. For cosmetic reasons, the skin incision is performed above the hyoid bone along the relaxed skin tension lines (Fig. 7.2.3).

One proceeds through the submental fat up to the floor of mouth musculature. Without damaging it, the muscles are sectioned down to the hyoid; then the thyroid cartilage is exposed. It is useful if the assistant or nurse pushes the larynx toward cranial with two fingers. For aesthetic reasons it is important to remove a sufficient amount of fat tissue (Fig. 7.2.4). Failure to do so will, as a result of the advancement of the hyoid, create an unattractive supralaryngeal wrinkle as a turkey-like appearance.

In contrast to the "standard method," Hörmann's modification needs only one triangular suture, which passes on both sides paramedial through the thyroid cartilage and medial around the hyoid. As suture, a monofilamentous grade 3 steel wire (Ethicon, Hamburg, Germany) is used. For this, first the suprahyoidal musculature is vertically separated

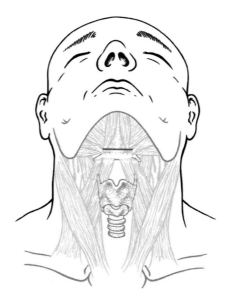

Fig. 7.2.3 Hörmann's technique of HS. Dermal incision

Fig. 7.2.4 Hörmann's technique of HS. Exposure of the hyoid bone and thyroid cartilage. Resection of redundant fat

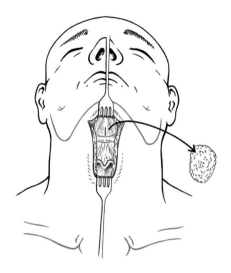

precisely in median, until a Langenbeck retractor can be applied (Fig. 7.2.4, red line). The fascia in the midline between each sternohyoid muscle is incised with electrocautery until the plane of the thyroid cartilage is reached. The blood supply to the thyroid cartilage is provided by the blood vessels of the perichondrium. Unnecessary elevation of the perichondrium should, therefore, be avoided to reduce the risk of necrosis. The muscles on both sides are retracted to expose the lateral parts of the thyroid cartilage. Now, starting at caudal, a sharp needle is pierced through the cartilage without drilling. The steel wire is fixed at the end of the needle, which comes out on the contralateral side of the thyroid cartilage (Fig. 7.2.5, left side). Then the hyoid body is encircled with the wire ligature until the tip of the needle appears on the Langenbeck retractor (Fig. 7.2.5, center). In order to prevent accidental opening up of the laryngeal tube by the wire, the assistant elevates the hyoid with a Joseph retractor. In order to prevent tearing of the suture, the distance to the upper edge of the thyroid cartilage should be at least 5 mm. Especially in older men, ossification of the thyroid cartilage may make piercing of it with the ligature difficult, respectively impossible. A surgical drill system as used in ear surgery is of help here.

Now the actual suspension takes place (Fig. 7.2.5, right side). One more time the hyoid is undergirded with the Joseph retractor. With one hand the assistant pulls the hyoid with this retractor toward anterior and caudal, while pushing the larynx with the other hand toward cranial. The surgeon now fixates the hyoid in this position on the larynx with the ligature by intertwining the two wire ends. In order to achieve an optimal result, it is important not to make a kink in the wire ligature, as otherwise it cannot be tightened. Finally the wire ends are twisted inwards in order to prevent painful piercing of the skin. A Redon drainage with suction is applied, and the wound is closed in layers.

This modification, which makes a myotomy and a cutting of the ligamenta stylohyoideum unnecessary, shortens the operating time, and reduces the invasiveness of the procedure (Fig. 7.2.6).

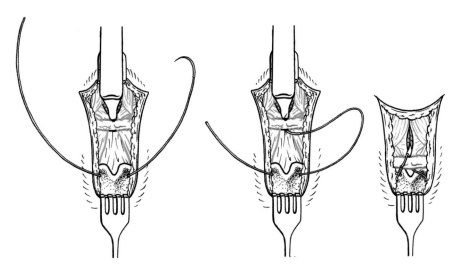

Fig. 7.2.5   Hörmann's technique of HS. (*Left*) Transfixing the thyroid cartilage with the steel wire suspension. (*Center*) Undermining the hyoid bone. (*Right*) Completion of suspension

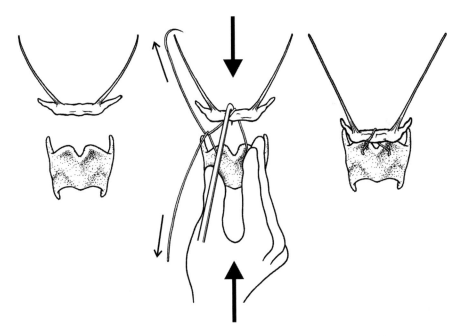

Fig. 7.2.6   Hörmann's technique of HS. (*Left*) Preoperative situation. (*Center*) HS without myotomy. (*Right*) Situation after surgery

7.2.3
Effectiveness for SDB

HS has an established place in the treatment of OSA due to retrolingual obstruction. Currently, no published data exist in regards to its usefulness for primary snoring due to retrolingual obstruction. In Amsterdam, we have until now not used it in primary snoring or upper airway resistance syndrome. In Mannheim, between January and May 2004, 26 patients with primary snoring or upper airway resistance syndrome were treated with at least HS; 25 of them (96%) reported a significant reduction in their snoring after operation.

Efficacy data in the therapy of OSA for isolated HS are also rare due to the fact that HS is almost always performed together with other procedures, either with mandibular osteotomy with genioglossus advancement (MO) (mostly in the USA) or radiofrequency of the tongue base (RFT TB), (mostly in Europe), or as part of multilevel surgery. The only existing published data are presented in Table 7.2.1.

The total success rate of these 60 patients lies for isolated HS with a severe OSA at slightly below 50% according to Sher's criteria. In the Amsterdam series, a clear difference was found between primary HS (71% success), and secondary HS (35%), as salvage after UPPP failure. In Amsterdam we routinely perform sedated endoscopy before surgery, and it is tempting to speculate that the good results are (in part) due to this form of patient selection.

Anyhow, the combined data suggest reasonable efficacy of isolated HS in the treatment of OSA. Still, controlled studies would be extremely interesting, and long-term data have not yet been published. In sum, both standard HS (Amsterdam) [143], and Hörmann's modification, has established itself as an essential and effective part of multilevel surgery [295, 766, 767].

However, although our experiences are encouraging, we have changed our policy after the reported series. Since it has been shown that radiofrequency of the tongue base as only procedure has a small but definite effect, and since radiofrequency of the tongue base is almost without adverse events and side effects (with applying antibiotics but no steroids, see Sect. 7.1) we now more or less routinely ("why not" – intervention) combine it with HS. Our results of combined HTP with RFT TB will be reported elsewhere later.

Table 7.2.1 Effectiveness of isolated hyoid suspension for OSA

Author	N	Follow-up (months)	AHI pre	AHI post	Success (%)	ESS pre	ESS post	EBM
Riley et al. [608]	15	3–6	44.7	12.8	53.3	No data	No data	4
den Herder et al. [115]	31	6	32.1	22.2	52	7.6	4.3	4
Stuck et al. [721]	14	2	35.2	27.4	40	9.1	6.1	4
All	60	2–6	35.97	21.06	49.53	8.07	4.86	C

AHI Apnea Hypopnea Index

7.2.4
Postoperative Care and Complications

HS is performed on an inpatient basis. The use of antibiotics is somewhat questionable. In Amsterdam no antibiotics are applied when HS is used as solitary procedure. If combined with RFT TB, we give 2 g of Amoxicillin during surgery and 3 times per day 625 mg orally for one week. In Mannheim, apart from the perioperative single-shot antibiotics; antibiotics are only indicated if inflammatory complications develop.

In Amsterdam we usually keep the patient for one night at the intensive care unit. Although in more than 100 procedures we have not had one case of severe respiratory distress in the night after surgery, it makes us still feel comfortable to have some extra monitoring in the first night. In Mannheim, intensive observation is usually not felt as necessary after HS.

The Redon drainage is removed if the wound fluid production is less than 10 mL per 24 h. This is usually after 1 or 2 days. Usually patients are dismissed after the drain has been taken out. In Amsterdam, patients can maintain their normal diet.

In order to protect the upper airway, several authors recommend in severe OSA routine nasal CPAP respiration during the postoperative phase after HS [413]. We continue CPAP respiration in patients who were using it preoperatively. In case a patient has not previously used an apparatus, it is decided, based on the observation in the first hours postoperatively in the recovery room whether CPAP therapy will be applied or not.

For further postoperative management after surgical procedures at the upper airway for severe OSA, see Chap. 13.

Neruntarat recently described self-limited aspiration as a complication after HS within the first three weeks after surgery [499]. In standard HS, in more than 100 cases we have had only one postoperative bleeding (in our third case) which necessitated tracheostomy and reopening of the neck in the first hours after surgery. Three cases developed in the first 6 months during follow-up fistulas which finally necessitated removal of the Mercilene stitches. In none of our patients, removal of stitches resulted in loss of the hyoidthyroidpexia.

In Hörmann's wire modification, the wire ligature occasionally can break, and might have to be removed.

7.2.5
Indications and Contraindications

HS is an invasive surgical method with potential complications. For the tongue base, a minimally invasive alternative exists in the form of RFT TB. We therefore see no primary indication for HS for primary snoring. Only in rare cases where RFT TB or other therapy failed or was otherwise not possible, HS could be considered in primary snoring.

In the case of mild OSA with suspected retrolingual collapse, HS competes with RFT TB. Due to the significantly lower invasiveness and postoperative morbidity we primarily choose RFT TB, and offer HS as salvage after failed RFT TB. For mild OSA oral appliances are a noninvasive alternative, albeit that approximately one-third of patients have a contraindication to oral appliance therapy. In mild-to-moderate OSA, mandibular advancement devices achieve a comparable cure rate and have a long-term acceptance rate of approximately 50%.

In the case of moderate-to-severe OSA, the success rates of both RFT TB and of dental splints decrease. For this indication, HS is superior to RFT TB. Therefore we consider moderate-to-severe OSA (AHI 20 up to 40) as a primary indication for the HS. If the obstruction site is suspected to lie solely in the retrolingual segment, an isolated HS presents itself as an option; it can also be combined with RFT TB upfront.

For more severe forms of OSA (AHI >40) it is assumed (and usually confirmed with sedated endoscopy, if this procedure is performed) that the complete airway (both retropalatal and retrolingual) is affected. For severe OSA, respiratory therapy is to be preferred in general. In case of CPAP failure, noncompliance, or simple refusal, a form of therapy remains indicated. Surgery then becomes necessary, but isolated HS with or without RFT TB is then often not sufficient. In case of severe OSA and multilevel obstruction, we therefore pursue primarily a single-stage multilevel concept which combines procedures at the soft palate and at the tongue base (see Chap. 10).

We have had several patients who had had Sistrunk's procedure for a thyroglossal cyst. The resulting missing of the corpus of the hyoid is a definite contraindication to HS.

Take Home Pearls

> In OSA due to retrolingual obstruction, HS can be considered as isolated procedure, but there is a trend to routinely combine it with radiofrequency of the tongue.
> There are several modifications, with and without cutting of the strap muscles, with and without cutting of the tendon of the stylohyoid muscle, with several forms of suture and steel wire. No data exist comparing the different techniques.
> The overall results of HS as isolated procedure in OSA and retrolingual obstruction are slightly above 50%, but in a small test series results of HS as only and as first procedure in retrolingual obstruction as assessed by sleep endoscopy are above 70%. Results of HS in OSA and retrolingual obstruction as salvage in UPPP failure lie only around 35%.
> The procedure is well-tolerated; the morbidity and complication rates are acceptable. It is an integral part of multilevel surgery in severe OSA, CPAP failure, and multilevel obstruction.

Tongue Base Resection

7.3

Joachim T. Maurer and Thomas Verse

Core Features

> The tongue base is resected by an internal or external approach.

> The neurovascular bundle has to be localized exactly before surgery.

> Resection of the lingual tonsil itself differs substantially from resection of the tongue base musculature.

> Success rates for moderate-to-severe OSA vary between 20 and 80%.

Before a minimally invasive surgical procedure at the tongue base in the form of RFT was available for the first time in the mid-nineties several surgical concepts already existed for the volume reduction of the tongue by directly resecting tissue. In cases where surgery was performed on the tongue base, a temporary tracheotomy often became necessary in order to secure the upper airway. A further problem was posited by painful swallowing impairments, which often lasted three or more weeks. As a result, these surgical techniques were always reserved for the severe cases of OSA which could not be treated with respiratory therapy. Still today, individual cases exist where such an invasive procedure can be indicated. Furthermore, some new techniques were introduced such as Coblation® via internal as well as external approach. Here, we will describe the essential techniques.

A second group of patients, for whom a partial tongue resection in the context of SDB may be indicated, are patients with a macroglossia, e.g., in the case of Down's syndrome. For this second group, only individual case studies are found in the literature; therefore, it is not possible to numerically describe the connection between OSA as a result of macroglossia and surgical therapies. Figure 7.3.1 shows one of our own cases, with intended resection borders. Coming out of the surgery of macroglossia in children with different malformation syndromes, several techniques for partial tongue resection in the anterior and medial tongue third are available [134, 336, 482].

K. Hörmann, T. Verse, *Surgery for Sleep Disordered Breathing*,
DOI: 10.1007/978-3-540-77786-1_7.3, © Springer Verlag Berlin Heidelberg 2010

Fig. 7.3.1 Partial tongue resection in a patient with Down's syndrome

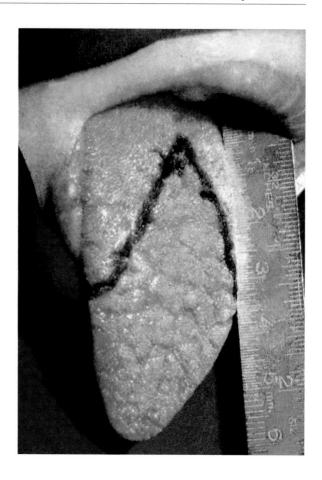

7.3.1
Surgical Technique

In principle, two different basic techniques can be made out which distinguish themselves by the surgical approach. The first description of a *transoral* tongue base resection in the medial area stems from the group around Djupesland [155, 156]. In the U.S., a laser surgery modification with partial epiglottis resection has been developed [225]. Recently, Robinson et al. [614] reported about resecting the lingual tonsil under endoscopic view using Coblation®. According to our own experience, this technique allows complete excision of the lingual tonsil as well as staying out of the tongue muscles at the same time.

These techniques are performed under general anesthesia in the operating theatre. Before treating the tongue base, a tracheotomy or a nasotracheal intubation is performed and anesthesia is administered through a laser-safe endotracheal tube if the laser is used. The tongue base is either exposed by use of a Davis mouth gag or a small adult or child No. 3 tongue

Fig. 7.3.2 Midline resection of the tongue base

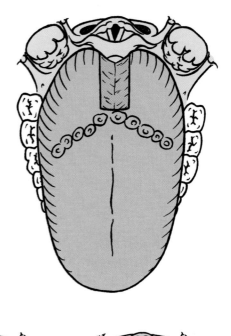

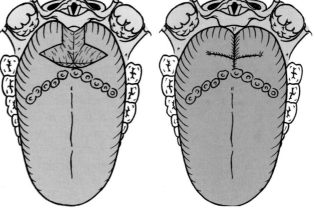

Fig. 7.3.3 Lingualplasty:
additional lateral wedge
resection according
to Woodson and
Fujita [823]

blade. The smaller blade allows prolapsing of the tongue base into the field [823]. A rigid
laser laryngoscope can be used as an alternative. A midline portion, approximately 2–2.5 cm
in width, beginning posterior to the circumvallatae papillae and extending toward the val-
lecula approximately 4–5 cm in length is deeply excised using a CO_2 or a KTP laser (Fig.
7.3.2). We prefer the CO_2 laser (20 W in a continuous wave mode). Care is taken to stay out
of the tongue musculature. Bleedings are coagulated with electrocautery.

Woodson and Fujita [823] recommend performing a so-called lingualplasty. Beginning
at the anterior corner of excision, an additional centimeter-long wedge of lateral tongue is
excised in order to create a defect (Fig. 7.3.3). It is important that the wedge resection
laterally is superficial to ensure preservation of neuromuscular structures.

Fig. 7.3.4   Additional resection of the majority
of the free portion of the epiglottis

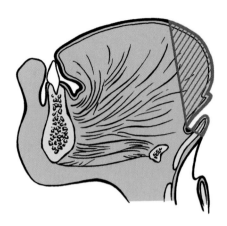

   After removal of the midline tongue, additional lingual tonsils and redundant tissue of
the epiglottis are removed via a laser laryngoscope. Finally, the defect is sutured using 2-0
absorbable sutures (i.e., Vicryl, Ethicon). This advances the tongue base (Fig. 7.3.3). Some
authors [465] always resect the majority of the free portion of the epiglottis, others only do
so in the case of an omega-shaped epiglottis [823] (Fig. 7.3.4).
   Woodson, Robinson, and Maturo, respectively, invented further techniques to reduce
the tongue volume in its middle and posterior third by transoral approaches using
Coblation®. These techniques are not yet sufficiently evaluated, but they are less invasive
than previous methods and will probably replace them in the future. They all have in common to localize and mark the neurovascular bundle before beginning surgery. Robinson
and Woodson [614] proposed a 5-cm midline incision in the middle third of the tongue
using a Bovie. After exposing the tongue musculature by retracting the wound edges laterally an Evac T&A Plasma Wand is used to remove tissue submucosally as close as 5 mm
to the neurovascular bundle markings. The incision is closed after the procedure. Robinson
extended this concept more laterally even exceeding the neurovascular bundles. He recommends placing a suprahyoid percutaneous drain after suturing the incision in order to avoid
postoperative hemorrhage as well as to optimize volume reduction [617]. Maturo [445]
described a small case series in children with extreme macroglossia making only a 1-cm
midline incision in the anterior third of the tongue. Then he proceeds posteriorly in the
midline to create a submucosal cavity using the same coblation wand as described above.
Further resection is monitored by a 0° irrigation endoscope. Transillumination allows control of the lateral resection margins. The anterior incision is left open. This procedure can
be performed in adults as well showing an increased efficacy and morbidity compared to
RFT of the tongue base [218].
   In contrast to the described transoral tongue base reductions, Chabolle and colleagues
[98] perform transcollar resections in severe sleep apneics via an *external* approach. Again
this technique is performed under general anesthesia with the patients intubated transna-
sally. A skin incision is made in a neck fold parallel to the lower border of the mandible,
between the hyoid bone and the mandible. The lower border of the submandibulary glands,
the anterior belly of the digastric muscles, the mylohyoid muscle, and the geniohyoid
muscles are exposed and sectioned. After identification of the neurovascular bundle the

Fig. 7.3.5 Transcollar tongue base resection according to Chabolle et al. [98]

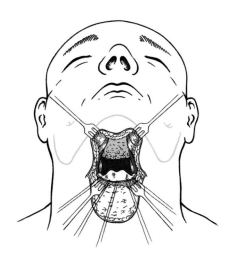

tongue base is exposed, and the pharynx is entered through the valleculae. Then the authors perform a resection of the tongue base that extends laterally to the lingual-tonsillary folds and anteriorly to the circumvallatae papillae (Fig. 7.3.5).

The procedure is usually combined with a hyoid suspension. The pharynx is finally closed with 1–0 nonabsorbable or absorbable sutures, and the skin is sutured in two layers.

A modification has been recently described by Robinson staying strictly submucosally and advancing the hyoid to the mandible by a strip of fascia lata [616].

He also [615] presented data on ultrasound-guided percutaneous submucosal tongue-base excision using Coblation® in 15 patients; 5 patients received UPPP as well. In addition, he advanced the tongue base mucosa into the submucous defect by a transmucosal suture. He resected large volumes of the tongue base, however avoiding tracheotomy in 14 cases. Using this technique one cannot directly expose the neurovascular bundle of the tongue during surgery. Therefore, ultrasound with doppler has to be used to clearly identify and preserve the hypoglossal nerve as well as the lingual arteries. We have no experience with this technique so far.

There are a few patients with normal-sized tongue and normal skeletal properties, whose retrolingual airway is solely constricted due to lingual tonsil hypertrophy. This is especially the case in patients who received a tonsillectomy in childhood. In these cases, a leveling of the lingual tonsil with the CO_2 laser (continuous wave oder superpulse mode; 8 W) via a laser laryngoscope suggests itself as an adequate procedure. We perform about 1–2 such procedures per year. In our experience, since the tongue musculature is not damaged, in almost all cases a trachetomy is not necessary. But in the case of a very prominent finding, one can proceed bilaterally, first leveling one side, then the other. If Coblation® is used instead of the CO_2 laser, retraction sutures or a Backhaus clamp placed in the middle third of the tongue may be a good alternative to expose the tongue base for endoscopic visualization with the 30°- or 70°-rigid endoscope. The Evac 70 coblation wand is bent in a way that the lingual tonsil can be completely ablated under endoscopic or direct visualization. The structure of the tonsil tissue can be distinguished easily from muscle tissue so that the muscle can be preserved. Coagulation can be achieved by switching to the coagulation mode of the coblation wand; electrocautery is rarely necessary. There is no suture necessary. We never had to tracheotomize a patient after this procedure so far.

7.3.2
Effectiveness for OSA

Since the partial resection of the tongue is an invasive surgical method with in some cases obligatory temporary tracheotomy, it is not astonishing that the literature exclusively provides data for the treatment of moderate-to-severe OSA. This data is compiled in Table 7.3.1.

It is notable that the results range between 20 and 80% success rate (Sher criteria). Altogether, data of 139 patients are available; 22 of these data sets stem from retrospective analyses. The methods and the amount of tissue resected vary substantially. The data situation therefore is heterogeneous, and still allows for a cautious inference. It appears that some patients with severe OSA due to a hypopharyngeal collapse do indeed profit from a partial tongue resection, especially if clinically only a macroglossia is manifest [465]. The amount of tissue resected is thought to be important in regard to the porbability of success. It can only be speculated in how far less severely affected sleep apneics achieve better results in regard to the clinical success rate. Long-term data is still lacking.

Table 7.3.1 Efficiency of tongue base reduction for OSA

Author	N	Add. proc.	Follow-up (months)	AHI pre	AHI post	Success (%)	ESS pre	ESS post	p ESS	EBM
Fujita et al. [225]	12	No	5–15	56.3	37	41.7	No data	No data	No data	4
Djupesland et al. [156]	20	UPPP	8.7	54	31	35	No data	No data	No data	3b
Woodson and Fujita [823]	14	No	1.5	50.2	8.6	78.6	No data	No data	No data	3b
Mickelson and Rosenthal [465]	12	No	2.4	73.3	46.6	25	No data	No data	No data	3b
Chabolle et al. [98]	10	UPPP	3	70	27	80	15	6	No data	4
Robinson et al. [615]	10	No	3	35.4	34	20	10.8	7.9	<0.05	4
Friedman et al. [218]	48	No	3	44.5	20.3	65	11.3	7.7	<0.05	3b
Robinson [616]	13	UPPP	3	54	28	39	8.5	6.2	>0.05	4
All	139		1.5–15	52.01	26.56	52.00	11.25	7.27		B

Add. Proc. additional procedures; *AHI* Apnea Hypopnea Index

Dünar and colleagues have presented a case study of an OSA caused by a massive enlargement of the lingual tonsil [165]. The authors removed the superfluous lymphatic tissue with the CO_2 laser. The Apnea Index was preoperatively 45.5 and could be reduced 2 months postoperatively to 2.5.

7.3.3
Postoperative Care and Complications

Due to the potential inflammations and postoperative bleedings, partial tongue resections ask for special postoperative observation and in several cases a tracheotomy. We observe our patients during the first postoperative night in an intensive care unit. If internal submucosal lingualplasty or glossectomy is performed, there is a risk of delayed hematoma due to bleeding of small branches of the lingual artery in the posterior third of the tongue which have been coagulated during the initial operation. Transnasal fiberoptic intubation or tracheotomy was necessary to secure the airway in two cases. A percutaneous suction drain as well as transmucosal sutures in the midline and ligaclips can reduce that risk [218, 615, 617].

As a result of the acute pain in swallowing, an effective analgesic management is necessary. Usually it is not sufficient to administer peripherally effective substances. Since the patients are also incapable of swallowing tablets, we administer alternatingly tramadol and metronidazol drops as base therapy. However, subjective pain is very different interindividually and an individual solution is warranted.

A gastral probe is placed intraoperatively. As soon as the patient is able to swallow, we switch to a porridge-based diet. Only very rarely is nourishment via the stomach probe necessary for more than 3 days.

Up to now, no severe complications have been reported after transoral tongue resections with the vast majority of patients receiving a tracheotomy to secure the upper airway within the first postoperative days. Woodson and Fujita report about one case of subcutaneous emphysema related to tracheotomy. Using the transcollar approach Chabolle and colleagues [98] described five early and three late abscesses (50%) in their series of patients, all requiring surgical intervention. Robinson reported no infection after the external submucosal approach, but a severe hematoma requiring tracheotomy. Three patients did not receive hyoid advancement and complained about aspiration due to a dehiscence of the mylohyoid muscle from the hyoid. This complication resolved after attaching the mylohyoid muscle to the hyoid bone and suspending the latter to the mandible [616].

As minor complications were reported minor bleedings (8–25%), prolonged odynophagia for up to 3 weeks (5–8%), tongue edema (5%), and short-term changes in taste sensation (8–56%) [155, 225, 465, 823]. According to our experience in this field, patients even more frequently develop prolonged odynophagia.

In the case of an isolated resection of the lingual tonsil neither we nor the literature has reported any severe postoperative bleedings or inflammations. Usually, a tracheotomy is not necessary. But we do observe the patients for an extended period in our recovery room and if swelling is relevant patients are kept in the intensive care unit during the first postoperative night. The symptomatic pain configuration is relatively less salient. Furthermore, we have as yet not observed any permanent other complications, such as long-term changes in taste sensation.

7.3.4
Indications and Contraindications

Due to the described invasiveness and postoperative morbidity of partial tongue base resection this surgical procedure is reserved for severe cases of OSA which cannot be sufficiently treated with a nasal ventilation therapy. In principle, we do not perform a partial tongue base resection in cases where the patient has not previously received a ventilation therapy. Since several cases call for a tracheotomy, this procedure has in our center been more and more relegated to the background. This is due to the fact that with hyoid suspension, radiofrequency surgery, and mandibular procedures in the case of skeletal anomalies, we have less morbidizing alternatives at our disposal which show at least a comparable efficacy.

Therefore, we today consider an indication for partial tongue base resection only as ultima ratio when conservative and surgical therapy options have been exhausted, and when a tracheotomy must be avoided under all circumstances. This might change if conclusive data are presented concerning submucosal glossectomy using coblation.

The situation is different in regards to the mere leveling of the lingual tonsil. This procedure is less painful, and needs no tracheotomy. For mild OSA, this procedure competes somewhat with RFT therapy at the tongue base; due to the latter's superiority in respect to postoperative morbidity, the former should only be used in the case of a massive enlargement of the lingual tonsil or for moderate-to-severe OSA.

Take Home Pearls

> Tongue base resection is an invasive procedure requiring tracheotomy in several cases.
> There are many different techniques available whereof none has prevailed.
> They seem to be effective for moderate-to-severe OSA.
> Long-term data are lacking.

Tongue Suspension

7.4

Boris A. Stuck and Thomas Verse

Core Features

> Tongue suspension is an alternative treatment of retrolingual obstruction and has been designed both for the treatment of snoring and obstructive sleep apnea.
> The principle of tongue suspension consists of a fixation of the tongue at the mandible via a suture that is passed through the tongue base and fixed to a screw at the mandible.
> Tongue suspension is performed as an inpatient procedure requiring general anesthesia.

In the case of an absence of other anatomical abnormalities such as skeletal malformations or tongue base tumors, snoring and airway obstruction can be caused or exacerbated by an airway obstruction at the level of the tongue base. During daytime, this phenomenon is prevented by the voluntary motor system. Already in 1992, a glossopexia was suggested in which the tongue base is fixated at the chin with the help of a tissue sling in order to prevent a retrolingual collapse as a result of the physiological muscle relaxation during sleep [191].

7.4.1
Surgical Technique

In the original technique, a glossopexy is combined with a resection of the tongue base [191]. For glossopexy, the authors use homologous fascia lata. The fascia lata is applied as a sling in the body of the tongue, the ends passed through two holes in the mandible and sutured to each other after maximal anterior suspension of the tongue (Fig. 7.4.1).

Due to the considerable amount of preparation and the necessity of harvesting fascia lata, this technique has not been able to establish itself. Yet this method has gained renewed

K. Hörmann, T. Verse, *Surgery for Sleep Disordered Breathing*,
DOI: 10.1007/978-3-540-77786-1_7.4, © Springer Verlag Berlin Heidelberg 2010

Fig 7.4.1 Original technique of glossopexy with fascia lata modified after Faye-Lund et al. [191]

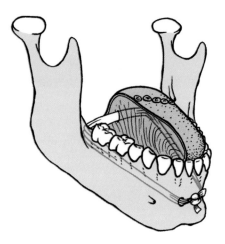

currency with the introduction of the Repose[R] system (Medtronic ENT, Jacksonville, USA), characterized as minimally invasive [151]. It comprises a surgical kit which includes, apart from surgical instruments, a nonresorbable suspension suture which is passed through the tongue base and then fixated with the help of a screw at the inner side of the chin. In contrast to the RFT of the tongue base, the Repose[R] system is a method requiring general anesthesia; we therefore consider it to be minimally invasive only to a certain degree.

The initial technique proceeded along the following lines [822]: First the included inserter was placed in the midline floor of the mouth posterior to the orifice of Wharton's duct. The screw was placed firmly against the mandible, with the screw perpendicular to the lingual cortex, and was then inserted. A suture passer was passed through the stab wound, and a doubled-looped suture was passed through the tongue lateral to the midline into the oropharynx. The point of insertion was approximately 1 cm from midline and 1 cm below the foramen coecum. A single strand of the suspension suture was then passed opposite the double loop with the suture passer. A curved Mayo needle was used to pass the suspension suture across the base of the tongue. The suspension suture was then passed into the looped suture strand and pulled anterior, finishing all three passes. Finally the suture was tied; care was taken to avoid cutting the suture on the incisor teeth (Fig. 7.4.2). Tightness of the suspension was assessed with the fingers where an indentation can be felt.

Meanwhile, the procedure has been slightly modified. The titanium screw with the attached sutures in now implanted into the posterior aspect of the lower mandible via a small submental skin incision. Via this approach, the risk of affecting the salivary glands and their ducts seems to be reduced.

The repose technique can also be combined with other surgical techniques. Several authors reported good results of a combination with a UPPP in the context of multilevel surgery [468, 524, 741, 743]. Fibbi and colleagues [196] combine the Repose tongue sling

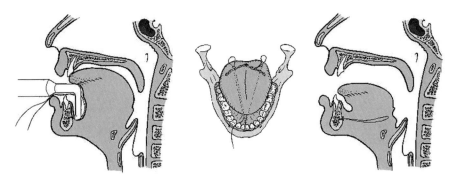

Fig 7.4.2   Tongue suspension suture with the Repose[R] system (initial surgical approach). (*Left*) Insertion of bone screw with Repose[R] Kit. (*Center*) Run of sutures through the tongue. (*Right*) Situation after surgery

with a genioglossus advancement in the case of clinically relevant tongue base constriction.

7.4.2
Efficiency for Simple Snoring

Until now, the technique has been employed both in the treatment of OSA and the treatment of simple snoring. Data for primary snoring stem from two multicenter studies [822, 832] which apparently to some extent contain the same patient data; therefore, we will only discuss the more recent study which includes a larger number of individuals.

Woodson [832] treated 14 primary snorers with the Repose[R] system. The AHI was at 9.2 preoperatively, and rose nonsignificantly to 15.6 two months after surgery. The other respiratory parameters also showed no statistically significant changes. Subjective outcome measures included Epworth Sleepiness Scale (ESS), functional outcomes of sleep (FOSQ), the quality-of-life questionnaire MO-SF36, and a 10-point Visual Analogue and Behavior-Based Scale of snoring and sleepiness. Two months after surgery, there were statistically significant improvements in all parameters but the Visual Analogue Scale for sleepiness.

According to this study, the Repose[R] system is successful in the treatment of snoring in the case of clinically attested tongue base constriction. Since further studies are not available, it is currently only possible to speak of a preliminary trend or informed opinion. In particular, special care has to be taken and intensified informed consent has to be obtained in primary snorers, as the method can be associated with relevant postoperative complications (see below) and requires general anesthesia. The authors are therefore particularly hesitant with regard to tongue suspension in snorers.

Table 7.4.1 Tongue suspension suture with the Repose^R system for OSA

Author	N	Follow-up (months)	AHI pre	AHI post	Success (%)	EBM
DeRowe et al. [151]	14	2	32.6	16.2	28.6	4
Woodson et al. [822]	9	2	32.2	17.9	No data	4
Woodson [832]	14	2	35.4	24.5	28.6	4
All	37	2–6	33.56	19.75	28.60	C

AHI Apnea Hypopnea Index; *EBM* evidence-based medicine

7.4.3
Efficiency for OSA

More study data are available for OSA; they are summarized in Table 7.4.1. The studies by Woodson partially comprise identical patient data; therefore, only the more recent publication was used for the calculation of the mean values.

The mean values for pre- and postoperative AHI as well as for the surgical success rate after Sher given in Table 7.4.1 are almost identical with those after isolated radiofrequency therapy at the tongue base (Chap. 7.1). Both techniques are used for the same indication, namely clinically evident obstruction at the tongue base level, and apparently both techniques are comparable in regards to their efficacy.

Thomas et al. [743] have compared the Repose^R tongue sling and the genioglossus advancement respectively each in combination with a UPPP in a randomized controlled study; they found slight advantages for the Repose procedure (57% success rate with Repose vs. 50% with genioglossus advancement). The subjective results in regards to daytime sleepiness and snoring were comparable.

Recently, Vicente et al. [781] have published their results of a combination of UPPP and tongue base suspension is a series of 55 patients with severe OSA (52.8 ± 14.9). After a follow-up period of 3 years, the surgical success rate was still reported as being 78% defined as a reduction in AHI of more than 50% with an AHI of below 20, together with an ESS below 11.

Data including a noncontrolled group or regarding long-term efficacy for isolated tongue suspension, however, are not available to date. The overall efficacy of the procedure is therefore difficult to evaluate.

7.4.4
Postoperative Care and Complications

It is generally recommended to treat the patients perioperatively with broad-spectrum antibiotics. In our center we use 2 g cephazoline as single shot. Steroids (dexamethasone 2 × 10 mg and prednisolone 40–60 mg for 3–5 days after surgery) and nonsteroidal anti-inflammatory drugs are administered by some authors [822]. Initially, swallowing disorders need to be taken into account; but in only a marginal number of cases do they call for a special diet. After a maximum of 3 days, all patients were again able to swallow in a normal fashion [196].

On a Visual Analogue Scale with the end points "0 = no pain" and "10 = maximal pain," the postoperative pain is given as 7.6 on the first postoperative day, and as 1.7 two weeks after surgery [822]. From our own experience we are able to report one patient where the suspension had to be removed due to persisting pain. Woodson and colleagues did not encounter such cases in the calculations of their success rates [832]. Fibbi and colleagues [196] report a case of prolonged odynophagia lasting for 3 weeks.

Postoperative complications include dehydration requiring intravenous rehydration several days after surgery (4.3%), delayed gastrointestinal bleeding requiring hospitalization (4.3%) [822, 832], and delayed floor-of-mouth sialadenitis (17.4%), the latter especially when the screw was placed via an intraoral approach. All complications resolved without sequela. During the first weeks, temporary swallowing and speech impediments are regularly reported.

In our own patient pool, we had two cases where the suspension suture spontaneously tore apart. The following night snoring and apneas recurred. Furthermore, we have the impression that the thread slowly cuts toward anterior through the tongue in some cases. This may not cause severe annoyance, but may over time lead to a reduction of the therapeutic effect.

7.4.5
Indications and Contraindications

Basically, the Repose tongue base suspension is potentially helpful in the treatment of airway obstruction at the level of the tongue base. For OSA, the results are comparable with RFT therapy at the tongue base. Apart from the costs, we believe there are two drawbacks to this method.

On the one hand, general anesthesia is necessary in order to place the suspension suture. We therefore do not agree with the estimation of the provider, who characterizes the procedure as minimally invasive. In our opinion, it should be possible to perform a minimally invasive surgical procedure for the therapy of SDB on an outpatient basis and under local anesthesia. Here RFT has clear advantages. On the other hand, and to our mind even more important, it is very difficult to achieve the correct tightness. Aim of the suspension suture is to prevent airway collapse during sleep without impeding the function of the tongue during the day, especially in respect to speech and swallowing. This technique consists in a tight-rope walk between sufficient suspension meaning effectiveness with regard to SDB and the unhindered functioning of the tongue during the day. On the other the concrete disadvantage of the method lies in the lack of a postoperative option to readjust the tightness. For this readjusting a second general anesthesia is necessary.

Very recently, a new surgical treatment has been presented trying to overcome this issue. Instead of a suture, a titanium anchor is placed in the back of the tongue, attached to a titratable spool which is fixed on the mandible [719]. After implantation, the tension on the system can be modified even months after surgery under local anesthesia. First clinical data are awaited.

Take Home Pearls

> Tongue suspension is less invasive than genioglossus advancement but more invasive than tongue base radiofrequency surgery, providing comparable results with regard to the treatment of OSA.
> With regard to the fact that the procedure requires general anesthesia and that relevant complications had been reported, the authors do not recommend this procedure for the treatment of snoring.
> Although the morbidity seems to be reduced by the modified approach via a submental skin incision, the problem with the correct adjustment of the tension on the suture remains and the clinical results are therefore hard to predict.
> The data regarding clinical efficacy is still limited to a small number of noncontrolled trials with limited number of patients.

8

Maxillofacial Surgeries

Genioglossus Advancement (GA)

8.1

Thomas Verse

Core Features

> The genioglossus advancement (GA) is used in combination with other surgical techniques for treatment of severe OSA. The surgical principle consists in mobilizing the whole area of this muscle insertion by incorporating the genial tubercle on the inner cortex via an osteotomy of the chin, and then moving it toward anterior.

> An isolated efficiency verification according to the principles of evidence-based medicine (EBM) is not available. In a meta-analysis of 80 patients who received a combination of GA and adjunctive procedures (e.g., hyoidsuspension), a success rate of 66% was reported.

In 1986, the inferior sagittal osteotomy of the mandible was used for the first time in the treatment of obstructive sleep apnea (OSA) by the Stanford research group [604]. The authors used this technique in combination with a hyoid suspension (HS) (Sect. 7.2 in Chap. 7) in patients with severe OSA. Since then the so-called mandibular osteotomy with genioglossus advancement (MO) has become part of several surgical protocols. Interestingly, the technique has until now only been used in combination with other techniques and not as an isolated procedure for treating OSA.

8.1.1
Surgical Technique

The genioglossus muscle has its origin at the oral side of the mandible. The surgical principle consists in mobilizing the whole area of this muscle insertion by incorporating the genial tubercle on the inner cortex via an osteotomy of the chin, and then moving it toward anterior (Fig. 8.1.1). In this new position, the bone segment is fixated osteosynthetically, either with a 24-gauge stainless steel wire or a screw. External cortex and cancellous bone are removed in order to prevent a cosmetically disagreeable protrusion of the chin.

K. Hörmann, T. Verse, *Surgery for Sleep Disordered Breathing*,
DOI: 10.1007/978-3-540-77786-1_8.1, © Springer Verlag Berlin Heidelberg 2010

The surgical approach is completely intraoral. The mucosal incision is made approximately 10–15 mm below the mucogingival junction and a subperiostal flap is developed to expose the symphysis. Exposure and identification of the mental nerves are unnecessary. In order to reduce the extent of the dissection, entailing a reduction of potential complications, Riley et al. have twice revised their technique of inferior sagittal osteotomy. Figure 8.1.2 shows the most recent technique [410] which we have adopted in our center. Miller et al. [467] recently recommended the use of the Genial Bone Advancement Trephine system (Stryker Leibinger Corp.; Kalamazoo) and reported good results.

A rectangular osteotomy encompassing the estimated location of the genial tubercle/genioglossus muscle complex is performed under copious irrigation. The superior horizontal bone is cut approximately 5 mm below the root apices to prevent incisor root injury and the inferior horizontal bone is cut approximately 10 mm above the inferior border (Fig. 8.1.2). Occasionally, the superior horizontal bone cut has to be made 1–2 mm above the incisor root apices because of the vertical position of the genial tubercle/genioglossus muscle complex [469]. Due to the elongated canine tooth roots that are often present, the vertical bone cuts are made just medial to the canine roots to avoid root injury. Before completing the osteotomy, a titanium screw is placed in the outer cortex to control and manipulate the bone flap. The amount of advancement depends on the thickness of the mandible. The bone flap is advanced and rotated about 30–45°, just sufficient to create bone overlap for a fixation screw.

Li et al. [410] control bleeding with electrocautery and a hemostatic agent such as Gelfoam R (Pharmacia and Upjohn Co, Kalamazoo). Bone wax is not recommended due to extrusion problems. These authors do not use surgical drains. In their hands, the procedure is routinely completed within 30–40 min.

In treating the hypopharyngeal site of obstruction, most authors combine the GA with a HS [499, 587, 608]. Fibbi et al. [196] recommend the combination of GA with a tongue suspension suture (Repose[R]) (Sect. 7.4 in Chap. 7). Furthermore, the GA is part of some multilevel surgery protocols as discussed in Chap. 10.

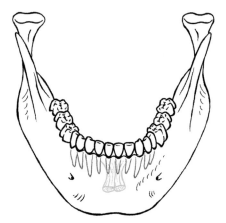

Fig. 8.1.1 Origin of the genioglossus muscle at the genial tubercle on the inner cortex of the mandible

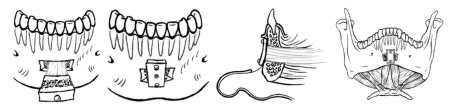

Fig. 8.1.2 Inferior sagittal osteotomy of the mandible. *Left*: bony segment pulled forward after rectangular osteotomy. *Center and right*: postoperative situation

8.1.1.1
Effectiveness for OSA

The GA is a therapy for OSA, but not for primary snoring. As mentioned above we have not been able to find any studies using polysomnographies in investigating the effectiveness of GA as an isolated procedure. Therefore, we have decided to summarize in Table 8.1.1 only the current data of studies performing combined procedures for tongue base obstruction.

Since most of these are noncontrolled data, and since all but two of them are also short-term data, a verification of the effectiveness according to the principles of evidence-based medicine (EBM) is still difficult. In addition, all authors performed additional procedures. This is why the effect of an isolated GA remains unclear.

In this context, the study by Neruntarat [499], who compares short- and long-term results, is of interest. All patients had received an uvulopalatal flap, an HS, and a GA in the framework of a multilevel surgery concept. In his retrospective analysis of 46 patients, a therapy success (Sher's criteria) of 78.3% after 6 months and of 65.2% after on average 39 months was found. Obviously this points to a decrease of the therapy effect over time. Unfortunately, it cannot be deduced which partial effect can be ascribed to the GA.

8.1.2
Postoperative Care and Complications

The GA is performed under general anesthesia on an inpatient basis. In cases where no further procedures involving the upper airway have been performed, a hospital stay of about 2 or 3 days is sufficient. We administer an intraoperative single-shot antibiosis with, e.g., 1×2 g cephazoline. The administration of corticoids is not necessary.

As GA is a used in severe OSA, some authors generally protect the upper airway with the routine use of nasal continuous positive airway pressure (CPAP) during the postoperative phase. We observe our patients in the recovery room for some hours and apply CPAP only in cases that show repeated apneas. If a CPAP therapy is necessary, the auto-CPAP mode is used. Observation in an intensive care unit is usually not necessary after MO.

Table 8.1.1 Effectiveness of GA for OSA

Author	N	Adjunctive procedure	Follow-up (months)	AHI pre	AHI post	Success rate (%)	EBM
Riley et al. [606]	5	HS	6	73.6	21	80	4
Riley et al. [605]	55	HS, UPPP	6	58.7	11.8	66.7	4
Riley et al. [608]	15	HS	3	44.7	12.8	53.3	3b
Johnson and Chinn [334]	9	UPPP	39	58.7	14.5	77.8	3b
Ramirez and Loube [587]	12	HS, UPPP	6	49	23	42	3b
Lee et al. [390]	33	UPPP	4–6	55.2	21.7	66.7	4
Fibbi et al. [196]	4	TBS	6	22.0	No data	75.0	4
Neruntarat [499]	46	HS, Flap	39.4	47.9	18.6	65.2	4
Miller et al. [467]	24	UPPP	4.7	52.9	15.9	66.7	4
Foltan et al. [205]	31	HM	7.3	20.9	10.3	74.0	3b
All	234			48.78	15.51	66.10	B

AHI Apnea Hypopnea Index; *EBM* level of evidence based medicine; *HS* hyoid suspension; *UPPP* uvulopalatopharyngoplasty; *TBS* tongue base suture; *HM* hyoid myotomy

As minor complication a wound dehiscence has been observed intraorally. It usually heals spontaneously without sequela. Furthermore, transient numbness of the lower lip and lower central incisors for several weeks [467], dysphagia for up to 1 week, and self-limiting aspiration have been reported [499]. In general, tooth root injuries, mental nerve injuries, and mandibular fracture as potential complications have been reported only very rarely [410]. In our own group of patients one subject developed a severe wound infection several days after surgery requiring surgical intervention. Similar cases have been reported by other authors as well [395, 605]. Speech or swallowing problems have neither been reported nor have they been seen in our own patients.

8.1.3
Indications and Contraindications

Like HS, GA is an invasive surgical method with potential complications. For the tongue base, a minimally invasive alternative exists in the form of radiofrequency treatment (RFT). We therefore see no primary indication for the HS for primary snoring, and mild OSA.

In the case of moderate and severe sleep apnea with tongue base obstruction, the GA is a surgical treatment option. In our center, we have completely ceased to perform this technique as we encountered several complications. We have had better experiences with HS. The latter can be performed more rapidly, is the only procedure which can be performed under local anesthesia, uses less osteosynthesis material, and is at least in our hands less prone to complications. Nevertheless, in the hands of an experienced surgeon GA may be a viable alternative in the treatment of moderate to severe OSA.

Take-Home Pearls

> The GA is used in combination with other surgical techniques for treatment of moderate and severe OSA. In our center we do not perform it anymore. Treatment options like hyoid suspension or laser-assisted excision of the tonsillar tissue at the tongue base are preferred.

Maxillomandibular Advancement (MMA) 8.2

Thomas Hierl

Core Features

> Maxillomandibular advancement (MMA) in severe sleep apneics is done as a secondary procedure after failure of a conservative (continuous positive airway pressure, CPAP) or multilevel surgery therapy. A simultaneous expansion of the naso, oro-, and hypopharyngeal airways is achieved.
> MMA is an invasive surgical technique with corresponding morbidity and complication rates.
> In high-selected patient groups, studies report a short-term success rate of 97% after 6 months and a success rate of 90% after 51 months.
> Complications after MMA are temporomandibular joint dysfunction, hypopharyngeal edema, velopharyngeal incompetence, and hypesthesia of the lower lip.

Maxillofacial surgery for the correction of malpostion of the upper and lower jaw was first suggested by Kuo et al. [378] as an alternative to tracheotomy in the treatment of obstructive sleep apnea (OSA). Today, MMA can be seen as the most successful surgical procedure after tracheotomy. On the other side, it must be said that it is an invasive surgical technique with corresponding morbidity and complication rates. Therefore, it is used as primary therapy in patients with relevant deformities of the face and the skull in most instances. For sleep apneics without a jaw anomaly, the Stanford 2 phase concept has become the standard treatment. In phase 1, it offers a multilevel surgery of the soft palate and tongue base, and if necessary of the nose in accordance with the procedures provided in Chap. 10; only in the case of therapy failure does it offer MMA as a secondary procedure.

The rationale of MMA is the simultaneous expansion of the naso-, oro-, and hypopharyngeal airways as soft palate, tongue, and lateral pharyngeal walls are advanced or stretched (Fig. 8.2.1).

K. Hörmann, T. Verse, *Surgery for Sleep Disordered Breathing,*
DOI: 10.1007/978-3-540-77786-1_8.2, © Springer Verlag Berlin Heidelberg 2010

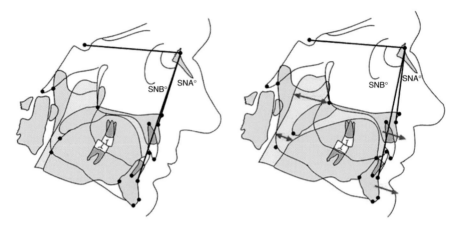

Fig. 8.2.1 *Left*: preoperative situation. Retropositioned maxilla and mandible with narrow pharyngeal airway space. *Right*: after MMA the widened pharynx, an anterior positioned tongue and soft palate can be seen. SNA° and SNB° which determine the sagittal position increase

8.2.1
Surgical Technique

Although MMA is a routine procedure in maxillofacial surgery, it is technically demanding and performed by a team of surgeons in a hospital environment under general anesthesia [581].

8.2.1.1
Surgery on the Upper Jaw

In order to advance the upper jaw it has to be freed from the upper parts of the midface and the cranial base, moved forward (and if necessary simultaneously up- respectively downward), and stabilized in the new position. The usual method consists in a transverse osteotomy of the maxilla (so-called Le Fort I osteotomy) [518]. The osteotomy lines (Fig. 8.2.2) resemble more or less the fracture lines analogous to the Le Fort I fracture.

While in 1970s–1980s, wire osteosyntheses, zygomatico-maxillary suspensions, and intermaxillary fixation (for approximately 6 weeks) were used, now miniplate osteosynthesis has become the standard procedure to hold the maxilla in its new position until bony union has occurred (Fig. 8.2.3). The extent of the maxillary advancement is determined individually depending on the amount judged necessary for relief of OSA, the new position of the mandible and the nutrition status during operation as excessive soft tissue stretching in the soft palate region may compromise vascularity. In most studies, 10 mm are suggested as some relapse (backward movement of the maxilla) has to be expected.

In case of stabilization with miniplates, intermaxillary fixation is not necessary in most instances; this is especially of relevance in the immediate postoperative phase in OSA patients. Furthermore, the amount of relapse will be minimized.

Fig. 8.2.2 Le Fort I osteotomy (*red line*). The
nasal septum and the pterygomaxillary junction
are detached with a chisel; the paranasal and
zygomatic buttresses are cut with a reciprocating
saw

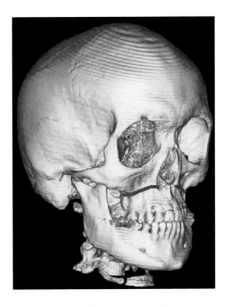

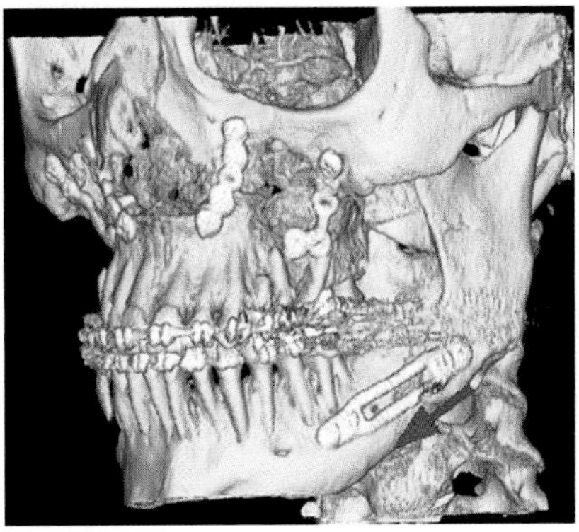

Fig. 8.2.3 Osteosynthesis technique using
titanium miniplates in orthognathic surgery.
Maxillary advancement in the Le Fort-I level
stabilized by way of four miniplates on the
paranasal and zygomatic buttresses.
Simultaneous mandibular advancement (see
red arrow) utilizing adjustable split-fix
miniplates (all Synthes®, Paoli, PA)

8.2.1.2
Surgery on the Lower Jaw

In principle, the advancement of the lower jaw can be performed almost anywhere in the
mandible ranging from an osteotomy in the mandibular body to the ascending ramus [574,
604]. The most common method is the bilateral sagittal split osteotomy (BSSO) according
to Obwegeser [519] with lateral corticotomy anterior to the mandibular angle [603, 604]
(Fig. 8.2.4).

In this procedure, the lingual bone separation proceeds horizontally between lingula
and incisura semilunaris. The osteotomy line on the buccal side proceeds vertically from
the molar region to the inferior border. The sagittal split is then performed using a chisel
(Fig. 8.2.4). It is crucial to take care that the inferior alveolar nerve remains lingual of the
chisel in order to prevent lesions. After aligning the mandible to a correct occlusion,

Fig. 8.2.4 Sagittal osteotomy of the
mandible with lateral corticotomy
anterior the mandibular angle
[according to 518]. *L* lateral

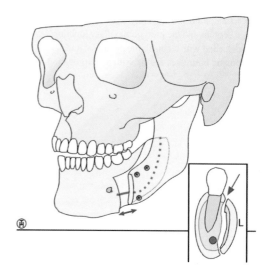

osteosynthesis is performed. Here wire sutures, or preferably position screws or miniplates can be used (Fig. 8.2.4).

In all cases of MMA surgery, some skeletal relapse has to be accepted. Factors determining the amount of relapse include osteosynthesis technique and the amount of advancement. In the maxilla and mandible 10–30% can be reckoned with. Thus in a 10 mm advancement a net forward movement of 7–9 mm will persist which is judged sufficient for OSA relief.

8.2.2
Efficiency of Maxillomandibular Advancement for OSA

MMA can be considered the most successful surgical procedure for the treatment of OSA after tracheotomy with respect to treatment outcome. Several controlled studies have demonstrated a comparable reduction of the Apnea Hypopnea Index (AHI) after MMA to continuous positive airway pressure (CPAP) therapy [284, 582, 607] (Table 8.2.1). Furthermore, an equivalent optimization of the sleep architecture compared to CPAP has been reported after MMA [123].

The successful results seem to be maintained for long follow-up periods. The Stanford studies report a short-term success rate of 97% after 6 months [607], and a success rate of 90% after 51 months [405].

Furthermore, Li et al. [402] were able to show by way of radiocephalometry and nasopharyngoscopic examinations that pharyngeal depth increased by 48% of the amount of the maxillary advancement and that pharyngeal length increased by 53% of the maxillary advancement in 5 patients after MMA.

Table 8.2.1 Multilevel surgery for OSA

Author	N	Adjunctive procedure	Follow-up (months)	AHI pre	AHI post	Success rate (%)	EBM
Waite et al. [788]	23	UPPP, GA, MLP	1.5	62.8	15.2	65.2	4
Riley et al. [607]	30	HS	6	72.0	8.8	96.7	3b
Hochban et al. [284]	38		2	44.4	2.5	97.4	3b
Prinsell [582]	50	HS	5.2	59.2	4.7	100	3b
Li et al. [405]	40		50.7	69.6	8.9	90	4
Bettega et al. [51]	20	Prior phase I	6	59.3	11.1	75	4
Goh and Lim [234]	11		7.7	70.7	11.4	81.8	4
Dattilo and Drooger [136]	15	Prior phase I	1.5	76.2	12.6	86.7	4
All	227		12.4	62.3	8.1	89.9	B

HS hyoid suspension; *GA* mandibular osteotomy with genioglossus advancement; *MLP* midline partial glossectomy

8.2.3
Postoperative Care and Complications

For patients suffering from severe OSA, it is recommended to start nasal CPAP at least 1 month before surgery to stabilize the cardiovascular system and reduce upper airway edema [51].

After surgery, extubation should be performed by the operating room staff with the patient being fully awake. MMA patients require careful monitoring, including continuous pulse oximetry, in an ICU environment [581]. Minor desaturations do not call for a CPAP therapy; yet frequent desaturations or apneas require CPAP ventilation therapy. When feasible, nonopioid drugs are used for postoperative analgesia (see Chap. 13).

Nutritional counseling emphasizing clear liquids during the first week, followed by a soft diet for 2 months, is recommended. Today, most authors do not favor prolonged intermaxillary fixation and use modern titanium plate systems for osteosynthesis. The usual hospital stay for MMA lies between 2 days [581, 607] and 1 week [51]. On average, patients return to their normal activities after 2–4 weeks. Patients should be asked to continue nasal CPAP until a follow-up polysomnography has confirmed the surgical success. Nasal decongestants should be administered for the first postoperative week as maxillary osteotomies lead to tearing of the nasal mucosa and edema with impaired nasal respiration.

Temporomandibular joint dysfunction is a potential complication after maxillomandibular surgery. Kerstens et al. [353] reported that 11.5% of the 480 patients who underwent surgery for dentofacial deformity developed temporomandibular joint symptoms after surgery. Similar data were given by White and Dolwick [814] (7.9%). However, temporomandibular joint problems can be often found in patients suffering from dento-facial deformities and the vast majority of the patients presenting preoperative tem-poromandibular joint symptoms reported improvement after surgery [409]. Here two patient groups have to be distinguished: firstly, patients with normal occlusion who undergo MMA for OSA treatment only and secondly, patients with marked maxillary/mandibular retrusion where MMA is intended for relief of OSA and to improve occlusal relationship.

Further complications are temporary mild-to-moderate hypopharyngeal edema (20%) and hypopharyngeal hematoma (5.7%), partly obstructing the airway [411]. In large maxil-lary advancements patients frequently develop velopharyngeal incompetence of a tempo-rary nature. Predominantly velopharyngeal incompetence is a phonetic deficit without liquid regurgitation. But there are also singular prolonged cases of velopharyngeal incom-petence with regurgitation up to a duration of maximally 12 months [412].

Hypesthesia of the lower lip is the typical complication of BSSO (anesthesia <1%; hypesthesia <5%) [51, 607]. A high percentage of resolution within the first months after surgery is reported. Recovery of full mandibular function (maximum mouth opening; bite force) will take some time and will not be gained in all instances. A further frequent com-plication is occlusion disturbances in up to 50% of the cases, requiring minor occlusial equilibration by way of orthodontics or prosthodontics [788].

Rare complications include local infection, perforation of the palate, and maxillary pseu-darthrosis [51]. Furthermore, severe complications like tooth loss, facial nerve paralysis, osteomyelitis, damage of the inferior alveolar nerve, and amaurosis have been reported.

The incidence rate for complications increases with higher patient age, especially after 45 years [51, 788].

Furthermore, the aesthetic effects of MMA should be pointed out. These should espe-cially be taken into consideration if the patient preoperatively presents no jaw malposi-tions, but is solely receiving surgery for the treatment of OSA. As a consequence, Goh and Lim [234] have recently suggested a modified procedure which includes partial resections of the upper and lower jaw in order to counteract the aesthetically disagreeable advance-ment of the jaws. It is debatable in how far these additional osteotomies can be justified with respect to purely aesthetic indication as complication rates should be expected to be significantly higher.

8.2.4
Indications and Contraindications

In addition to the sleep lab diagnosis radiocephalometry is necessary in order to determine the indication and amount of MMA. In general, the parameters given in Fig. 8.2.5 are analyzed. In case the SNA angle (angle measurement from Sella (S) to nasion (N) to sub-spinale (A)) is at least 82°, and the SNB angle (angle measurement from Sella (S) to nasion (N) to supramentale (B)) at least 80°, a maxillomandibular deficiency can be ruled out.

Fig. 8.2.5 Basic radiocephalometric landmarks for sagittal and vertical maxillomandibular relationships. (*S* sella; *N* nasion; *Ba* basion; *A* subspinale; *B* supramentale; *Pg* pogonion; *Gn* gnathion; *Tgo* tangent point gonion; *Pm* pterygomaxillare; *Ar* articulare; *Sp* anterior nasal spine; *NSL* nasion-sella line; *NL* nasal line; *OL* occlusal line; *ML* mandibular line). Special OSA parameters are not included

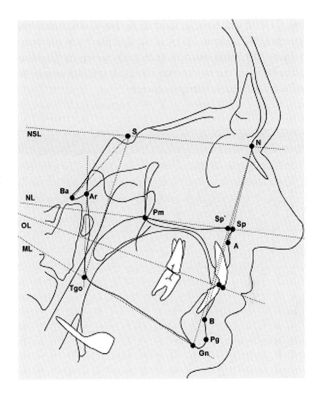

While in the case of a maxillomandibular deficiency MMA may already be used as a primary therapy of OSA, the indication is more difficult in the case of a regularly shaped facial skull. Most authors, including ourselves, see the indication for surgery only in those cases in which a respiratory therapy has either been abandoned or refused, or is not possible. In principle, an obstruction both in the retropalatal as well as the retrolingual segment is demanded as precondition for the MMA. A posterior airway space (PAS) <11 mm is generally considered as a positive selection criterion for MMA. Hochban et al. [284] determine the PAS at the level of the mandibular plane, whereas Prinsell [581] suggests measuring the PAS at its narrowest place instead of strictly defined anatomical landmarks.

It is also being debated, whether after the failure of a respiratory therapy less morbidizing and aggressive surgical procedures should be performed initially, or whether MMA should be considered primarily in the case of normal maxillofacial dimensions, too. The opinions on this are quite varied. Hochban et al. posit the indication very generously. One argument is that soft palate surgery prior to MMA may increase the chance of postoperative velopharyngeal incompetence. Most other study groups [51, 136, 607], in accordance with the Stanford 2 phase model, posit the MMA indication only secondarily, namely after failed UPPP with tonsillectomy as well as hyoid suspension and RFT of the tongue. Other groups [788] perform MMA in the first place and combine the operation with pharyngeal surgery. We believe that in each study group an interdisciplinary dialogue should take place between the otorhinolaryngologist and the maxillofacial surgeon in order to determine a constructive therapy concept.

Take-Home Pearls

> Maxillomandibular advancement (MMA) is a treatment option for high-selected patients with a severe sleep apnea and a maxillomandibular deficiency. Studies report for these high-selected patients as high success rates as after tracheotomy.

Distraction Osteogenesis (DOG)

8.3

Thomas Hierl

Core Features

> Distraction osteogenesis (DOG) has become an accepted procedure in the treatment of severe maxillomandibular deficiency in syndromic and nonsyndromic patients. Obstructive sleep apnea (OSA) is often found in these cases. Mandibular and maxillary-midfacial DOG are performed. Most publications on DOG in OSA patients include only small numbers or are case reports.

> Avoiding or ending tracheostomy is the major treatment objective in this patient group and DOG is the most effective procedure.

Since its introduction into maxillofacial surgery by McCarthy et al. [454], distraction osteogenesis (DOG) has become an accepted procedure in the treatment of severe maxillomandibular deficiency in syndromic and nonsyndromic patients. As a grossly retropositioned mandible or midface causes a narrow pharyngeal airway, obstructive sleep apnea (OSA) is often found in these cases. Thus DOG will be the procedure of choice where conventional maxillomandibular advancement (MMA) cannot be performed or is expected to lead to unstable results. This is especially true for neonates and young children in whom MMA is rarely performed [43].

In DOG, an osteotomy of the mandible or midface without advancement is followed by a short latency period of 4 days. Then the two or more bony segments are slowly moved apart (in most instances at 1 mm/day) using some kind of distraction device. Thus the unmineralized tissue filling the osteotomy gap is slowly stretched until – after cessation of distraction – it will turn into bone during the 4–10 weeks lasting consolidation period. Now the device will be removed and orthodontic appliances will act against relapse and help achieve proper occlusion.

K. Hörmann, T. Verse, *Surgery for Sleep Disordered Breathing*,
DOI: 10.1007/978-3-540-77786-1_8.3, © Springer Verlag Berlin Heidelberg 2010

8.3.1
Mandibular Distraction Osteogenesis

The first devices designed for mandibular distraction have been extraoral distractors which are fixed to the bone by way of percutaneous pins. Initially unidirectional devices prevailed (i.e., distraction only in one direction), now most companies offer multidirectional distractors which allow correction of the distraction vector during treatment (Fig. 8.3.1).

Extraoral devices are mainly used in syndromic neonates and infants where placement of internal distractors is difficult (e.g., Pierre-Robin sequence, Nager syndrome; Stickler syndrome, velocardiofacial syndrome, Pfeiffer syndrome, Treacher-Collins syndrome).

In less complicated cases, intraoral unidirectional distractors might be used (Fig. 8.3.2). These are inconspicuous and avoid facial scars. Most companies offer internal distractors with 15–25 mm distraction range, thus for larger advancements extraoral devices are still the matter of choice.

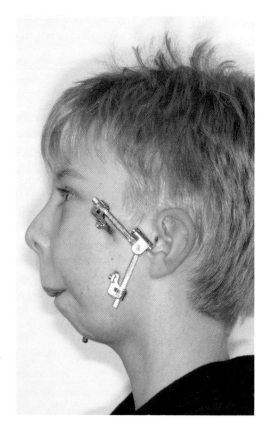

Fig. 8.3.1 Thirteen-year-old boy suffering from mandibular hypoplasia and retrusion due to trauma in infancy. Severe pharyngeal narrowing and OSA. Distraction of the mandible with multidirectional distractors on both sides (Multiguide; Stryker-Leibinger Co, Kalamazoo, MI)

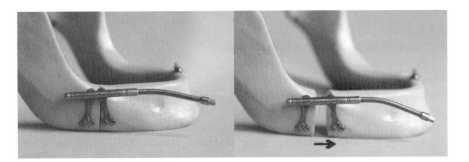

Fig. 8.3.2 Internal mandibular distractor: *right* situation after osteotomy and device placement. *Left* during activation (here maximum 15 mm). The flexible activation rod lies in the buccal sulcus (Zurich mandibular distractor, Martin Co., Tuttlingen, Germany). Notice the transverse osteotomy in contrast to the sagittal split in MMA. Fixation of the device is achieved with 1.5 mm diameter monocortical microscrews

8.3.1.1
Surgical Technique

DOG is a technically complicated procedure performed under general anesthesia after nasotracheal intubation in a clinical setting (in adults, local anesthesia is possible but rarely used). Perioperative antibiotics are preferable.

In neonates and children, a lateral corticotomy in the area of the mandibular angle or ascending ramus is performed via an intraoral buccal sulcus incision. The upper and inferior borders are cut with burs or reciprocating saws. Then the pins are fixed bicortically via stab incisions and a greenstick resp. full fracture is done with a chisel. Lastly, the distractor is attached to the pins and the mobility of the segments is tested by distractor activation.

Regarding internal devices, the operation starts with a buccal sulcus incision and the distractors are temporarily fixed with micro- or miniscrews. Now the osteotomy line is marked. Then the distractor is removed and a full osteotomy is performed. The distractors are reattached and the mobility of the segments is tested by turning the distractor. Finally, the intraoral incision is closed. Fixation of the device can be performed via transbuccal stab incisions or preferably with a contra-angle handpiece and screwdriver.

Contrary to the sagittal split osteotomy in MMA, the osteotomy is at right angle to the outer cortical border. Care has to be taken not to cut the inferior alveolar nerve during the outer corticotomy or to place bicortical pins through the nerve canal. To prohibit violation of tooth buds or roots, preoperative radiologic diagnostic is necessary. In syndromic patients, CT-scans are obtained in most instances to get an understanding of the individual pathology. Reformatting and volume-rendering software allow to examine all important structures and visualize the upper airways. In nonsyndromic adult cases, OPT and lateral cephalogram are sufficient in most instances.

8.3.2
Maxillary-Midfacial Distraction Osteogenesis

Maxillary-midfacial DOG includes advancements at the Le-Fort I to the Le-Fort III levels. Internal and external devices are both available. All procedures are performed under general anesthesia in a hospital environment. Several syndromes are associated with sleep-related breathing disorders due to the pharyngeal narrowing caused by midfacial retrusion. These include Crouzon's disease, Apert syndrome, Weber–Christian disease, achondrodysplasia, and to some extent cleft lip and palate. In case of severe preoperative airway obstruction temporary tracheostomy has to be considered.

8.3.2.1
Surgical Technique

In the Le-Fort I level, surgery is similar to MMA. The only differences are that the osteotomized bone is not advanced and that distractors instead of plates are inserted. Here the osteotomy design has to keep in mind that there must be enough bone cranially to fix the distractor. Furthermore, distractor placement on both sides should be parallel and aligned to the planned distraction vector. Mistakes will lead to unwanted movements with potentially unacceptable results. In the Le-Fort III level, access is gained via a bicoronal incision. The lateral orbital rim, the nose, and the zygoma are freed from above. Pterygomaxillary disjunction is done via an intraoral incision or through the bicoronal incision. Most internal Le-Fort III distractors are fixed in the transition from zygomatic arch to the zygoma (Fig. 8.3.3) and the activation rods leave through the bicoronal cut. Alternatively to internal devices, extraoral haloborne distractors may be used. The major advantages are that there is no need for parallel alignment of the distractors and the osteotomy cuts can be freely designed as no bone for distractor anchorage is needed superior to the bone cut. Furthermore, the distraction vector can be

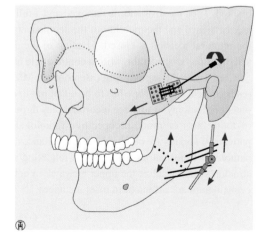

Fig. 8.3.3 Mandibular DOG using an external device (cf. Fig. 8.3.1). *Dotted black line* represents the typical osteotomy line in the mandibular angle area (the bone cut may be placed almost anywhere). In the midface a Le-Fort III advancement by way of an internal distractor is shown (*red dotted line*). The activation rod passes through the skin in the region of the bicoronal incision necessary for the osteotomy. *Red arrows* symbolize distractor activation and segment movement

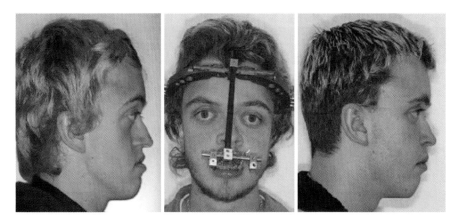

Fig. 8.3.4   Midfacial distraction in a Crouzon`s disease case. External halo-borne distractor (RED; Martin Co. Tuttlingen, Germany) used to advance the midface after a quadrangular osteotomy (i.e., Le-Fort III minus the nasal part). *Left*: Preoperative situation. *Center*: During distractor activation. *Right*: 6 months after removal of the device (16 mm advancement). The connection of the midface to the extraoral distractors can be achieved via orthodontic splints or miniplate retention systems

changed during treatment (Fig. 8.3.4). The only drawback is its rather clumsy appearance being extraoral. Internal distractors are removed after a consolidation period of 6–12 weeks, external devices after 3–8 weeks.

8.3.2.2
Efficiency of DOG for OSA

Most publications on DOG in OSA patients include only small numbers or are case reports. Concerning neonates or children exact polysomnographic pre- and postoperative data are not given in the majority of reports. However, avoiding or ending tracheostomy is the major treatment objective in this patient group and DOG is the most effective procedure. Only in cases of central apnea, decannulation could not be achieved (Table 8.3.1).

As can be seen in Tables 8.3.1–8.3.3, most studies deal with syndromic patients resp. cases with TMJ-ankylosis which can be considered as most difficult to treat surgically. Looking at the 3D pharyngeal airway changes induced by DOG, major improvement in OSA should be expected when treating these malformations. Figures 8.3.5 and 8.3.6 demonstrate a typical OSA case.

No data regarding the long-term outcome are available as of now. As DOG leads to stable skeletal results, a similar outcome in adults as in MMA has to be expected. In syndromic children, there is only limited skeletal relapse, too. As the affected midface shows no or only little growth after DOG, a midfacial retrusion (and perhaps OSA) will reappear. Further surgery on the midface is therefore a part of the treatment scheme.

A fascinating option during DOG is to perform multiple sleep studies during the advancement of the upper or lower jaw. Thus the efficacy and the average length needed

Table 8.3.1   Mandibular DOG for OSA in infants and children

Author	N	Age	Diagnoses	Distraction length (mm)	Success
Moore et al. [480]	1	6 years			Decannulation
Williams et al. [818]	4	Ø 2.7 years	TC-S, Nager	15–27	Decannulation in 3/4
Schierle et al. [648]	3	7–15 months	Nager, Down	15–20	Decannulation in 2/3
Morovic and Monasterio [483]	7	1–18 months	PR-S, TC-S	10–25	Decannulation, "reduced" AHI
Sidman et al. [674]	11	2 weeks to 5.5 years	PR-S, Down, Nager	10–22	Decannulation, relief of OSA in 10 patients
Denny et al. [147]	5	6–26 days	PR-S	Ø 12.4	Decannulation, no OSA
Villani et al. [783]	2	2/3 months	PR-S	15/20	Decannulation
Ortiz-Monasterio et al. [527]	15	Ø 3 years	PR-S		AHI 28 → 0
Perlyn et al. [558]	4	15–64 months	Nager, TC-S	8–25	Decannulation
Izadi et al. [319]	15	Ø 8.5 days	PR-S, TC-S, Stickler, Nager	12–15	14/15 Avoidance of tracheostomy
All	67				64/67

TC-S Treacher-Collins syndrome; *PR-S* Pierre-Robin sequence; *Nager* Nager syndrome; *Stickler* Stickler syndrome; *Down* Down syndrome. Exact data on pre- and posttreatment sleep lab data is missing as do follow-up reports with respect to OSA. Decannulation: decannulation and closure of tracheostomy was successful; Ø Mean

to treat OSA can be analyzed [543, 824]. This could help in defining the advancements that are needed to treat OSA effectively and investigate on the relation of morphologic changes and OSA.

8.3.2.3
Complications and Postoperative Care

Most potential problems of MMA may be encountered in DOG (cf. Sect. 8.2). Beside these, DOG has further intricacies which will be listed up below. First of all, DOG is a technically demanding procedure (more difficult than MMA) where surgery and the postoperative period are equally important. Device malposition or improper vector planning may lead to therapy failure and a high learning curve has been stated [475]. Thus the overall complication rate will be higher than in MMA. Some orthodontic therapy will be needed in most cases to achieve proper occlusion. One of the problems is to decide when to remove

Table 8.3.2 Mandibular DOG for OSA in adults

Author	N	Age	Diagnoses	Distraction length (mm)	Success
Karakasis et al. [343]	1	48	TMJ ankylosis	20	RDI: 52.8 → 10.7
Paoli et al. [543]	1	44	OSA	12	AHI: 87.9 → 23.3[a]
Li et al. [403]	5	26–68 years	1/5 Hemifacial microsomia	5.5–12.5 (Ø 8.1)	RDI: 49.3 → 6.6
Wang et al. [797]	28	3–60 years. (Ø 21.2 years)	21/28 TMJ ankylosis	9–30 (Ø 8.1)	23/28 cured, 5/28 improved AHI: 58 → 3.2
Harada et al. [264]	1	31	OSA	15	AI: 29.9 → 4.1
Woodson et al. [824]	1	48	OSA	37	RDI: 38 → 2
All	37			9.5	

TMJ ankylosis ankylosis of the temporo-mandibular joint. Follow-up data is only on behalf of the skeletal stability

[a]After DOG, a maxillary advancement was performed, final AHI: 6.6

the device. The bony regenerate should be still "ductile" to end up in satisfactory occlusion by way of intermaxillary elastics but strong enough to prevent relapse. This is an important issue as perfect occlusion will not be achieved by DOG alone in most cases (in contrary to MMA). Compared to MMA, a higher percentage of open bite will be seen.

A major issue is the cost of DOG as distractors belong to the most expensive hardware. Thus financing therapy can be difficult. Relapse does not seem to be a major problem in most reports, thus a stable skeletal situation can be expected. Unwanted aesthetic effects play no major role as all patients treated by DOG will suffer from extreme maxillomandibular malformations, thus DOG will lead to a normalized facial appearance (Fig. 8.3.4).

8.3.2.4
Indications and Counter Indication

Indications for DOG are given by the underlying skeletal malformation to be treated. DOG solely for the cure of OSA will be an exception in patients with severe mandibular retrusion where conventional mandibular advancement bears the risk of an unstable skeletal situation. Thus the majority of patients will suffer from syndromic diseases, cleft lip and palate, and posttraumatic deformities.

Ancillary soft tissue operations as RFT can be debated where maximum advancement can not be achieved or in cases of tonsillar hyperplasia and macroglossia. As the airways are extremely constricted in syndromic patients, isolated soft tissue therapy will not be the

Table 8.3.3 Maxillary-midfacial DOG for OSA

Author	N	Age	Diagnoses	DOG-level	Distraction length (mm)	Success	Follow-up
Uemura et al. [755]	1	2.5 years	Crouzon	LF-III	16	AI: 16.4 → 2.6	12 months
Cedars et al. [95]	7	4–13 years	Crouzon, Apert	LF-III	16–27	3/7 initial cure of OSA, recurrence in 2; 1/7 partial improvement, 1/2 decannulated	0–2.5 years
Meling et al. [458]	2	4–5 years	Pfeiffer, Crouzon	LF-III	23–25	Improvement of OSA, tracheostomy avoided	
Cohen [117]	4	0.7–10 years	Apert, cleidocranial days	LF-III; monobloc LF-I	17–25	Improvement of OSA	
Elwood et al. [172]	2	3–6 years	Achondrodysplasia	LF-I	25	Decannulation	18 months
Satoh et al. [642]	1	13 years	Hajdu-Cheny-s	LF-III	20	Improvement	
All	17				16–25		

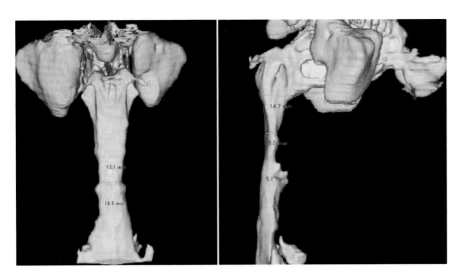

Fig. 8.3.5 CT-based volume rendering of the pharyngeal airways in a 53-year-old nonsyndromic male OSA patient. Preoperative situation displaying narrowing in the retrovelar pharynx (software: Vworks; Cybermed, Korea)

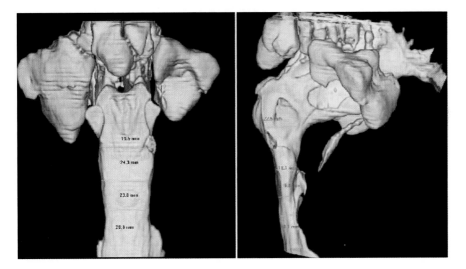

Fig. 8.3.6 Same patient as in Fig. 8.3.5. Postoperative situation after 16 mm advancement in the Le-Fort I level. Significant sagittal and also transversal widening of the naso- and oropharynx. AHI reduction from 39 to 9 in a 2 year follow-up PSG

procedure of first choice. Avoiding or ending tracheostomy will be the major aim in children and close cooperation between craniofacial-, maxillofacial-, ENT-surgeon, neurosurgeon and pediatrician will be necessary.

Take Home Pearls

> With distraction osteogenesis, underlying skeletal malformations are treated.
> For these patients, DOG has a positive influence on OSA.
> A close cooperation between craniofacial-, maxillofacial-, ENT-surgeon, neurosurgeon, and pediatrician is necessary.

Laryngeal OSA

9

Thomas Verse

Core Features

> Laryngeal obstructive sleep apnea (OSA) is a rare condition. It occurs in adults and children. Laryngeal OSA has to be diagnosed endoscopically during sleep or sedation.

> In children, laryngeal OSA is caused by malformations, tumors, and laryngomalcia; the latter especially in preterm infants.

> In adults, laryngeal OSA mainly occurs in elder men due to a floppy epiglottis. More rare conditions are laryngeal and hypopharyngeal tumors and other disorders in this anatomical region.

> In children, laser surgery may help to provide tracheostomy. Various techniques have been described as being effective.

> In adults, treatment depends on the underlying illness.

The most frequent sites of obstruction are situated behind the soft palate and/or behind the tongue. Nevertheless, the larynx may contribute to the genesis of obstructive sleep apnea (OSA): As early as in 1981 Olsen et al. [522] described a case of OSA caused by a laryngeal cyst. Removal of the cyst yielded the disappearance of apneas. Since then, several case reports and small case series have been published, but it is still not possible to determine the concrete incidence of laryngeal OSA. Basically, there are two forms of laryngeal OSA: the pediatric and the adult form. In the following discussion, they will be considered separately.

9.1
Pediatric Laryngeal OSA

During childhood, malformations, complex malformation syndromes, tumors, or laryngomalacia may be considered as possible causes of a laryngeal OSA. In the case of newborns a further aspect can make matters worse: the immaturity of the respiratory control is

K. Hörmann, T. Verse, *Surgery for Sleep Disordered Breathing*,
DOI: 10.1007/978-3-540-77786-1_ 9, © Springer Verlag Berlin Heidelberg 2010

often responsible for repetitive apneas and periodic breathing in early postnatal life. Consequences of this unstable breathing on blood gases and heart rate can lead to severe cerebral hypoxia and be life threatening, especially in preterm infants [160, 681, 702].

Malformations that lead to a laryngeal OSA have been documented in various case studies. Ruff et al. [632] describe the case of a previously healthy 13-year-old boy who developed OSA and bilateral vocal cord dysfunction secondary to type I Chiari malformation. He subsequently underwent a tracheostomy, a posterior fossa craniectomy, and C1-laminectomy. Four months after surgery he returned to school but still continued to require his tracheostomy. Two other case reports [59, 599] document that a congenital aplasia of the epiglottis may result in laryngeal OSA. Both children developed daytime sleepiness as a result of their OSA. One child underwent tracheostomy after she had developed heart failure. She was decannulated at the age of 7. Recently Chan et al. [100] presented an unusual case of a child with adenoid hypertrophy and occult supraglottic lymphatic malformation that manifested as laryngeal OSA.

Up to now, an epiglottic cyst [509], neurofibromas [673], and laryngeal papillomatosis [324] have been described as causes of OSA during childhood. We ourselves have recently treated a childhood OSA resulting from a hemangioma of the larynx of a 4-year old. The therapy consists in a resection or treatment of the tumors. Depending on tumor entity, size, and location, a temporary or permanent tracheotomy may become inevitable.

Laryngomalacia, or congenital laryngeal stridor, is a relatively benign, self-limiting condition first described in 1843 [40]. It seems to be the most common laryngeal congenital anomaly of all [290, 843]. It plays a significant role in the pathogenesis of laryngeal OSA in the case of the newborn, and especially for the preterm infant. In order to diagnose this dysfunction a fiberoptic laryngoscopy is essential. McSwiney et al. [457] described three anatomic abnormalities that cause laryngomalacia: (1) the epiglottis may be long and curled upon itself (the so-called omega-shaped epiglottis), and it prolapses posteriorly on inspiration; (2) the aryepiglottic folds may be short; and (3) the arytenoids may be more bulky than normal and prolapse forward on inspiration. Additionally, a mild subglottic edema may be present [843].

In mild cases, attentive observation is still the method of choice. Improvement always occurs before 12–18 months of age, and the outcome of these patients is invariably good [457]. In more severe cases, either a tracheotomy or laryngeal surgery may become necessary.

9.1.1
Surgical Techniques

Three principle types of surgery for laryngeal OSA can be distinguished. These are employed depending on the individual anatomic situation of each child.

The technique first to be described consists in a partial resection of the epiglottis. Zalzal et al. [843] first described a case series of 10 patients who underwent epiglottoplasty. This procedure addresses both the epiglottis and the mucosa of the aryepiglottic folds and the arytenoids. The epiglottis is grasped with cup forceps, and scissors are then used to trim the lateral edges of the epiglottis and the aryepiglottis folds. The mucosa of the arytenoids and corniculate cartilages is trimmed in a similar fashion. The author described the bleeding as minimal. Perioperative antibiotics are recommended.

Golz et al. [237] perform partial laser epiglottidectomy both in infants and adults if the epiglottis is found to be unusually long and flaccid. This technique solely addresses the epiglottis. As we, the authors use a Kleinsasser laryngoscope, a Riecker-Kleinsasser chest support, and the CO_2-Laser (continuous wave or superpulsed mode, 6–10 W). The extent of the resection was individualized for each patient in this series according to the anatomic abnormality causing the obstruction. The authors perform a U-shaped excision leaving the lateral sides of the aryepiglottic folds intact. Bourolias et al. [64] recently described their technique of reshaping the epiglottis with the CO_2 laser.

The second principle technique is called supraglottoplasty. Its characteristic consists in the resection of supraglottal mucosa. Senders and Navarrete [657] differentiate between four types of laser-assisted supraglottoplasty depending on the individual laryngeal finding (Figs. 9.1–9.4). The authors use the CO_2 laser adapted to a microscope micromanipulator (100–200 ms pulse sequences; 5–8 W). The authors excise either the supra-arytenoidal mucosa (arytenoidoplasty, Fig. 9.1), the mucosa of the aryepiglottic folds (aryepiglottoplasty; Fig. 9.2), the posterior edges of the epiglottis (epiglottoplasty; Fig. 9.3), or the lingual mucosal surface of the epiglottis (epiglottopexy; Fig. 9.4). Depending on the anatomical situation, every combination of the four techniques can be performed.

The amount of redundant mucosa that should be resected is most suitably identified using the "suction test" [571]. Instead of the CO_2 laser, laryngeal microinstruments can be used as well. We prefer the CO_2 laser because of its additional hemostatic effect. For relatively minor cases we have found it advantageous to punctually vaporize the mucosa with a defocused laser beam, instead of excising it.

A third technique deals with the problem of the shortened aryepiglottal fold. Here the problem is not the redundant mucosa, which prolapses into the glottis during inspiration, but rather a too short distance between arytenoid and epiglottis root. We and other study groups [424, 656] treat these cases with a V-formed, 3–4 mm deep incision into both of the aryepiglottal folds. Already, intraoperatively the laryngeal entrance in the anterio-posterior dimenstion becomes visibly wider. For this procedure, we also prefer the CO_2-laser (continuous wave or superpulsed mode; 6–8 W).

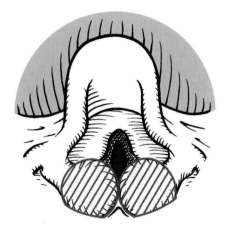

Fig. 9.1 Arytenoidoplasty according to Senders and Navarrete [657]. Coagulation of redundant mucosa of the arytenoids with a defocused laser beam

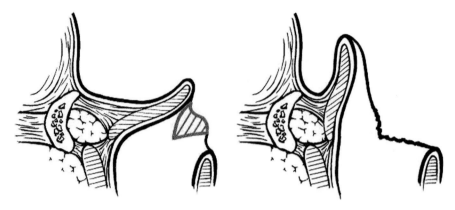

Fig. 9.2 Aryepiglottoplasty according to Senders and Navarrete [657]. Opening of a too short aryepiglottic fold

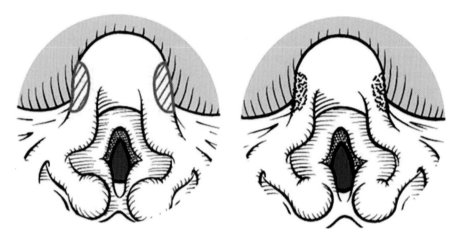

Fig. 9.3 Epiglottoplasty according to Senders and Navarrete [657]. Reduction of the too big epiglottis

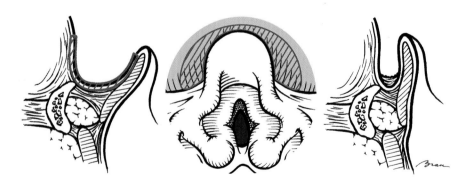

Fig. 9.4 Epiglottopexy according to Senders and Navarrete [657]. Scarring approximates the epiglottis to the base of tongue

In principle, according to the individual anatomical situation, combinations of the three basic techniques are also possible. Toynton et al. [747] combined an incision of the arytenoid fold with a removal of redundant supraglottal mucosa.

9.1.2
Efficiency for SDB

Unfortunately, up to now no studies exist which present clean sleep lab data before and after larynx surgery. On the other hand, there are many therapy studies which use as primary variables the daytime symptoms of laryngomalacia. The following Table 9.1 summarizes the results of several recent studies.

It is difficult to compare the studies in Table 9.1 since they deal with different techniques, employ different success criteria, and in part treat very different kinds of patients. From a few of the studies [148, 657] it can be deduced that patients who have not been successfully treated with larynx surgery, are those who display significantly more frequently complex or additional malformations.

Due to the fact that these are solely retrospective studies, it needs to be mentioned that an evidence proof according to Cochrane criteria has as yet not been established. Nevertheless, we do feel justified to infer a tendency to the effect that for a high percentage rate children with a severe laryngomalacia can be spared a tracheotomy with the help of an individually adapted larynx procedure.

9.1.3
Postoperative Care and Complications

Despite the high success rate, in 11.6% of the cases an initial deterioration of the stridor and in 4.7% the necessity of a reintubation or tracheotomy (1.2%) must be anticipated. These risks further increase in those cases which do not present an isolated laryngomalacia but complex malformations [657]. In any case, we regard an observation of the children in an accordingly furnished intensive care unit during the first postoperative night as necessary. In cases where the parents or other supervising persons are present, a monitoring of the respiration may be sufficient. In any case, this procedure should be performed on an inpatient basis.

Most authors [148, 657] routinely use corticoid therapy (beclomethasone, 125 µg/kg) within the first 3–5 days postoperatively, as we do in our center. In contrast to other recommendations we do not routinely use anti-inflammatory drugs or antibiotics.

Overall, the complication rate of the described surgical procedures is quite low, and does not vary significantly between the various techniques. The overall complication rate is given as between 5.8 [747] and 7.4% [148]. There is no difference concerning the complication rate in patients with isolated laryngomalacia compared to those having additional congenital anomalies [148].

As minor complications, aspiration of early feeds (7.0%), granulomas (1.5%) that had to be removed under general anesthesia, significant edema (1.5%), minor intra-operative hemorrhage (1.2%), and a posterior fibrous web between the arytenoids (0.7%) which required division with microscissors or laser, have been described.

Table 9.1 Effectiveness of surgery for severe laryngomalacia in children

Author	N	Procedure	Follow-up	Success rate (%)	Definition of success	EBM
Golz et al. [237]	12	Partial laser epigottidectomy	14–52 months	100	Subsiding of stridor	4
Senders and Navarrete [657]	23	Laser supraglottoplasty	No data	78 82.6	Immediate relief of symptoms avoidance of tracheotomy	4
Toynton et al. [747]	91	Aryepiglottoplasty	1 month	54.9 94.5	Relief of stridor improvement of stridor	4
Reddy and Matt [593]	106	Supraglottoplasty	No data	95.7	Relief of symptoms	4
Denoyelle et al. [148]	136	Laser supraglottoplasty	3 days to 60 months	79	Relief of symptoms	4
Zafereo et al. [842]	10	Laser supraglottoplasty	2–29 weeks	100 90 20	Successful extubation Significant improvement Complete resolution	4
All	378			55–100		C

Major complications were seen in up to 3.7% of the patients. These consisted in recurrence of disease, need for tracheotomy, supraglottic stenosis, fibruous intralaryngeal webs, and one case of non-airway related perioperative death [148, 747].

9.1.4
Indications and Contraindications

The diagnosis of the laryngeal OSA is performed with the help of an endoscopic examination. In the case of tumors and complex malformations the therapy depends on the primary disease. Laryngomalacia is a disease of the perinatal phase, and is especially salient in the case of preterm infants. In minor cases, waiting is the therapy of choice. A close cooperation with the child's pediatrician is necessary.

In severe cases, an endoscopy needs to be employed in order to determine whether a shortening of the epiglottis, a removal of redundant supraglottal mucosa, an incision of the aryepiglottal fold, or a combination of the three procedures is indicated. In the case of a correct indication, in over 80% of the cases the children can be spared a tracheotomy or a decannulation becomes possible. We do not consider a minimum age restriction to be in effect for these procedures.

The alternative to a surgical procedure consists in a noninvasive respiration therapy [190].

9.2
Adult Laryngeal OSA

In contrast to children, laryngomalacia plays only a minor role in adults. The only exception to this is the so-called floppy epiglottis. The floppy epiglottis is a relatively rare anatomic finding in adults. Nevertheless, Catalfumo et al. [94] found this condition in 12 of 104 patients who failed a UPPP procedure. We relatively frequently observe a floppy epiglottis in older male patients [773]. One explanation for this may be the fact that apart from the pinna of the ear the epiglottis is the only organ of the head and neck consisting exclusively of elastic cartilage. Pellnitz [553] has shown a significant increase in the length, breadth, and weight of the epiglottis in males, while females show reductions for the same parameters. Histological study of 500 epiglottal specimens obtained at autopsy shows that size increases in the male epiglottis is due to secondary intercellular deposits of byproducts of the metabolism. There were sex-specific differences in the perichondrium. Pellnitz postulated specific hormonal influences in connection with these findings, since the growth of the larynx is considered a secondary sexual characteristic. Nevertheless, a floppy epiglottis has also been described in younger men and, rarely, in women [22, 820].

In contrast to pediatric laryngeal OSA, the removal of redundant supraglottic mucosa is not a treatment option for adults. The condition also rarely occurs in adults, probably as a result of repeated exposure to subatmospheric pressure [585]. Nasal continuous positive airway pressure (CPAP) ventilation is the treatment of choice in these cases.

Tumors as cause of a laryngeal OSA are much more frequently a possibility in the case of adults than in children. Specifically, the following tumor entities have been reported as inducing OSA: supraglottic cyst [104], squamous cell carcinomas of the oral vestibule [820], the epiglottis [237], the glottis [624, 784], the whole larynx [703], and superior laryngeal nerve schwannoma [796]. Additionally, laryngeal OSA has been observed after irradiation therapy [109, 276] and after partial and reconstructive laryngectomy for glottic carcinoma [318, 624].

Acquired laryngomalcia has furthermore been described as a consequence of laryngeal trauma [820], sarcoidosis [228, 660], Hunter's syndrome [525], acromegalia [23], and mast cell pharyngitis [86]. More recent publications describe a correlation between apnea severity and laryngeal inflammation due to extraesophageal reflux [329, 550]. However, causality has not yet been proven.

A far larger group is made up of neurological diseases. Especially the Shy-Drager syndrome [232, 346], and vocal cord paralysis (due to other reasons) [23, 287, 816] are to be considered. An OSA can also occur after closure of a tracheostoma, even if no OSA existed prior to the tracheotomy. Especially in the elderly, laryngeal pathologies may facilitate the development of OSA after surgery. Therefore, postoperative reevaluation is recommended for all elderly patients with laryngeal abnormalities after operative closure of the tracheostomy [772].

9.2.1
Surgical Techniques

The surgical techniques are basically the same as those used in children. First, an exact diagnosis is necessary which ideally is obtained via endoscopy [30, 146]. In the case of tumors or more complex disorders the therapy is determined by the primary disease.

If a floppy epiglottis is manifest, the partial resection via a laser laryngoscope and the shortening of the glosso-epiglottic ligament are indicated [237, 773]. In contrast to the situation in children, difficulties may arise in the cutting of the cartilage. We therefore employ the CO_2 laser in continuous wave mode and set it at an input rate of 10–12 W. In individual cases the additional use of relevant microinstruments can be of advantage. Furthermore, the use of curved rotating microdissection monopolar scissors as used in laparoscopic surgery has been recommended [523]. We ourselves have not had any experience with these instruments. In both cases the major part of the free epiglottis is resected (Fig. 9.5).

9.2.2
Efficiency for SDB

Apart from one exception, the literature only offers case studies dealing with this topic. It is therefore not possible to determine the efficacy of the presented surgical procedures in

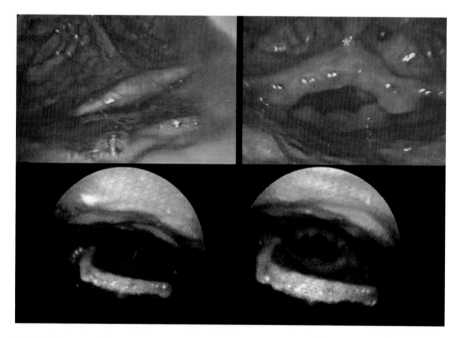

Fig. 9.5 Laser partial epiglottectomy. *Left*: preoperative situation with complete occlusion of the larynx. *Right*: situation after surgery with larynx wide open. *Asterisk*: shorted glosso-epiglottic ligament. *Bottom*: another postoperative example after partial epiglottectomy

relation to the OSA. Golz and colleagues [237] retrospectively reported on a series of 27 patients after partial laser resection of the epiglottis. Preoperatively the mean Apnea Hypopnea Index (AHI) was at 45 ± 14.6. Follow-up polysomnographies were performed at least 1 year after surgery. The AHI fell down to 14 ± 5.1. A statistically significant decrease was achieved in 21 patients (77.8%). Unfortunately, no raw data are presented. Therefore it is not possible to calculate the success rate using Sher's criteria.

In summary, the described surgery of the larynx appears to achieve successful results in a carefully selected patient pool. But for the evidence according to Cochrane criteria grade V must be assumed.

9.2.3
Postoperative Care and Complications

The patients undergo extubation immediately postoperatively. A follow-up respiratory treatment or tracheotomy is not necessary. We recommend the perioperative administration of 500 mg dexamethason intravenously. In contrast to children, an observation in an intensive care unit is not necessary if the option of either an extended (several hours) postoperative observation in the waking room or cardiopulmonary monitoring is available. In our center a perioperative antibiotics prophylaxis with 2 g cephazolin is performed. Since usually no major dysphagic problems arise, no special postoperative diet is necessary. The analgetic regimen depends on the individual case.

In contrast to children, as far as we know, postoperative supralaryngeal stenoses have not been described in the case of adults. From the few case studies no major complications can be inferred. From our own experience we can report mild dysphagia, which regularly occurs especially during the swallowing of fluids in the first week postoperatively; but parenteral nutrition did not become necessary in any of these cases.

9.2.4
Indications and Contraindications

Also for adults a precise endoscopical diagnosis is the precondition for a therapy. We always perform a fiberoptic endoscopy in flat position. In individual cases, an additional sleep endoscopy under sedation or, even better, during natural sleep, can be helpful [277, 278].

In the case of a floppy epiglottis a respiration therapy is frequently not possible due to the fact that the CPAP presses the epiglottis onto the larynx entrance, comparable to a lid on a pot [773]. In these cases, no alternative to surgery exists. From tumor surgery we know that in contrast to a partial resection of the tongue base a partial resection of the epiglottis frequently does not produce any significant dysphagia. Therefore, the partial resection of the epiglottis with the CO_2 laser is overall not very stressful for the patient; as a result we quite generously posit the indication for surgery. Yet it must be said that a floppy epiglottis is in our experience a rare occurrence. We perform a partial resection of the epiglottis only about twice per year. Of the annually more than 700 patients who undergo surgery in our center for sleep medical indication, these cases make up merely 0.3%.

In less severe cases, it is possible that already a hyoid suspension or a genioglossus advancement is sufficient in order to move or suspend the epiglottis far enough toward anterior so that a larynx occlusion no longer occurs. The decisive criterion here is not the size of the epiglottis but its stiffness. The laxer the epiglottis is the more one should consider a partial resection. But if the epiglottis is shifted toward dorsal due to an enlarged tongue base, then we are of the opinion that the hyoid suspension, if necessary in combination with a radiofrequency treatment (RFT) of the tongue base, should be preferred.

For all other disorders of the larynx the therapy depends on the primary disease. But for vocal cord palsies it should be noted here that they – even bilateral paralysis – can be very favorably treated with a respiration therapy [816, 844].

Take Home Pearls

> Laryngeal OSA is a special form of OSA, which every surgeon should be aware of. In case of doubt a sleep endoscopy will help to diagnose this condition.
> Main risk factor in children is immaturity in newborns. In these cases laser surgery can help to avoid tracheostomy.
> In adults a floppy epiglottis, mostly seen in the elder man, is the most common reason for laryngeal OSA. Again, laser surgery can help to resolve the problem.
> Apart from the mentioned conditions all other diseases of the larynx and hypopharynx may cause laryngeal obstruction. Treatment depends on the underlying disease.

Multilevel Surgery

10

Thomas Verse

Core Features

> Multilevel surgery addresses the level of the soft palate (SP) and the level of the hypoharynx concurrently within the same operation.
> Minimally invasive, multilevel surgery combines only minimally invasive techniques, such as palatal implants and interstitial radiofrequency treatments (RFT) of the SP, base of tongue, and tonsils.
> Minimally invasive multilevel surgery can be performed as outpatient procedure.
> Invasive multilevel surgery is needed to address moderate and severe obstructive sleep apnea (OSA). In patients with an AHI>30, it should only be performed as a second-line treatment after unsuccessful continuous positive airway pressure (CPAP) therapy.
> Invasive multilevel surgery requires an inpatient setting and special peri and postoperative care.
> In children, multilevel surgery can help to avoid tracheotomy. However, it needs to be reserved to comprehensive centers with sufficient clinical experience.

A multilevel procedure for the surgical therapy of obstructive sleep apnea (OSA) was presented for the first time in 1989 by Waite and colleagues [788]. The authors combined nasal surgery with an uvulopalatopharyngoplasty (UPPP), transoral tongue surgery, a genioglossus advancement (GA), and a maxillomandibular advancement osteotomy (MMA). Basically, the classification of the upper airway into different levels of obstruction stems from Fujita [226], who distinguished between retropalatal, retrolingual, and combined retropalatal and retrolingual obstruction. On the basis of this distinction, Riley et al. [609] defined the term and concept of multilevel surgery.

In the meantime, first studies have been published concerning virtually every possible combination of soft palate (SP) and tongue base (TB) procedures. For the sake of giving some structure to these data, we will distinguish in the following between minimally invasive concepts for mild OSA and more invasive concepts for moderate and severe OSA.

K. Hörmann and T. Verse, *Surgery for Sleep Disordered Breathing*
DOI: 10.1007/978-3-540-77786-1_10, © Springer Verlag Berlin Heidelberg 2010

Multilevel surgery is also performed on children with severe OSA on the basis of various primary illnesses in order to avoid an otherwise necessary tracheotomy. These concepts are discussed in a separate section.

10.1
Surgical Concepts

10.1.1
Effectiveness of Minimally Invasive Multilevel Surgery for Mild-to-Moderate OSA

Of the procedures employed, only the isolated interstitial radiofrequency treatments (RFT) and the SP implants can be regarded as minimally invasive techniques. Prerequisite for inclusion of the data into the following Table 10.1 is the application at least at the SP and TB, as well as the presentation of raw data for the calculation of the various parameters (Table 10.1).

A series of trials has been published regarding combined radiofrequency surgery at the TB and the SP. Steward et al. have treated a series of 29 patients with TB and SP radiofrequency surgery and have documented a statistically significant improvement in Apnea Hypopnea Index (AHI) and daytime somnolence [708]. The success rate was reported to be 59% (at least 50% reduction in AHI with postoperative values below 20). Comparable results have been published by Stuck et al. in 2004 where a statistically significant reduction in AHI and daytime somnolence was reported in a group of 20 patients [723]. Woodson et al. have published a remarkably designed trial comparing multilevel radiofrequency surgery at the TB and the SP with continuous positive airway pressure (CPAP) and placebo (sham-CPAP) [828]. Although the changes in the AHI in the radiofrequency group were not statistically significant compared to baseline and to placebo, subjective and functional

Table 10.1 Minimally invasive multilevel surgery for obstructive sleep apnea (OSA)

Author	N	Application sites	Follow-up (months)	AHI pre	AHI post	Success [%]	ESS pre	ESS post	EBM
Fischer et al. [201]	15	RFT SP + TB + Tons	4.8	32.6	22.0	20.0	11.1	8.2	4
Woodson et al. [828]	26	RFT SP + TB	1	21.3	16.8	No data	11.9	9.8	2b
Stuck et al. [723]	18	RFT SP + TB	2	25.3	16.7	38.9	9.3	6.1	4
Steward et al. [708]	22	RFT SP + TB	2.5	31.0	18.8	59.0	11.4	7.0	3b
Friedman et al. [214]	122	Pillars, RFT TB	12.2	23.2	14.5	47.5	9.7	6.9	4
All	177		1–12.2	24.7	16.0	45.7	10.2	7.3	B

AHI Apnea Hypopnea Index; *EBM* evidence based medicine; *RFT* interstitial radiofrequency treatment; *SP* soft palate; *TB* tongue base; tons, tonsils; pillars: soft palate implants outcome measures improved in statistical significance and there were no differences between the radiofrequency group and CPAP regarding these measure.

The data in the table are still very sparse. Yet we believe that it is possible to deduce two trends. On the one hand, the combined treatment of TB plus SP does not appear to significantly improve the results of an isolated TB treatment in respect to the AHI. In our clinical experience, the advantages of a combined treatment lie more in an additional effect upon the respiratory noises during sleep. We have recently been able to demonstrate [723] that the postoperative morbidity and complication rate after combined treatment and after isolated TB treatment are identical. Moreover, since the TB probes can also be used without difficulty at the SP, no significant further costs are created by an expansion of the therapy to the SP. Since snoring is frequently more of a burden to the patients than the health impediment caused by the often mild OSA, we almost exclusively perform combined treatments, even if the obstruction is assumed to be located solely at the TB.

Yet the relatively low success rate of the study by Fischer et al. [201] (RFT at the SP, TB and tonsils) is difficult to adequately interpret, since for other surgical procedures an unambiguously positive effect of tonsil reduction on the severity of the OSA has been demonstrated. The authors themselves use somewhat different success criteria and describe a success rate of 33%. According to our experience (Sect. 6.1.2) and that of other authors [495] RFT at the lymphatic tonsil tissue produces a pronounced volume effect; therefore we would have assumed a stronger effect on the AHI. Further studies will be needed to clarify this issue.

We see a second trend in the limitation of RFT to cases of mild OSA with an AHI of maximally 20. This trend is corroborated by the results of the currently single existing placebo-controlled study on this topic. Woodson et al. [828] treated 30 patients respectively either with CPAP, with combined RFT at SP and TB, and with a sham operation. Unfortunately, the authors did not provide any raw data; therefore, this study could not be included in Table 10.1. As expected, CPAP respiration was found to be superior to RFT, and RFT in turn superior to the sham operation. Yet in regards to the subjective results, which were measured with various validated test instruments for the assessment of life quality, no differences were found in the comparison of CPAP with RFT surgery. This means multilevel minimally invasive surgery is a valid option for selected patients with mild OSA with the understanding that they may require secondary treatment [214].

10.1.2
Effectiveness of Multilevel Surgery for Moderate-to-Severe OSA

On the level of the SP, invasive therapy concepts include either a UPPP or an uvulopalatal flap. For the treatment of the hypopharyngeal obstruction different procedures have been recommended. Table 10.2 summarizes the existent data. In the case of a relevant clinical diagnosis, several authors additionally perform nasal surgery. Recently, we were able to demonstrate that additional nasal surgery does not have a positive effect on the severity of the OSA [766, 767]. This result is in line with the information we gathered in Chap. 4 in regards to isolated nasal surgery in the case of OSA.

Altogether, data of 1,600 patients (EBM 4 to 2b) exist so far. For the present study situation, this results in grade B evidence according to the Oxford Center for Evidence-based Medicine Levels of Evidence [535]. The success rate according to Sher et al. [665] lies at almost 54%. All studies dealt with on average moderate or severe forms of OSA. We are of the opinion that a sufficient amount of data exist to validate the efficacy of multilevel surgery in the case of moderate and severe OSA.

Difficulties arise in attempting to evaluate the divergent concepts against each other. For the area of the SP, all study groups either perform the conventional UPPP or more rarely the uvulaflap, always including tonsillectomy. The extended uvulopalatal flap (EUPF) is a modification described in Sect. 6.3. We consider these techniques to be comparable. Therefore, the concepts differ from one another in respect to the therapy of the hypopharyngeal constriction of the upper airway. Two study groups [156, 167] recommend in somewhat dated publications a partial resection of the tongue. With 32 and 44% respectively the success rates lie below average. A more recent study [298] does not provide data for surgical success. Furthermore, as shown in Sect. 7.3, partial TB resection is a procedure with a relatively high postoperative morbidity and complication rate. We therefore regard this procedure to be historical.

A much less invasive approach is to limit tongue surgery to the lingual tonsil [401]. Laser lingual tonsillectomy (LLT) does not require temporary tracheostomy. Postoperative pain can be handled with painkillers. We, ourselves have encouraging experiences with this kind of surgery. Li and colleagues combined LLT with UPPP plus tonsillectomy in severe sleep apneics. The results are about 10% below the average in Table 10.2. Further data need to document the efficiency of this approach.

Seven working groups [35, 180, 212, 494, 712, 763, 767] solely employ the minimally invasive RFT at the TB. Baseline AHI varies from 22.9 [180] to 43.9 [212], with most studies including moderate sleep apneics. The success rates were given from 40 [767] to 52% [712]. Undoubtedly, of all the TB procedures presented here the RFT has the lowest postoperative morbidity and complication rate. But we infer from the data a tendency indicating that solely a RFT at the TB, combined with the UPPP, may not in itself be sufficient for properly treating a severe OSA with surgical means.

Four working group used the tongue base suspension (TBS) [468, 524, 697, 781]. Severity of OSA was in between an AHI of 38.7–52.8. Surgical success rates vary extensively between 20 and 81.8%, a fact that makes it very difficult to evaluate the efficiency of TBS properly. Furthermore, the Repose System used by all authors, has substantial disadvantages (see Sect. 7.4). This is why we ourselves do not use the system any longer.

The majority of studies employ for the therapy of the hypopharyngeal constriction either the mandibular osteotomy with GA or the hyoid suspension (HS) or both. Currently, the data do not provide information as to which combination is superior. It presumably depends more on the surgeon with which technique he or she achieves the best results.

Initially, we followed the Stanford [609] concept. Yet after the mandibular osteotomy with GA several complications occurred in our patient pool, such as infections of the oral floor with abscess formation and loosenings of the osteosynthesis; therefore, we have searched for alternatives with fewer complications. We believe to have found the solution in a combination of RFT and HS [766]. In the context of this concept, tonsillectomy and HS have shown themselves to be the most effective elements of our multilevel concept.

Table 10.2 Multilevel surgery for OSA

Author	N	Soft palate	Hypopharynx	Follow-up (months)	AHI pre	AHI post	Success [%]	ESS pre	ESS post	EBM
Riley et al. [605]	55	UPPP	GA, HS	3.0	58	23.2	67.3	No data	No data	4
Djupesland et al. [156]	19	UPPP	GP	8.7	54.0	31.0	31.6	No data	No data	4
Riley et al. [609]	223	UPPP	GA, HS	9.0	48.3	9.5	60.1	No data	No data	4
Johnson and Chinn [334]	9	UPPP	GA	39.0	58.7	14.5	77.8	No data	No data	4
Ramirez and Loube [587]	12	UPPP	GA, HS	6.0	49.0	23.0	41.7	No data	No data	4
Powell et al. [573]	67	Flap/UPPP	GA, HS	3.0	30.5	No data	No data	No data	No data	3b
Elasfour et al. [167]	18	UPPP	MLP	3–21	65.0	29.2	44.4	No data	No data	3b
Lee et al. [390]	35	UPPP	GA	4–6	55.2	21.7	66.7	No data	No data	4
Bettega et al. [51]	44	UPPP	GA, HS	6.0	45.2	42.8	22.7	No data	No data	4
Hsu and Brett [299]	13	UPPP	GA, HS	12.6	52.8	15.6	76.9	18.2	6.4	4
Hendler et al. [275]	33	UPPP	GA	6.0	60.2	28.8	45.5	No data	No data	4
Nelson [494]	10	UPPP	RFT	2.0	29.5	18.8	50.0	12.7	6.5	3b
Vilaseca et al. [782]	20	UPPP	GA, HS	6.0	60.5	44.6	35.0	12.0	7.9	4
Miller et al. [468]	15	UPPP	TBS	3.8	38.7	21.0	20.0	No data	No data	4
Neruntarat [498]	31	Flap	GA, HS	8.0	48.2	14.5	71.0	14.9	8.2	4
Neruntarat [500]	32	Flap	HS	8.1	44.5	15.2	78.0	14.1	8.2	4
Neruntarat [499]	46	Flap	GA, HS	39.4	47.9	18.6	65.2	No data	No data	4
Friedman et al. [212]	143	UPPP	RFT	No data	43.9	28.1	41.0	15.2	8.3	3b
Sorrenti et al. [697]	15	UPPP	TBS	4.0	44.5	24.2	40.0	11.2	6.6	4
Thomas et al. [742]	9	UPPP	TBS	4.0	46.0	No data	55.6	12.1	4.1	2b
	8	UPPP	GA	4.0	37.4	No data	50.0	13.3	5.4	2b
Sorrenti et al. [698]	8	UPPP	TBR	3.0	55.1	9.7	87.5	14.3	5.3	4
Miller et al. [467]	24	UPPP	GA	4.7	52.9	15.9	66.7	No data	No data	4
Dattilo and Drooger [136]	37	UPPP	GA, HS	1.5	38.7	16.2	70.3	10.0	7.5	4

(continued)

Table 10.2 (continued)

Author	N	Soft palate	Hypopharynx	Follow-up (months)	AHI pre	AHI post	Success [%]	ESS pre	ESS post	EBM
Hörmann et al. [295]	66	UPPP/Flap	RFT, HS		38.9	19.3	57.6	9.6	6.4	4
Li et al. [401]	6	EUPF	MLG	6.0	50.7	14.3	83.3	No data	No data	4
	6	EUPF	LLT	6.0	56.2	62.8	0.0	No data	No data	4
Verse et al. [766]	45	Flap	RFT, HS	4.7	38.3	20.6	51.1	10.4	7.1	4
Omur et al. [524]	22	UPPP	TBS	6.0	47.5	17.3	81.8	13.9	5.4	4
Hsieh et al. [298]	6	EUPF	MLG	6.0	50.7	11.6	No data	No data	No data	4
Bowden et al. [65]	29	UPPP	HS	12.0	36.5	37.6	17.2	13.8	10.9	4
Liu et al. [420]	44	UPPP	GA	3.0	62.0	29.6	52.3	14.3	6.3	4
Baisch et al. [35]	67	Flap	RFT, HS	1.0	38.3	18.9	59.7	9.7	6.6	3b
	16	Flap	RFT	1.0	28.6	21.7	No data	9.7	4.9	3b
Verse et al. [767]	45	Flap	RFT, HS	4.3	38.9	20.7	51.1	9.4	7.2	3b
	15	Flap	RFT	5.9	27.8	22.9	40.0	9.1	4.1	3b
Jacobowitz [320]	37	UPPP	RFT, HS, GA	3.0	46.5	14.9	70.3	12.1	6.7	4
Vicente et al. [781]	55	UPPP	TBS	36.0	52.8	14.1	78.0	12.2	8.2	4
Teitelbaum et al. [736]	47	UPPP	GA, HS	6.0	No data	No data	21.2	No data	No data	4
Stripf et al. [712]	25	UPPP	RFT	No data	39.2	16.5	52.0	No data	No data	4
Yin et al. [840]	18	UPPP	GA, HS	6.0	63.8	21.4	67.0	No data	No data	4
Richard et al. [600]	22	UPPP	RFT, HS, GA	No data	48.7	28.8	45.5	8.6	3.6	4
van den Broek et al. [763]	37	UPPP	RFT	No data	No data	No data	48.6	No data	No data	3b
Eun et al. [180]	66	UPPP	RFT	6	22.9	13.9	No data	11.4	7.5	4
All	1,600			1–39.4	44.56	20.54	54.18	12.19	7.18	B

AHI Apnea Hypopnea Index; *EBM* grade of evidence based medicine; *UPPP* uvulopalatopharyngoplasty; *flap*: uvulopalatal flap; *EUPF* extended uvulopalatal flap; *GA* mandibular osteotomy with genioglossus advancement; *HS* hyoid suspension; *GP* glossopexia; *MLP* midline laser partial glossectomy; *RFT* interstitial radiofrequency treatment of the tongue base; *TBS* tongue base suspension; *LLT* laser lingual tonsillectomy

With the exception of the studies by Johnson and Chinn [334], Neruntarat [499] and Vicente et al. [781], who present long-term data over a postoperative span of 3 years, Table 10.1 only includes short-term data. Therefore, a long-term evaluation of on average 51 months coming out of Stanford [610] of 40 patients with primary surgical success has received special attention. After more than 4 years 90% (36/40) still enjoyed treatment success. Four patients had again developed an OSA. In this group, the AHI was preoperatively 83.3, 6 months postoperatively 10.5, and after 4 years 43. But it should be mentioned that in the meantime these patients had experienced a significant weight increase (body mass index (BMI) preoperative, 28.7 kg/m²; short-term follow-up 28.0 kg/m²; long-term 30.6 kg/m²).

Similar results have recently been also described by Shibata et al. [667]. Additionally to the improvement of the AHI, these authors were able to demonstrate a postoperative normalization of the arterial hypertension for 31 patients.

Additionally, Friedman and coworkers [219] were able to show a positive effect on CPAP therapy in patients who had persistent symptoms of OSA after multilevel surgery. Compliance with CPAP therapy significantly increased from a mean of 0.02 ± 0.14 h per night prior to surgery to a 3.2 ± 2.6 h per night following surgery. The effective CPAP pressure decreased from 10.6 ± 2.1 cm H_2O before multilevel surgery to 9.8 ± 2.1 cm H_2O postoperatively.

Obviously, the best success rates are found for staged concepts, which provide as a second, additional surgical stage a bimaxillary advancement in the case of the nonresponders. This dividing up into two phases also goes back to the Stanford study group [609] and has gained acceptance in many places. The available data are presented in Table 10.3.

As already presented in Sect. 8.2, the MMA is also in the context of multilevel surgery an eminently successful treatment in regards to the severity level of the OSA. This is apparently also the case for morbidly obese patients. In a series of 23 obese sleep apneics with a mean BMI of 45 kg/m² the Stanford 2 phase concept achieved a success rate of 82.6%. In this series, the mean AHI fell from preoperatively 83 to 10.6, 6 months postoperatively. But it needs to be mentioned that the patients had also slightly reduced their weight. The average BMI was postoperatively 43 kg/m². The authors conclude from their data that counseling in regards to weight reduction and avoidance of weight gain will improve treatment outcomes.

Table 10.3 Staged concepts of multilevel surgery for OSA

Author	N stage 1	Nonresponse stage 1	N stage 2 (MMA)	Response stage 2 (MMA)	AHI pre stage 1	AHI post stage 2	EBM
Riley et al. [609]	223	89 (40%)	24	23 (97%)	75.1	8.4	4
Lee et al. [390]	33	11 (33.3%)	3	3 (100%)	74.0	5.0	4
Bettega et al. [51]	44	34 (77.3%)	20	15 (75%)	59.3	11.1	4
Li et al. [409]	No data	No data	19	18 (94.7)	63.6	8.1	4
Hendler et al. [275]	33	18 (54.5%)	7	4 (57.1%)	90.1	16.5	4
All	333	152 (45.6%)	73	63 (86.3%)	69.2	9.7	C

MMA bimaxillary advancement; *AHI* Apnea Hypopnea Index; *EBM* evidence-based medicine

It is striking that only a relatively small number of patients have actually chosen an MMA, as can be seen in two series [390, 609]: in both of the studies only 27% of the candidates chose the option MMA. The reason for this remained unanswered in the studies. Apparently, the indications for and staging of MMA, with respect to the many procedures available, are unsettled and often limited to severe OSA, dentocraniofacial deformities, and when other surgeries have failed. Due to the potential risks involved, MMA is not a surgical option for the majority of sleep apneics. For more details please refer to Sect. 8.2.

10.2
Postoperative Care and Complications

Multilevel surgery for OSA is an inpatient treatment. With the exception of isolated RFT it should not be performed on an outpatient basis. As a rule, the duration of the hospitalization is 3–7 days. Due to the fact that the patients are for the most part severe sleep apneics, already special perioperative measures are necessary; these are described in Chap. 13.

In general, the perioperative risk during and after multilevel surgery is increased as compared to isolated palatal surgery [357]. However, even in the case of severe sleep apneics postoperative observation in an intensive care unit is not required if an observation option exists for the first postoperative hours in the recovery room [541]. If events here are without complications, the patient can be brought into a normal care unit. If the patient has already preoperatively received a CPAP respiration device, he or she should be encouraged to continue using it postoperatively for several days, until the postoperative inflammations have reliably subsided. If the patient does not possess a CPAP device, we apply one. A pressure of 10 cm H_2O is usually sufficient.

For 5 days, we perform in our patients a postoperative antibiotics prophylaxis. Intraoperatively we administer once 1.5 g Cefuroxim, and postoperatively we administer 2 × 500 mg Cefuroxim per orally for 5 days. In principle, the use of more cost-efficient broadband antibiotics is of course also possible. We do not consider a routine administration of corticosteroids for necessary.

The most painful part of the multilevel surgery comprises the SP procedures and the tonsillectomy. In order to keep the pain postoperatively as low as possible, it is important to take care that intraoperatively the sutures at the SP are knotted tightly, but that the soft tissue is not squeezed. A loose adaptation of the wound edges should be attempted, since postoperatively in some cases a significant edema is to be expected. Even after adequate surgery the period of pain requiring analgesics lasts in our experience an average of 12 days. But since the pain varies strongly interindividually, an individualized pain treatment plan with relevant controls is needed. Routinely we give Diclofenac 3 × 50 mg/ day as effervescent tablet in combination with Metamizol 4 × 250 mg as drops. Tablets are difficult to swallow within the first postoperative days. Persistent pain despite adequate analgesics may indicate the beginning of a wound infection. In these cases an antibiosis, e.g., with Amoxicillin, can quickly alleviate the condition.

Apart from pain, the possibility of serious dysphagia must be taken into account. In the first 3 days, some patients need to receive parenteral nutrition. In some cases a one-time administration of corticosteroids (e.g., 250–500 mg Methylprednisolon) is sufficient. In virtually all cases, oral nutrition can be resumed after 3 days, even without the administration of cortisone. After tonsillectomy we prescribe the usual diet.

The complications after multilevel surgery consist on the one hand in the sum of the complications of the individual procedures. These have already been discussed in the relevant chapters. On the other hand, it is of course conceivable that the effects of several simultaneous surgical treatments at the upper aerodigestive tract are amplified. In this context Altman and colleagues [10] were able to demonstrate abnormal objective swallowing in 9 of 15 patients 18 months after multilevel surgery for OSA. Six of fifteen demonstrated normal objective swallowing. Of these, five reported subjective change. This study is in accordance with the results stemming from our multilevel therapy protocol. Almost all of our patients initially suffer from dysphagia, which in some cases persists for up to 3 weeks. Up to now, in the context of our concept we have not observed a continued dysphagia with impediment of food intake lasting over several months.

10.3
Indications and Contraindications

Minimally invasive multilevel surgery in the form of an isolated radiofrequency therapy is not yet scientifically sufficiently validated. Yet in analogy to the results concerning the isolated use at the SP and at the TB we are of the opinion that we can posit a legitimate indication both for primary snoring as well as for mild forms of OSA. Patients need to be informed that they might need secondary treatment. It remains to be seen how far the additional treatment of the tonsils, as suggested by Fischer et al. [201], will broaden the indication. Yet currently we assume that above an AHI of 20 more invasive techniques achieve better success rates.

For moderate and severe OSA a variety of combinations has been described. At the SP, UPPP with tonsillectomy is the preferred procedure. For no other surgical procedure does a comparable amount of data exist. Some study groups, including ours, like using the uvulopalatal flap (Sect. 6.3). Since the techniques are somewhat similar, it is ultimately up to the surgeon with which technique he or she feels most comfortable.

In our opinion, partial resections of the tongue muscles are obsolete as routine procedures. They often require a temporary tracheotomy, and should be restricted to special cases. Isolated resections of the lingual tonsil seem to be a much less invasive surgery. So far, the preliminary data do not allow a concluding evaluation.

The surgical kits for tongue suspension are currently under development. The Repose System has a lot of disadvantages; that is why we ourselves do not use it any longer.

This leaves mandibular osteotomy with GA, HS and RFT for the therapy of a hypopharyngeal constriction. As described above, we feel justified to infer from the data in Table 10.2 that an isolated RFT at the TB in combination with the UPPP + TE is not sufficient for the treatment of severe OSA. This combination might be appropriate for moderate OSA, as it prevents the patient from a certain amount of postoperative morbidity. For severe OSA, the SP procedure should be combined with a HS and/or a GA. Which combination is ultimately the most successful, can as yet not be inferred from the available data. The largest Stanford series [609] uses both techniques in combination. This protocol with a success rate of 60% after Sher is currently regarded as the standard procedure.

In our daily practice, we have replaced the GA with a radiofrequency therapy, and we perform a UPPP with tonsillecztomy, an HS and a radiofrequency therapy of the TB. In patients after prior tonsillectomy, we perform an uvulopalatal flap instead of UPPP, as in this condition the dissection within the scar to divide the two tonsillar pillars as needed for an UPPP is troublesome and time consuming. With the help of this newly devised protocol we have been able to significantly reduce the postoperative morbidity and complication rate. With the Mannheimer multilevel surgery concept we achieve a success rate of 51.1–59.7% after Sher [35, 767]; this result situates us at the average level of the cited studies. We believe that with this less morbidizing surgical concept we are acting in the interest of our patients, even if combinations with mandibular osteotomy and GA may furnish somewhat higher success rates.

In the case of those patients who even after a multilevel surgery continue to suffer from an OSA in need of respiratory treatment, yet continue to not tolerate the respiration therapy, it should be tested whether an MMA is an option. Otherwise these patients have to retry CPAP.

Finally, multilevel airway reconstruction seems to be an effective treatment for moderate and severe OSA – even in the morbidly obese patient [408]. Careful patient selection and identifying potential coexisting obesity-hypoventilation syndrome, as well as counseling on weight reduction and avoiding continual weight gain will improve treatment outcomes.

10.3.1
Multilevel Surgery in Children

The study group around Cohen and Burstein reports good success for surgical multilevel treatment in the case of children with neurological disorders [114] and children with other disorders such as Down`s syndrome, hemifacial microsomia, Pierre Robin sequence, and various craniofacial disorders [115]. In these series, the authors were able to spare respectively 83 and 90% of the children who had undergone surgery a previously recommended tracheotomy. Tonsillectomy, adenoidectomy, turbinectomy and/or septoplasty, tongue hyoid advancement, UPPP, conventional mandibular advancement, distraction osteogenesis of the mandible, and tongue reduction were combined with each other. But the authors do not mandate a rigid therapy concept. Rather, the specific combination of single operations is determined by the individual clinical diagnosis, which is classified into four levels (Fig. 10.1) [83].

In any case, multilevel surgery in children is a multidisciplinary task requiring excellent interdisciplinary cooperation. In our opinion pediatric multilevel surgery should be reserved to few specialized centers.

Fig. 10.1 Functional and anatomic airway zones in infants and children according to Burstein et al. [83]. (1) nares to velum; (2) lips to hypopharynx; (3) epiglottis to trachea; (4) subglottis to bronchii

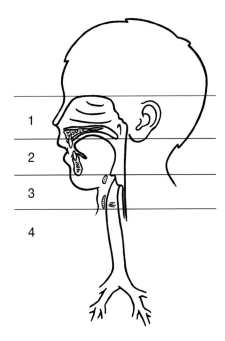

Take Home Pearls

> Minimally invasive multilevel surgery is a treatment for snoring and mild OSA. Patients should be informed that they might require secondary treatment.
> Invasive multilevel surgery requires an inpatient setting with special perioperative care.
> In the case of severe OSA patients should undergo CPAP treatment first. Surgery is limited to those severe sleep apneics that cannot tolerate CPAP.
> In adults with an AHI≤30 invasive multilevel surgery can be offered as a first-line treatment.
> In children multilevel surgery is a multidisciplinary task requiring excellent interdisciplinary cooperation. It should be reserved to specially qualified centers.

Tracheotomy

11

Thomas Verse and Wolfgang Pirsig

Core Features

> Before the introduction of CPAP-ventilation and uvulopalatopharyngoplasty (UPPP) in 1981, tracheotomy was the only effective treatment for severe obstructive sleep apnea (OSA). Even today, it remains one of the most effective treatment modalities for severe OSA.
> Due to its potential complications and its negative effect on the general quality of life, tracheotomy is rarely used today, particularly as there are various other treatment modalities with less impairment of well-being.
> However, there still are indications for tracheotomies in sleep medicine. Temporary tracheotomies are used to protect the upper airway perioperatively after invasive surgeries. Permanent tracheotomies are performed in cases with severe craniofacial malformations, excessive overweight, and in the case of patients that cannot be intubated.

Tracheotomy was the first effective treatment for patients with severe OSA [376, 635, 678], and even today it remains the method of last resort. In children, a tracheotomy is much more often indicated as some malformations can only be corrected at a later point in a child's anatomical development, which makes it necessary to wait for the best point in time to perform surgery.

11.1
Surgical Technique

Tracheotomy is a standard technique performed by every general, ENT, or maxillofacial surgeon. We always perform a complete mucocutaneously anastomized tracheostomy to avoid granulation and difficulties when changing the tubes. However, patients who require a tracheotomy for OSA often are morbidly overweight. Standard-sized tracheostomy

K. Hörmann, T. Verse, *Surgery for Sleep Disordered Breathing*,
DOI: 10.1007/978-3-540-77786-1_11, © Springer Verlag Berlin Heidelberg 2010

tubes often are too short because of increased submental or anterior cervical girth. The surgeon has two options to overcome the problem: modify the tracheostomy tube or recontour the neck to accommodate a standard tube. As the patients are supposed to be able to handle the tracheostomy tube on their own, we prefer the latter approach. Gross et al. [244] described their surgical technique and retrospectively estimated their complication rate after 23 months as 43%, including wound infections, neck abscess, and hemorrhage.

Today an increasing number of percutaneous dilating tracheotomies are performed especially in intensive care units. It is a promising tool for patients who require their tracheotomies for short-term periods. In the treatment of OSA, there are two groups of patients requiring tracheotomies. For the first group, tracheotomies are performed to protect the upper airway during the immediate postoperative period after invasive procedures within the upper airway. Most surgeons perform conventional surgical tracheostomies in these patients as they are already in the operation theater. This is what we also recommend and do. The other group of patients needs their tracheostomies for long-term periods. This points to a clear advantage for the conventional surgical approach.

11.2
Effectiveness for OSA

Partinen et al. [546] studied the survival rates of 198 patients with OSA, of whom 71 were treated with tracheotomy, while the rest were managed conservatively with weight reduction. Over a follow-up period of 5 years, there were 14 deaths, all of them in the group undergoing conservative therapy.

Ledereich et al. [389] compared 30 patients with permanent tracheostomies with 71 patients who had received other therapies (temporary tracheotomy, UPPP, tonsillectomy, nasal operations, or conservative treatment with medications stimulating respiration). Patients were observed for 5 years. Excessive daytime sleepiness was reported by only 24% of those in the tracheostomy group but by 59% of those who had undergone other treatments. Apnea phases were recorded in 3% of the tracheotomized patients and in 35% of the other patients. Snoring was reported by 13% of patients with tracheostomy but by 58% of the comparison group.

Data providing polysomnographic figures is summarized in Table 11.1. Although there are no randomized, controlled studies, tracheotomy can be regarded as a very effective treatment modality for OSA.

In a study by Kim et al. [360] all patients that were classified as nonresponders after tracheotomy showed evidence of cardiopulmonary decompensation as defined by an initial $PaCO_2$ greater than 45 mmHg already prior to surgery.

Cohen et al. compared 13 pediatric tracheostomy patients with 50 children who had undergone other kinds of sleep apnea surgery. Clinical success was achieved in 100% after tracheostomy and in 59% of the sleep apnea surgery group [116]. However, the tracheotomized children showed impaired quality of life for 95% of the items investigated.

Table 11.1   Effect of tracheotomy on the severity of obstructive sleep apnea

Author	N	Follow-up (months)	Age (years)	AHI pre	AHI post	Success rate (%)	Def. of success	EBM grade
Guilleminault et al. [252]	50	9–72 (mean 32)	12–66	No data	No data	100	AI < 5	4
Haapaniemi et al. [256]	7	30–108	41–64	56.3% (O_2 min)	82.9% (O_2 min)	100	No data	4
Kim et al. [360]	23	No data	22–77	58.2 (37.2)	19.8 (26.0)	73.9	AHI < 20	3b
Thatcher and Maisel [742]	79	3–240	25–70	81	No data	100	No data	4
All	159	3–240	22–77			96.2		C

AHI Apnea Hypopnea Index; *Def.* definition; *EBM* Evidence-based medicine.

Thatcher and Maisel [742] observed a decannulation in 16 out of 79 patients 2 months to 13 years after tracheostomy for OSA: 5 patients chose CPAP-ventilation, 3 grew intolerant of their tracheotomies, 3 underwent successful UPPP, and 2 experienced significant weight loss.

11.3
Postoperative Care and Complications

Guilleminault et al. [252] followed 50 tracheotomized OSA patients over a period of on average 32 months (range: 9 months to 6 years). Following tracheotomy, all patients exhibited an Apnea Index below 5, but all experienced persistent central respiratory events during the first postoperative year. Kim et al. [360] report that in patients with cardiopulmonary decompensation, tracheotomy led to improvement but not elimination of OSA in seven of 13 patients studied. One reason cited was the increased incidence of central respiratory events, while another related to the occlusion of the tracheostomy by chin and neck adipose tissue. A similar case with occurrence of severe central sleep apnea 4 years after initially successful tracheostomy for OSA was reported by Fletcher [203].

Conway et al. [124] followed 11 patients over 90 months and reported three categories of complications: granulation, stenoses, and psychosocial problems. Fewer complications were seen with the cervical skin flap technique; therefore, the authors favor this technique. Thatcher and Maisel [742] recorded 14 deaths within a 20-year period after tracheotomy in 79 patients. Average age at time of death was 62 years. Five deaths were cardiopulmonary, four were from cancer, two were from postoperative complications of unrelated surgeries, and one from aspiration. Tracheostomy-related mortality included one postoperative mycardial infarction and one tracheal-innominate fistula.

OSA may also recur following closure of a tracheostoma [772]. This occurs not only in patients who have undergone tracheotomy for the treatment of OSA but also in those who have been tracheotomized for completely unrelated reasons. Primarily responsible are laryngeal changes in advancing age, which promote the development of OSA following closure of a tracheostoma. Elderly adults with pathologic changes in the larynx should be followed postoperatively in order to recognize the possible recurrence of OSA following closure of their tracheostomas. Five similar cases were reported by Kim et al. [360]. Likewise, polysomnography with occluded tracheostomy is recommended before surgical closure in children [750].

11.4
Indications and Contraindications

Basically, it is necessary to differentiate between a temporary and a permanent tracheotomy (Table 11.2). While we occasionally still employ the former in the context of other invasive procedures on the upper airway in order to secure the airway during the postoperative phase, we have not performed a permanent tracheotomy in adults for the past 3 years.

Different is the situation in the case of children. Especially for children with congenital malformations a permanent tracheotomy may become necessary [11] For example in the case of laryngomalacia after successful tracheotomy one can wait for the stabilization of the laryngeal skeleton and relevant growth [11, 657]. But also prematurity, cardiovascular malformations, neurological and congenital/chromosomal abnormalities predispose a higher risk to require tracheotomy. Some malformations can be corrected surgically. Quite a few of these cases initially require a tracheotomy to gain time to await the optimal occasion to perform the necessary surgery. The following inherent dysfunctions are known to predispose to OSA, sometimes requiring a tracheotomy in children: Shy-Drager syndrome [346], Crouzon syndrome [680], congenital laryngeal anomalies (laryngomalacia, subglottic stenosis, glottic web, vocal cord paralysis, laryngeal stenosis, subglottic hemangioma) [11], congenital tracheal abnormalities (tracheomalcia, anterior compression, tracheal stenosis, tracheooesophageal fistula) [11], cerebral palsy [437], CHARGE association [619], Chiari type I malformation [632], achondroplasia [236], Canavan disease [207], and Duchenne muscular dystrophy [434].

Table 11.2 Comparison of the possible indications for a temporary or permanent tracheotomy

Temporary tracheotomy	Permanent tracheotomy
For the postoperative securing of the airways after	As ultima ratio
Laryngeal surgery	Therapy failures with CPAP or BIPAP masks in the case of excessive obesity
Tongue base surgery	Surgically not curable pharyngeal obstruction
Oral surgery on upper and lower jaw	Patients that cannot receive intubation or for children with Congenital malformations, which cannot or only after puberty be surgically corrected

Although tracheotomy is still the gold standard of care for these patients with malformations, we always have to keep in mind that this procedure causes a great deal of postoperative morbidity for both patient and family [116]. A variety of newer treatment modalities, such as distraction osteogenesis of the mandible and mid-face, or multilevel surgery today offer sufficient alternatives in specific cases [115].

Take Home Pearls

> Tracheotomies still play a role
> In the temporary protection of airway after invasive surgeries in the head and neck.
> As permanent tracheotomies in adult patients with excessive overweight, that cannot tolerate CPAP treatment, patients that cannot be intubated and pediatric patients with severe craniofacial deformities.

Bariatric Surgery

12

Helge Kleinhans and Thomas Verse

Core Features

> Obesity, a widespread and increasing health problem within the US and Europe, is, among others, associated with OSA.
> Bariatric surgery encompasses a variety of surgeries. The most important ones are adjustable gastric banding, vertical banded gastroplasty, sleeve gastrectomy, intragastric balloons, jejunal bypass, biliopancreatic diversion, and Roux-en-Y gastric bypass.
> A significant reduction in BMI is associated with a comparable significant decrease in sleep apnea severity.
> Bariatric surgery is recommended for patients with a BMI > 35 kg/m^2 and an obesity related concomitant disease or for patients with a BMI > 40 kg/m^2.

Currently, 32.9% of US adults and 13% of US children hold a body mass index above 30 kg/m^2 and are obese by definition. In Europe, 15.7% of adults and 4% of children and adolescents are obese. In Germany, 22.9% of adults are obese, while the rate is 6.3% for children and adolescents.

Obesity is increasing worldwide. It is estimated that more than 300 million people are obese [269]. Morbid obesity is growing twice as fast as diabetes mellitus prevalence and will overtake it soon [206, 208, 269, 325, 379, 421–423, 557].

The rise in the prevalence of obesity is also associated with increases in comorbidities (for instance, type 2 diabetes, hypertension, obstructive sleep apnea (OSA), heart disease, stroke, asthma, weight bearing degenerative problems, several forms of cancer, depression, etc.), which are responsible for more than 2.5 million deaths per year worldwide [487, 534, 836].

In the case of extreme obesity (BMI $\geq$ 45 kg/m^2) in young adulthood, life expectancy is reduced by 13 years in men and 8 years in women.

The incidence of OSA has been underestimated in obese patients. A 10% increase in body weight in 4 years is associated with a sixfold higher risk of developing OSA [554]. There is an ongoing debate on whether the correlation between obesity and OSA occurs exclusively because of anatomic factors [652, 713].

K. Hörmann, T. Verse, *Surgery for Sleep Disordered Breathing*,
DOI: 10.1007/978-3-540-77786-1_12, © Springer Verlag Berlin Heidelberg 2010

Obese OSA patients show 42% more fat in their cervical region as compared with normal individuals [484], thereby causing pharyngeal lumen narrowing and resulting in increased risk of developing OSA [634].

A study has shown that bodyweight loss is related to increase of airway transversal diameter, which could result in Apnea Hypopnea Index (AHI) improvement [630].

Furthermore, obesity may also be involved in the genesis of OSA because of metabolic activity of adipose tissue [780].

12.1
Techniques

Bariatric surgical procedures reduce caloric ingestion by modifying the anatomy of the gastrointestinal tract. These operations can be divided into either restrictive, malabsorptive, or combined varieties.

The restriction is usually done by reduction of the gastric reservoir with a narrow outlet to delay emptying. For this purpose, the neo gastric volume is reduced to approximately 20–25 mL.

Examples of restrictive procedure are the adjustable gastric banding, vertical banded gastroplasty, endoluminal vertical gastroplasty, sleeve gastrectomy, or the intragastric balloon.

12.1.1
Adjustable Gastric Banding (Fig. 12.1)

This laparoscopic procedure divides the upper stomach into a small pouch and a large residual region by placing an adjustable band around the fundus. It consists of a soft silicon ring connected to a port system, placed in the epigastric subcutis. Worldwide, the adjustable band is used in 24% of the surgical procedures with a preponderance to European countries [80]. With an estimated rate of 0–0.5%, it has the lowest mortality rate of all bariatric procedures [517]. Long-term results of a 10-year observation period refer to a 13.2% reduction of the initial weight [682]. Short-term studies, however, suggest much higher reduction rates. Complications such as "band slippage," pouch complications, and decompression of the esophagus might lead to a reoperation rate up to 17% [804].

12.1.2
Vertical Banded Gastroplasty (Fig. 12.2)

In this restrictive procedure, the fundus region is divided by a vertical staple line. Additionally, the outlet is wrapped by a band. Long-term weight loss is higher compared to the Adjustable gastric banding [517]. Revision rates of 20–56% mostly affect staple line and band disruption, stomal stenosis, and pouch dilatation [38, 45, 764].

Fig. 12.1 Adjustable gastric banding. *P* pouch; *S* stomach

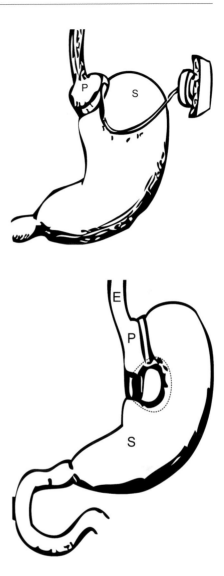

Fig. 12.2 Vertical banded gastroplasty. *E* esophagus; *P* pouch; *S* stomach

12.1.3
Sleeve Gastrectomy

The laparoscopic procedure was originally used as a first-line treatment for super obese patients. It consists of a partial gastrectomy in which the great curvature is stapled off the stomach. As a result of the restrictive technique, the stomach becomes a tube like formation. In addition, ghrelin producing cells of the gastric mucosa are reduced. Compared to adjustable gastric banding, the sleeve gastrectomy results in better hunger control and weight loss. Disadvantage is the irreversible loss of gastric tissue.

12.1.4
Intragastric Balloon

The intragastric balloon (IB) is a temporary device for weight loss in moderate obesity [443]. A balloon is placed endoscopically into the stomach and filled with 500 mL of saline solution. Extensive testing is going on; long-term results are still missing. Nausea, abdominal pain, and balloon migration are adverse effects.

Malabsorptive procedures reduce the caloric intake by shortening the transit time and mucosal surface of the intestine. In general, weight loss with malabsorptive procedures tends to be greater than weight loss with restrictive procedures [80]. Though weight loss is excellent, these procedures are associated with multiple complications such as malnutrition, vitamin, and electrolyte deficiencies, as well as liver failure [141, 241]. Therefore, patients undergoing malabsorptive surgery have to be monitored in a lifetime follow-up.

12.1.5
Jejunal Bypass (Fig. 12.4)

The operation was the first bariatric procedure performed in 1969. It is an end-to-side anastomosis of jejunum to terminal ileum, bypassing most of the small bowel, with the cause of massive malabsorption. Due to its high complication rate and need of revision, the role in up-to-date bariatric surgery is minor.

12.1.6
Biliopancreatic Diversion (Fig. 12.6)

There are two biliopancreatic diversion (BPD) surgeries: A BPD and a BPD with a duodenal switch (DS) (Fig. 12.3). The BPD consists of a partial gastrectomy and a gastroileostomy. A long segment of the small intestine receives food only; the short common channel receives food and biliopancreatic secretions. The use is limited due to high rates of protein loss, anemia, and stomal ulceration.

In a BPD with duodenal switch (BPD/DS), a smaller portion of the stomach is removed, the remaining stomach remains attached to the proximal duodenum and is connected in terms of an "alimentary limb" to a 150 cm small intestine segment. The remaining duodenum is connected to the lower part of the small intestine variable at length ("enzyme limb"). The common channel in which food and enzymes encounter measures 100 cm.

These procedures are reserved for patients with super morbid obesity (BMI > 50 kg/m^2).

12.1.7
Roux-en-Y Gastric Bypass (Fig. 12.5)

The Roux-en-Y gastric bypass (RYGB) is a typical practice of a combined malabsorptive and restrictive procedure and the most common bariatric operation performed in the US.

Fig. 12.3   Biliopancreatic diversion with
duodenal switch. *A* alimentary limb;
B biliopancreatic portion; *C* common
channel; *S* stomach

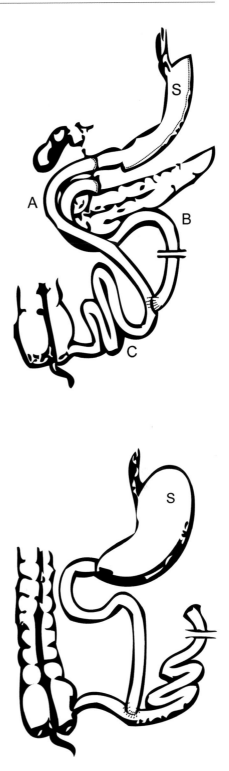

Fig. 12.4   Jejunal bypass. *S* stomach

Fig. 12.5 Roux-en-Y gastric bypass (RYGB).
A alimentary limb; *B* biliopancreatic portion;
C common channel; *P* pouch; *S*. Stomach

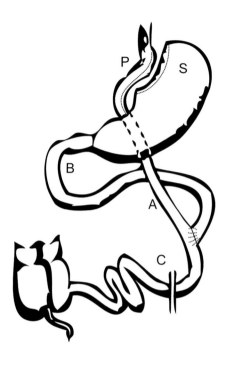

The stomach is narrowed by creating a small 25 mL pouch at the fundus region. The smaller stomach is connected directly to the 150 cm measuring "alimentary" jejunal portion of the small intestine, bypassing the rest of the stomach and the upper 50 cm "biliopancreatic" portion of the small intestine. Digestion and absorption occur in the common channel (100–150 cm of length) [73, 111].

Early weight loss is rapid, reaches a plateau usually after 2 years. Long-term reduction of 25% body weight is reported in a 10-year observation study [682].

By now, two-third of all bariatric procedures are performed laparoscopically [79]. These techniques provide many advantages compared to open surgery. A lower incidence of hernia, wound infection, and shorter hospital stay are some proven aspects [153, 428, 505, 811].

12.2
Effectiveness for OSA

A metaanalysis has documented the effects of bariatric surgery in 2,399 OSA patients submitted to surgery. For approximately 86% of the cases, OSA was improved or resolved [126]. Continuous positive air pressure (CPAP) treatment could be withdrawn in most patients. As seen in adult patients, pediatric studies generally report good OSA-related outcome after bariatric surgery [342].

Fig. 12.6 Biliopancreatic diversion.
A alimentary limb; *B* biliopancreatic portion;
C common channel; *S* stomach

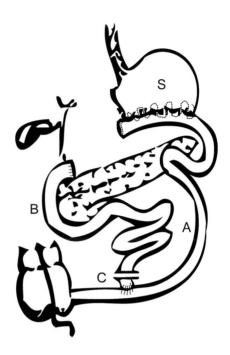

The mean BMI changes in OSA patients after bariatric surgeries seem to be similar to patients without sleep apnea [246].

On the other hand, it has to be mentioned that in the long run there are cases of recurrence of sleep apnea without concomitant weight increase, as described in 14 cases 7.5 years after successful weight reduction surgery [563].

The currently still limited polysomnographic data on the effect of bariatric surgery for OSA are listed in Table 12.1.

12.3
Indications and Contraindications

Unfortunately, diet therapy, with and without supportive organizations, is relatively ineffective in treating obesity at long sight [515, 516]. According to the National Institutes of Health guidelines for surgical treatment for obesity and obesity-associated comorbid conditions, patients with a BMI of 35 kg/m^2 or greater and an obesity-related comorbid condition (including OSA) or patients with a BMI of 40 kg/m^2 or more are recommended for surgical treatment [508].

The potential benefit of bariatric surgery for patients with mild obesity (BMI of 30–35 kg/m^2) remains unclear. Patients should have made previous attempts to lose weight, should be free of medical and psychological contraindications, and should be

Table 12.1 Effect of gastric surgery on the severity of obstructive sleep apnea

Author	N	Surgery	Follow-up (month)	BMI pre	BMI post	AHI pre	AHI post	p-Value	EBM
Peiser et al. [552]	15	GBP (AI)	2–8	48.3	33.1	82.0	15.3	No data	4
Charuzi et al. [102]	13	GBP	6	70.8	55.0	88.8	8.0	<0.05	4
Charuzi et al. [101]	46	GBP or VBG (AI)	6	47.5	32.1	58.8	7.8	<0.001	4
Summers et al. [729]	1	VBG	6	54.0	37.0	40.0	5.0	No data	Case report
Sugerman et al. [725]	40	GBP or VBG or HG	69.6	56.0	40.0	64.0	26.0	<0.001	4
Pillar et al. [563]	14	GBP	90	45.0	35.0	40.0	24.0	<0.05	4
Scheuller and Weider [647]	15	GBP or VBG	12–144	160 kg	105 kg	96.9	11.3	<0.0001	4
Rasheid et al. [591]	11	GBP	3–21	62.0	40.0	56.0	23.0	<0.05	4
Guardiano et al. [246]	8	GBP	28	49.0	34.0	55.0	14.0	<0.01	4
Valencia-Flores et al. [761]	28	GBP	13.7	56.5	39.2	53.7	8.6	<0.01	4
Busetto et al. [85]	17	IB	6	55.8	48.6	52.1	14.0	<0.01	4
Dixon et al. [154]	25	LAGB	17.7	52.7	37.2	61.6	13.4	<0.01	4
Fritscher et al. [223]	12	GBP	24.2	51.5	34.1	46.5	16.0	<0.05	4
Haines et al. [260]	101	GBP	11	56.0	38.0	51.0	15.0	<0.001	4
All	331		3–144	54.51	38.39	57.91	14.80		C

AHI Apnea Hypopnea Index; *VBG* vertical banded gastroplasty; *GBP* gastric bypass; *HG* horizontal gastroplasty; *LAGB* laparoscopic adjustable gastric banding; *IB* intragastric balloon

supervised by a multidisciplinary team with experience in bariatric surgery and perioperative care.

It has been shown that patients with a BMI above 50 kg/m^2 do not benefit from a restrictive bariatric procedure because after gastric banding they still stay for a period of 2 years within the range of morbid obesity [81, 476]. Upon the presentation of type 2 diabetes, combined malabsorptive and restrictive bariatric procedures outmatch simply restrictive techniques [682, 801].

Secondary causes of obesity should be considered, although they do not usually cause severe obesity. Routine screening for Cushing's syndrome and hypothyroidism is not necessary unless clinical suspicion is high. [709] An accurate medication history should be obtained; oral contraceptives, antidepressants and oral hypoglycemic pharmaceuticals are associated with weight gain [269].

A majority of patients presenting for bariatric procedures have one or more psychiatric disorders [337]. Other psychosocial factors that have been associated with a suboptimal surgical outcome include disturbed eating habits [492]. These facts point out the importance of an appropriate psychological evaluation of the candidates presenting for bariatric surgery.

Specific contraindications to bariatric surgery are few. They include mental or cognitive disorders that limit the patient's ability to understand the procedure. Severe coexisting medical conditions such as unstable coronary artery disease or liver cirrhosis may eliminate the possibility of surgery. Contraindications for sole restrictive procedures are eating disorders like "binge- or sweet-eaters," as well as an insufficient lower esophageal sphincter [726, 802].

12.4
Postoperative Care and Complications

Perioperative care of patients undergoing bariatric surgery requires specialized expertise and institutes. Studies have demonstrated that the chance of postoperative complications is significantly associated with surgical record [506, 806].

Unfortunately, many patients do not receive systematic perioperative care, and may have suboptimal outcomes [267, 598].

Sleep apnea patients usually have more airway-related problems in the postoperative period, as well as pulmonary complications such as severe hypoxemia, apnea, or atelectasis [597].

In a retrospective study in patients submitted to joint replacement, OSA patients have shown more adverse outcomes than matched control subjects, mostly within the first 72 h after the procedure. One-third of those patients with OSA developed substantial respiratory or cardiac complications, including arrhythmias, myocardial ischemia, unplanned intensive care unit transfers, and reintubation. The length of hospital stay was higher for sleep apnea patients compared with control subjects [255].

Those patients with severe OSA who undergo major surgery with a significant amount of anesthesia should be monitored closely for potential upper airway collapse. The use of opioids during anesthesia or postoperative analgesia may account for pharyngeal collapse [584].

Postoperative CPAP provides obstruction free ventilation, improves oxygenation, prevents the development of respiratory complications, and reduces hemodynamic fluctuations [594].

Operative mortality is 0.1% for purely restrictive procedures, 0.5% in patients undergoing gastric bypass procedures, and 1.1% in patients undergoing BPD or DS procedures [80]. Common causes of death among patients undergoing bariatric surgery include pulmonary embolism and anastomotic leaks. Factors that have been found to contribute to increased mortality include lack of experience on the part of the surgeon or the program, advanced patient age, male sex, and severe obesity (BMI $\geq$ 50) [195, 204, 506, 572].

Take Home Pearls

> The surgical treatment of obesity is superior toward conservative treatment in terms of long-lasting weight control and improvement of comorbidities.

> Bariatric surgery is an effective treatment for OSA in patients with clinically significant obesity.

> Regarding weight loss and reduction of comorbidities, gastric bypass is superior to gastric banding.

> Patient screening for bariatric surgery has to be done in an interdisciplinary team. Postoperative supervision usually lasts a lifetime.

> Patients with severe OSA who undergo major surgery with a significant amount of anesthesia should be monitored closely for potential upper airway collapse.

Anesthesiologic Airway Management

13

Harald V. Genzwuerker

Core Features

> Airway maintenance in patients with obstructive sleep apnea (OSA) can be challenging; therefore, profound preoperative evaluation and preparation are mandatory.

> Decisions for anesthesiologic airway management focus on awake fiberoptic intubation vs. induction of general anesthesia, and on the preservation of or the return to spontaneous ventilation.

> The strategies differ based on preoperative knowledge of intubation difficulties and airway abnormalities.

> The recovery phase after the end of the surgery calls for the same alertness as the initial management of airway difficulties.

> Close cooperation of surgeon and anesthesiologist in the pre, intra, and postoperative period will help reduce airway-related morbidity and mortality.

13.1
Implications in Patients with OSA

Obstructive sleep apnea (OSA) is, by definition, a problem of the upper airway. Its presence indicates an increased likelihood of difficult intubation and airway maintenance under anesthesia. Three different groups of patients undergoing general anesthesia can be defined, each requiring different strategies for managing the airway: patients who have been diagnosed for OSA, patients with symptoms suggesting sleep apnea, and patients who lack signs of the syndrome or in whom such features are missed preoperatively. Surgical procedures can be OSA-related or for any other diagnosis with varying invasiveness. The common goal in all cases will be to avoid inadequate ventilation and oxygenation resulting in hypoxemia or hypercarbia and any associated hemodynamic changes (e.g., tachycardia, arrhythmia, and hypertension) leading to increased morbidity and mortality. Death, brain injury, and cardiopulmonary arrest, are amongst the most severe adverse events associated with difficulties in airway management, with airway trauma and damage to teeth as additional risks [106].

K. Hörmann, T. Verse, *Surgery for Sleep Disordered Breathing*,
DOI: 10.1007/978-3-540-77786-1_13, © Springer Verlag Berlin Heidelberg 2010

Widespread guidelines for management of the difficult airway have been introduced by the American Society of Anesthesiologists (ASA) in 1992 and have been published in revised form in 2003 [20]. A difficult airway is defined as the clinical situation in which a conventionally trained anesthesiologist experiences difficulty with face mask ventilation, difficulty with tracheal intubation, or both. The purpose of the ASA guidelines is to reduce the likelihood of adverse outcomes. the main goal is to ensure adequate oxygenation whenever difficulties occur. As D.B. Scott wrote more than 20 years ago: patients do not die from "failure to intubate," but from failure to stop trying or from undiagnosed esophageal intubation [654].

The first step in managing the difficult airway is to identify any patient at risk in the preoperative period. Evidence on prediction of difficult airways is inconclusive, but any patient with a diagnosed OSA or presenting clinical signs such as obesity, limited mouth opening or a large tongue should be treated as a patient with a difficult airway until proven otherwise. The description of a difficult airway in previous anesthesia records or in an anesthesia pass issued by an anesthesiologist offers clinically suggestive evidence that the difficulty may reoccur. Whenever possible, an airway history should be obtained prior to the initiation of anesthetic care in all patients. Focused medical history, physical examination, and review of medical records may improve the detection of a difficult airway in patients with OSA, therefore enabling the anesthesiologist to prepare the patient and the anesthesia team for the occurrence of airway difficulties. In some patients, additional evaluation may be indicated to further judge the likelihood of the anticipated airway difficulty.

It is widely accepted that preparatory effects will help in minimizing the risk in patients presenting with a difficult airway. In case of a known or suspected difficult airway, the patient should be informed of the special risks and procedures for management of the difficult airway. An additional experienced anesthesiologist should be available, specialized equipment for difficult airway management should be prepared, and a strategy as well as a backup strategy based on an institutional algorithm for establishing a secure airway should be defined (Fig. 13.1). Preoxygenation should be performed for 3 or more minutes and supplemental oxygen should be administered whenever possible during the process of establishing a secure airway and also after extubation.

There are several basic management choices when faced with a suspected or known difficult airway: awake intubation vs. induction of general anesthesia followed by intubation attempts, the preservation vs. the ablation of spontaneous ventilation, noninvasive vs. invasive techniques for the initial approach to intubation.

13.2
Strategies for Intubation in Patients with a Known or Suspected Difficult Airway

One important strategy in patients with a known or suspected difficult airway may be the avoidance of the necessity for invasive airway management. Whenever feasible, local anesthesia infiltration or regional blockades should be preferred in these patients.

Fig. 13.1   Algorithm "airway management"

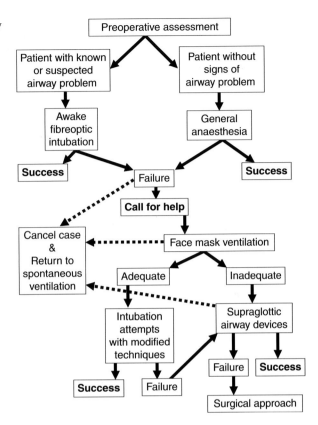

In patients with OSA, awake intubation may be attempted with a fibreoptic broncho-scope after application of local anesthetics. Once the glottis has been successfully identified, the tracheal tube can be advanced and general anesthesia can be inducted. If the procedure fails due to lack of patient cooperation, difficulties in identifying the glottic aperture caused by anatomical aberrations or massive secretion, the attempt may be canceled, the feasibility of local or regional anesthesia may be considered, or the decision for invasive airway access may be made. The latter might be considered as first choice in some patients with the options of surgical or percutaneous tracheostomy and surgical or needle cricothyrotomy with the option of jet ventilation.

When general anesthesia is induced in patients with a known or suspected difficult airway, tracheal intubation will still be successful in a number of patients without problems, especially when performed by an experienced anesthesiologist. If the initial intubation attempt fails, an additional anesthesiologist should be called if not already present, and the option of awakening the patient and returning to spontaneous ventilation should be considered based on the urgency of the surgical procedure. The possibility of face mask ventilation is the key issue for all further proceedings: when face mask ventilation and oxygenation of the patient are possible, repeated attempts at tracheal intubation can be attempted, with modified techniques where necessary. Alternative

Fig. 13.2 Bonfils intubation fiberscope

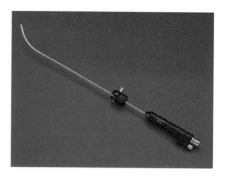

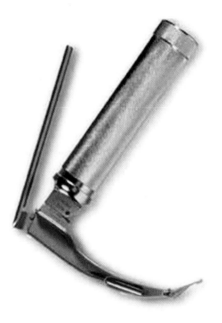

Fig. 13.3 McCoy-Blade with option of leverage
of the epiglottis

approaches may be the use of a fibreoptic bronchoscope, possibly in combination with
a supraglottic airway device, the use of rigid fiberscopes such as the Bonfils [58] (Fig.
13.2), of special larnygoscope blades such as the McCoy-blade with the option of additional leverage of the epiglottis (Fig. 13.3), or the use of an intubation stylet. The
Bonfils allows overcoming a major problem in many OSA patients, passage of the big
tongue and visualization of the vocal chords even when the epiglottis cannot be lifted
sufficiently with the laryngoscope. This device has become an integral part of managing airway difficulties in our department ever since it was introduced. In many patients,
correct positioning of the head will further aid in achieving the goal of tracheal intubation. Pressure on the cricoid cartilage by an assistant, ideally backward, upward, and
toward the right ("BURP" – backward, upward, rightward pressure) may also facilitate

identification of the glottis. Any "blind" intubation attempts without visualization of the glottis should be avoided for they may lead to trauma and swelling, interfering with further management of the airway.

Whenever face mask ventilation is difficult or impossible in a patient after induction of general anesthesia, with or without a failed intubation attempt, supraglottic airway devices such as a laryngeal mask (Fig. 13.4, left side) or a laryngeal tube (Fig. 13.4, right side) should be inserted to ensure oxygenation of the patient while reconsidering intubation strategies. One approach can be to attempt fibreoptic intubation via the supraglottic device, direct or with a tube exchange catheter, after preoxygenation of the patient.

Fiberoptic intubation may be facilitated by using the Intubating Laryngeal Mask Airway or LMA-Fastrach™ (LMA Deutschland GmbH, Germany) (Fig. 13.5), which provides a curved steel shaft guiding the fiberscope toward the glottis. Another option is to reconsider the necessity of tracheal intubation vs. the possibility of maintaining the airway with a supraglottic airway device for the surgical procedure.

Newer alternatives to tracheal intubation and face mask ventilation such as the LMA-ProSeal™ (LMA Deutschland GmbH, Germany). (Fig. 13.6a) or the laryngeal tube suction (LTS II) (Fig. 13.6b) provide an additional lumen, allowing placement of a gastric tube and suctioning, and should be preferred over the standard devices in obese patients since the airway seal achieved is also better.

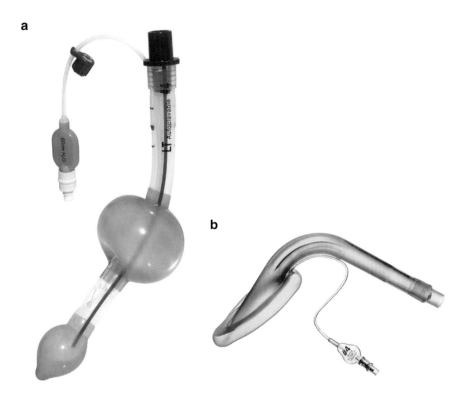

Fig. 13.4   *a*: laryngeal mask airway. *b*: laryngeal tube

Fig. 13.5 Intubating laryngeal mask airway
(LMA-Fastrach™)

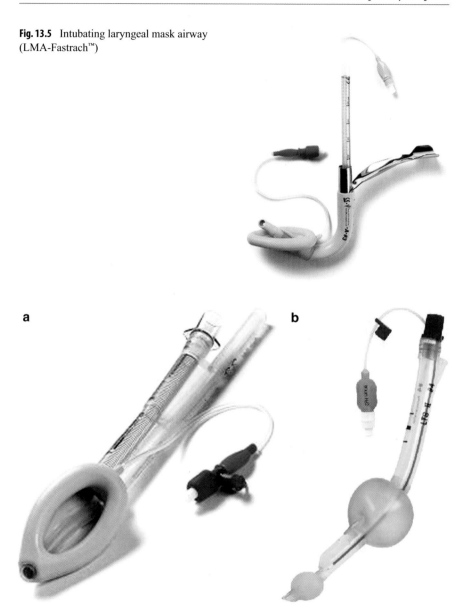

a   b

Fig. 13.6 *a*: ProSeal laryngeal mask airway. *b*: laryngeal tube suction (LTS II)

13.3
Life-Threatening Situations

In any situation requiring urgent airway maintenance, the presence of a preformulated
strategy to ensure oxygenation, adequate ventilation – and possibly intubation – is absolutely mandatory.

The anesthesiologist may be faced with two different scenarios: a patient presenting with severe obstruction, cyanosis, and/or hypoxemia who requires urgent intubation and cannot be ventilated with a face mask or one who cannot be intubated (or a combination of both). In other patients, general anaesthesia may be induced and the team is then surprised by difficulties maintainig the airway in a patient who lacks signs of a difficult airway or in whom such features were missed preoperatively.

The emergency airway management should be basically the same as above, but the choice of the options and strategies should be narrowed down to the techniques the anesthesiologist is most acquainted with. In any patient requiring urgent oxygenation, supraglottic airway devices should be inserted early on, even when face mask ventilation is possible, since the airway seal with these devices is superior and not only the delivery of oxygen to the lungs is better, but also the rate of gastric insufflation is therefore lower. Fibreoptic intubation via these devices or the use of a newer supraglottic alternative providing access to the alimentary tract for suctioning should be considered. However, if the problem is caused by airway obstruction on the glottic level, this strategy fails and options such as translaryngeal jet ventilation, surgical or needle cricothyrotomy, or an emergency tracheostomy must be considered early on, especially when oxygenation is difficult or not possible. Close cooperation with the ENT specialist is mandatory, not only in these critical incidents, but in the pre and perioperative management of all patients with OSA.

13.4
Extubating the Difficult Airway

After successful management of a difficult airway, several considerations should guide the decisions for the postoperative phase. The surgical procedure, the condition of the patient, as well as any documented or suspected trauma to the upper airway due to manipulations during the process of securing the airway will influence the anesthesiologist's strategy for extubating the patient with a difficult airway. While removal of the tracheal tube will not be a problem, reinsertion in case of any airway obstruction will not be easier than during the first attempt. On the contrary, edema and secretions will increase the risk of hypoxemia should airway maintenance be necessary.

Immediately after a patient with a difficult airway has been successfully intubated, the equipment for airway management must be rechecked and completed as necessary to allow adequate reaction on any peri and postoperative airway problems. The use of steroids to reduce mucosal swelling of glottis and upper airway induced by manipulation during repeated intubation attempts is recommended.

In general, patients with a known difficult airway must be awake and communicative for extubation, and airway reflexes must have returned. Spontaneous ventilation must be sufficient, allowing an adequate tidal volume and oxygenation. After profound suctioning of the pharynx to remove secretions, the cuff of the tracheal tube should be deflated and the tube should be closed to test whether swelling may cause airway obstruction after removal of the tube. If no breathing sounds are noticed around the tracheal tube, there is a high risk of complete airway obstruction and the patient should be taken to an intensive care unit for prolonged weaning. If the swelling persists, tracheostomy must be considered. In all patients in whom breathing sounds around the tube can be heard, extubation may be attempted with the complete equipment and personnel for difficult intubation present.

13.5
Negative Pressure Pulmonary Edema

Patients with OSA are at risk to suffer from upper airway obstruction and are therefore extubated in our department only after insertion of an oropharyngeal tube (Guedel) to reduce the risk of negative-pressure pulmonary edema (NPPE), also addressed as postobstructive pulmonary edema [6]. NPPE presents in most cases as a complex of symptoms with rapid onset, consisting of acute respiratory failure with dyspnea, tachypnea, and strained respiratory efforts. Additional signs are paradox ventilation, pink frothy sputum, stridor, and severe agitation. Upper airway obstruction (UAO) produces extreme reduction of intrathoracic pressure during spontaneous ventilation, consecutively causing increase in venous return to the right ventricle and increase in intrathoracic blood volume, resulting in elevated hydrostatic pressures and interstitial transudation of fluids.

13.6
Postoperative Care

In the postoperative phase, patients with OSA often show respiratory depression and repetitive apneas even after successful surgery. Respiratory disorders can be induced by posttraumatic swelling of the upper airways leading to a mechanical obstruction. Postoperative edema formation can be prevented by administering steroids during the operation. Another aspect of postoperative respiratory problems is the apnea or hypopnea induced by perioperative opioids. There are many reports demonstrating the coincidence of postoperative apneas and the use of opioids, but the correction of upper airway annomalities is very painful and leads to the obligatory use of opioids in combination with nonopioid analgetics. Furthermore, the use of clonidine seems to be helpful because of the coanalgetic effect of the substance and the reduction of blood pressure. Elevated blood pressure levels often can be seen after surgery leading to a higher risk of postoperative bleeding.

To avoid postoperative respiratory complications and episodes of high blood pressure it seems necessary to monitor these patients for at least 2 h. Admission to the intensive care unit is not a standard in these patients. Interdisciplinary cooperation as well in the recovery area as during the further in-hospital course ensures patient safety. Mechanisms to detect respiratory and hemodynamic problems must be implemented.

13.7
Documentation

The presence and nature of airway difficulties should be documented in the patient's file. In addition, an anesthesia pass should be issued describing the problem and the strategy that led to successful management. The patient or a responsible person should be informed and instructed to carry the pass at all times and show it whenever surgical procedures are planned to facilitate future medical care.

Take Home Pearls

> Patients presenting for surgery related to sleep-disordered breathing should be presented to the anesthesiologist as soon as the decision for a surgical intervention is made, in order to allow adequate examination and preparation.
> Algorithms and procedures to manage known and unsuspected airway difficulties must be implemented and followed. Additional personnel and equipment is necessary to successfully achieve airway maintenance should problems arise.
> Hypoxia and apnea are essential risks in the postoperative period. Upper airway obstruction may lead to negative pressure pulmonary edema.

References

1. Abdu MH, Feghali JG. Uvulopalatopharyngoplasty in a child with obstructive sleep apnea. A case report. J Laryngol Otol 1988;102:546–548
2. Afzelius LE, Elmquist D, Hougaard K, Laurin S, Nilsson B, Risberg AM. Sleep apnea syndrome – an alternative treatment to tracheotomy. Laryngoscope 1981;91:285–291
3. Agren K, Nordlander B, Linder-Aronsson S, Zettergren-Wijk L, Svanborg E. Children with nocturnal upper airway obstruction: postoperative orthodontic and respiratory improvement. Acta Otolaryngol 1998;118:581–587
4. Ahlquist-Rastad J, Hultcrantz E, Svanholm H. Children with tonsillar obstruction: indications for and efficacy of tonsillectomy. Acta Pediatr Scand 1988;77:831–835
5. Aland JW Jr. Retropharyngeal lipoma causing symptoms of obstructive sleep apnea. Otolaryngol Head Neck Surg 1996;114:628–630
6. Alb M, Tsagogiorgas C, Meinhardt JP. Negative-pressure pulmonary edema (NPPE). Anasthesiol Intensivmed Notfallmed Schmerzther [in German] 2006;41:64–78
7. Albu S, De Min G, Forti A, Babighian G. Nd:YAG laser-assisted uvulopalatoplasty for snoring. Acta Otolaryngol Belg 1998;52:69–73
8. Ali NJ, Pitson D, Stradling JR. Sleep disordered breathing: effects of adenotonsillectomy on behaviour and psychological functioning. Eur J Pediatr 1996;155:56–62
9. Al-Jassim AH, Lesser TH. Single dose injection snoreplasty: investigation or treatment? J Laryngol Otol 2008;122:1190–1193
10. Altman JS, Halpert RD, Mickelson SA, Senior BA. Effect of uvulopalatopharyngoplasty and genial and hyoid advancement on swallowing in patients with obstructive sleep apnea syndrome. Otolaryngol Head Neck Surg 1999;120:454–457
11. Altman KW, Wetmore RF, Marsh RR. Congenital airway abnormalities requiring tracheotomy: a profile of 56 patients and their diagnosis over 9 year period. Int J Pediatr Otorhinolaryngol 1997;41:199–206
12. American Academy of Sleep Medicine ICSD-2- International classification of sleep disorders Diagnostic and coding manual, 2nd edn. American Academy of Sleep Medicine, 2005: pp 51–59
13. American Academy of Sleep Medicine ICSD-2- International classification of sleep disorders Diagnostic and coding manual, 2nd edn. American Academy of Sleep Medicine, 2005: pp 204–205

14. American Sleep Disorders Association. ASDA standards of practice. Practice parameters for the use of portable recording in the assessment of obstructive sleep apnea. Sleep 1994;17: 372–377

15. American Sleep Disorders Association. ASDA standards of practice. Portable recording in the assessment of obstructive sleep apnea. Sleep 1994;17:378–392

16. American Sleep Disorders Association. Practice parameters for the indications for polysomnography and related procedures. Sleep 1997;20:406–422

17. American Sleep Disorders Association. Practice parameters for the treatment of obstructive sleep apnea in adults: the efficacy of surgical modifications of the upper airway. Sleep 1996; 19:152–155

18. American Sleep Disorders Association. Practice parameters for the use of laser-assisted uvulopalatoplasty. Standards of Practice Committee of the American Sleep Disorders Association. Sleep 1994;17:744–748

19. American Sleep Disorders Association: International Classification of Sleep Disorders (ICSD): Diagnostic and Coding Manual. American Sleep Disorders Association, Rochester, Minnesota, 1997: pp 21–24

20. American Society of Anaesthesiologists Task Force on Management of the Difficult Airway (2003). Practice guidelines for management of the difficult airway: an updated report by the American Society of anaesthesiologists task force on management of the difficult airway. Anesthesiology 2003;98:1269–1277

21. Amin R, Anthony L, Somers V, Fenchel M, McConnell K, Jefferies J, Willging P, Kalra M, Daniels S. Growth velocity predicts recurrence of sleep-disordered breathing 1 year after adenotonsillectomy. Am J Respir Crit Care Med 2008;177:654–659

22. Andersen APD, Alving J, Lildholdt T, Wulff CH. Obstructive sleep apnea initiated by a lax epiglottis. Chest 1987;91:621–623

23. Anonsen C. Laryngeal obstruction and obstructive sleep apnea syndrome. Laryngoscope 1990;100:775–778

24. Antila J, Sipilä J, Tshushima Y, Polo O, Laurikainen E, Suonpaa J. The effect of laser-uvulopalatopharyngoplasty on the nasal and nasopharyngeal volume measured with acoustic rhinometry. Acta Otolaryngol 1997; (Suppl 529): 202–205

25. Ariyasu L, Young G, Spinelli F. Uvulectomy in the office setting. Ear Nose Throat J 1995; 74:721–722

26. Astor FC, Hanft KL, Benson C, Amaranath A. Analysis of short-term outcome after office-based laser-assisted uvulopalatoplasty. Otolaryngol Head Neck Surg 1998;118:478–480

27. Atef A, Mosleh M, Hesham M, Fathi A, Hassan M, Fawzy M. Radiofrequency vs laser in the management of mild to moderate obstructive sleep apnoea: does the number of treatment sessions matter? J Laryngol Otol 2005;119:888–893

28. Aubert-Tulkens G, Hamoir M, van den Eeckhaut J, Rodenstein DO. Failure of tonsil and nose surgery in adults with long-standing severe sleep apnea syndrome. Arch Intern Med 1989;149: 2118–2121

29. Ayas NT, FitzGerald JM, Fleetham JA, White DP, Schulzer M, Ryan CF, Ghaeli R, Mercer GW, Cooper P, Tan MC, Marra CA. Cost-effectiveness of continuous positive airway pressure therapy for moderate to severe obstructive sleep apnea/hypopnea. Arch Intern Med 2006;166: 977–984

30. Bachar G, Feinmesser R, Shpitzer T, Yaniv E, Nageris B, Eidelman L. Laryngeal and hypopharyngeal obstruction in sleep disordered breathing patients, evaluated by sleep endoscopy. Eur Arch Otorhinolaryngol 2008;265:1397–1402

31. Bäck LJ, Palomäki M, Piilonen AK, Ylikoski J. Sleep-disordered breathing: radiofrequency thermal ablation is a promising new treatment possibility. Laryngoscope 2001;111: 464–471

32. Bäck LJ, Tervahartiala PO, Piilonen AK, Partinen MM, Ylikoski JS. Bipolar radiofrequency thermal ablation of the soft palate in habitual snorers without significant desaturations assessed by magnetic resonance imaging. Am J Respir Crit Care Med 2002;166:865–871

33. Baer GA, Rorarius MG, Kolehmainen S, Selin S. The effect of paracetamol or diclofenac administered before operation on postoperative pain and behaviour after adenoidectomy in small children. Anaesthesia 1992;47:1078–1080

34. Baisch A, Maurer JT, Hörmann K, Stuck BA. Combined radiofrequency assisted uvulopalatoplasty (RF-UPP) in the treatment of snoring. Eur Arch Otorhinolaryngol 2009;266: 125–130

35. Baisch A, Maurer JT, Hörmann K. The effect of hyoid suspension in a multilevel surgery concept for obstructive sleep apnea. Otolaryngol Head Neck Surg 2006;134:856–861

36. Balcerzak J, Przybylowski T, Bielicki P, Korczynski P, Chazan R. Functional nasal surgery in the treatment of obstructive sleep apnea [in Polish]. Pneumonol Alergol Pol 2004;72:4–8

37. Ballester E, Badia JR, Hernandez L, Carrasco E, de Pablo J, Fornas C, Rodriguez-Roisin R, Montserrat JM. Evidence of the effectiveness of continuous positive airway pressure in the treatment of sleep apnea/hypopnea syndrome. Am J Respir Crit Care Med 1999;159: 495–501

38. Balsiger BM, Poggio JL, Mai J, Kelly KA, Sarr MG. Ten and more years after vertical banded gastroplasty as primary operation for morbid obesity. Gastrointest Surg 2000;4:598–605

39. Barthel SW, Strome MS. Snoring, obstructive sleep apnea, and surgery. Med Clin North Am 1999;83:85–96

40. Barthez E, Rilliet F. Traité clinique et practique des maladies des enfants [in French]. Paris. G. Bailliere, 1843:484–488

41. Bassiouny A, El Salamawy A, Abd El-Tawab M, Atef A. Bipolar radiofrequency treatment for snoring with mild to moderate sleep apnea: a comparative study between the radiofrequency assisted uvulopalatoplasty technique and the channeling technique. Eur Arch Otorhinolaryngol 2007;264:659–667

42. Battagel JM, Johal A, Kotecha B. A cephalometric comparison of subjects with snoring and obstructive sleep apnoea. Eur J Orthod 2000;22:353–365

43. Bell RB, Turvey TA. Skeletal advancement for the treatment of obstructive sleep apnea in children. Cleft Palate Craniofac J 2001;38:147–154

44. Belloso A, Morar P, Tahery J, Saravanan K, Nigam A, Timms MS. Randomized-controlled study comparing post-operative pain between coblation palatoplasty and laser palatoplasty. Clin Otolaryngol 2006;31:138–143

45. Benotti PN, Forse RA. Safety and long-term efficacy of revisional surgery in severe obesity. Am J Surg 1996;172:232–235

46. Benumof JL. Obstructive sleep apnea in the adult obese patient: implications for airway management. J Clin Anesth 2001;13:144–156

47. Berger G, Finkelstein Y, Ophir D. Histopathologic changes in the soft palate after laser-assisted uvulopalatoplasty. Arch Otolaryngol Head Neck Surg 1999;125: 786–790

48. Berger G, Finkelstein Y, Stein G, Ophir D. Laser-assisted uvulopalatoplasty for snoring: medium- to long-term subjective and objective analysis. Arch Otolaryngol Head Neck Surg 2001;127:412–417

49. Berger G, Stein G, Ophir D, Finkelstein Y. Is there a better way to do laser-assisted uvulopalatoplasty? Arch Otolaryngol Head Neck Surg 2003;129:447–453

50. Bertrand B, Eloy P, Collet S, Remarque C, Rombeaux P. Effect of nasal valve surgery by open-septorhinoplasty and lateral cartilage grafts (spreader grafts) on snoring among a population of single snorers. Preliminary report. Acta Otorhinolaryngol Belg 2002;56:149–155

51. Bettega G, Pepin JL, Veale D, Deschaux C, Raphael B, Levy P. Obstructive sleep apnea syndrome. Fifty-one consecutive patients treated by maxillofacial surgery. Am J Respir Crit Care Med 2000;162:641–649

52. Biermann E. Nasal CPAP therapy in obstructive sleep apnea syndrome: does functional rhinosurgery improve compliance [in German]? Somnologie 2001;5:59–64

53. Birkent H, Soken H, Akcam T, Karahatay S, Gerek M. The effect of radiofrequency volumetric tissue reduction of soft palate on voice. Eur Arch Otorhinolaryngol 2008;265:195–198

54. Blumen MB, Coquille F, Rocchicioli C, Mellot F, Chabolle F. Radiofrequency tongue reduction through a cervical approach: a pilot study. Laryngoscope 2006;116:1887–1893

55. Blumen MB, Dahan S, Fleury B, Hausser-Hauw C, Chabolle F. Radiofrequency ablation for the treatment of mild to moderate obstructive sleep apnea. Laryngoscope 2002;112: 2086–2092

56. Blumen MB, Dahan S, Wagner I, De Dieuleveult T, Chabolle F. Radiofrequency versus LAUP for the treatment of snoring. Otolaryngol Head Neck Surg 2002;126:67–73

57. Blunden S, Lushington K, Kennedy D, Martin J, Dawson D. Behavior and neurocognitive performance in children aged 5–10 years who snore compared to normal controls. J Clin Exp Neuropsych 2000;22:554–568

58. Bonfils P. A new method for difficult intubation in Pierre-Robin-children: the retromolar route. Anaesthesist 1983;32:363–367

59. Bonilla JA, Pizzuto MP, Brodsky LS. Aplasia of the epiglottis: a rare congenital anomaly. Ear Nose Throat J 1998;77:51–55

60. Boot H, van Wegen R, Poublon RML, Bogaard JM, Schmitz PIM, van der Meche FGA. Long-term results of uvulopalatopharyngoplasty for obstructive sleep apnea syndrome. Laryngoscope 2000;110:469–475

61. Borowiecki B, Pollak CP, Weitzman ED, Rakoff S, Imperato J. Fibro-optic study of pharyngeal airway during sleep in patients with hypersomnia obstructive sleep-apnea syndrome. Laryngoscope 1978;88:1310–1313

62. Boudewyns A, de Cock W, Willemen M, Wagemans M, de Backer W, van de Heyning PH. Influence of uvulopalatopharyngoplasty on alpha-EEG arousals in nonapneic snorers. Eur Respir J 1997;10:129–132

63. Boudewyns A, van de Heyning P. Temperature-controlled radiofrequency tissue volumetric reduction of the soft palate (Somnoplasty®) in the treatment of habitual snoring: results of a European multicenter trial. Acta Otolaryngol 2000;120:981–985

64. Bourolias C, Hajiioannou J, Sobol E, Velegrakis G, Helidonis E. Epiglottis reshaping using CO_2 laser: a minimally invasive technique and its potent applications. Head Face Med 2008;4:15

65. Bowden MT, Kezirian EJ, Utley D, Goode RL. Outcomes of hyoid suspension for the treatment of obstructive sleep apnea. Arch Otolaryngol Head Neck Surg 2005;131:440–445

66. Brausewetter F, Hecht M, Pirsig W. Antrochoanal polyp and obstructive sleep apnoea in children. J Laryngol Otol 2004;118:453–458

67. Brietzke SE, Gallagher D. The effectiveness of tonsillectomy and adenoidectomy in the treatment of pediatric obstructive sleep apnea/hypopnea syndrome: a meta-analysis. Otolaryngol Head Neck Surg 2006;134:979–984

68. Brietzke SE, Mair EA. Acoustical analysis of snoring: can the probability of success be predicted? Otolaryngol Head Neck Surg 2006;135:417–420

69. Brietzke SE, Mair EA. Extended follow-up and new objective data. Otolaryngol Head Neck Surg 2003;128:605–615

70. Brietzke SE, Mair EA. Injection snoreplasty: how to treat snoring without all the pain and expense. Otolaryngol Head Neck Surg 2001;124:503–510

71. Brietzke SE, Mair EA. Injection snoreplasty: investigation of alternative sclerotherapy agents. Otolaryngol Head Neck Surg 2004;130:47–50

72. Brodsky L, Adler E, Stanievich JF. Naso- and oropharyngeal dimensions in children with obstructive sleep apnea. Int J Pediatr Otorhinolaryngol 1989;17:1–11

73. Brolin RE, Kenler HA, Gorman JH, Cody RP. Long-limb gastric by pass in the superobese. A prospective randomized study. Ann Surg 1992;215:387–395

74. Brooks LJ, Stephens BM, Bacevice AM. Adenoid size is related to severity but not the number of episodes of obstructive apnea in children. J Pediatr 1998;132:682–686

75. Brosch S, Matthes CH, Pirsig W, Verse T. Uvulopalatoplasty changes fundamental frequency of voice – a prospective study. J Laryngol Otol 2000;114:113–118

76. Brouillette RT, Hanson D, David R. A diagnositic approach to suspected obstructive sleep apnea in children. J Pediatr 1984;105:10–14

77. Brouillette RT, Manoukian JJ, Ducharme FM, Oudjhane K, Earle LG, Ladan S, Morielli A. Efficacy of fluticasone nasal spray for pediatric obstructive sleep apnea. J Pediatr 2001;138: 838–844

78. Brown DJ, Kerr P, Kryger M. Radiofrequency tissue reduction of the soft palate in patients with moderate sleep-disordered breathing. J Otolaryngol 2001;30:193–198

79. Buchwald H, Avidor Y, Braunwald E, Jensen MD, Pories W, Fahrbach K, Schoelles K. Bariatric surgery: a systematic review and meta-analysis. JAMA 2004;292: 1724–1737

80. Buchwald H, Williams SE. Bariatric surgery world wide 2003. Obes Surg 2004;14: 1157–1164

81. Buchwald HA. Bariatric surgery al gorithm. Obes Surg 2002;12:733–750

82. Burgess LPA, Derderian SS, Morin GV, Gonzalez C, Zajtchuk JT. Postoperative risk following uvulopalatopharyngoplasty for obstructive sleep apnea. Otolaryngol Head Neck Surg 1992; 106:81–86

83. Burstein FD, Cohen SR, Scott PH, Teague GR, Montgomery GL, Kattos AV. Surgical therapy for severe refractory sleep apnea in infants and children: application of the airway zone concept. Plast Reconstr Surg 1995;96:34–41

84. Busaba NY. Same-stage nasal and palatopharyngeal surgery for obstructive sleep apnea: is it safe? Otolaryngol Head Neck Surg 2002;126:399–403

85. Busetto L, Enzi G, Inelmen EM, Costa G, Negrin V, Sergi G, Vianello A. Obstructive sleep apnea syndrome in morbid obesity: effects of intragastric balloon. Chest 2005;128:618–623

86. Butterfield JH, Marcoux JP, Weiler D, Harner SG. Mast cell pharyngitis as a cause of supraglottic edema. Arch Otorhinolaryngol 1988;245:88–91

87. Cahali MB, Formigoni GG, Gebrim EM, Miziara ID. Lateral pharyngoplasty versus uvulopalatopharyngoplasty: a clinical, polysomnographic and computed tomography measurement comparison. Sleep 2004;27:942–950

88. Cahali MB. Lateral pharyngoplasty: a new treatment for obstructive sleep apnea hypopnea syndrome. Laryngoscope 2003;113:1961–1968

89. Caldarelli DD, Cartwright R, Lilie JK. Obstructive sleep apnea: variations in surgical management. Laryngoscope 1985;95:1070–1073

90. Carenfelt C, Haraldsson PO. Frequency of complications after uvulopalatopharyngoplasty. Lancet 1993;341:437

91. Carenfelt C. Laser uvulopalatopharyngoplasty in treatment of habitual snoring. Ann Otol Rhinol Laryngol 1991;100:451–454

92. Cartwright R, Venkatesan TK, Caldarelli D, Diaz F. Treatments for snoring: a comparison of somnoplasty and an oral appliance. Laryngoscope 2000;110:1680–1683

93. Cassisi NJ, Biller HF, Ogura JH. Changes in arterial oxygen tension and pulmonary mechanics with the use of posterior packing in epistaxis: a preliminary report. Laryngoscope 1971;81: 1261–1266

94. Catalfumo FJ, Golz A, Westerman T, Gilbert LM, Joachims HZ, Goldenberg D. The epiglottis and obstructive sleep apnoea syndrome. J Laryngol Otol 1998;112:940–943

95. Cedars MG, Linck DL, Chin M, Toth BA. Advancement of the midface using distraction techniques. Plast Reconstr Surg 1999;103:429–441

96. Celenk F, Bayazit YA, Yilmaz M, Kemaloglu YK, Uygur K, Ceylan A, Korkuyu E. Tonsillar regrowth following partial tonsillectomy with radiofrequency. Int J Pediatr Otorhinolaryngol 2008;72:19–22

97. Chabolle F, de Dieuleveult T, Canabes J, Séquert C, Dahan S, Drweski P, Engalenc D. Long-term results of surgical pharyngectomy (uvulo-palato-pharyngoplasty) versus office CO_2 laser (L.A.U.P.) for the treatment of uncomplicated snoring [in French]. Ann Otolaryngol Chir Cervicofac 1998;115:196–201

98. Chabolle F, Wagner I, Blumen M, Séquert C, Fleury B, de Dieuleveult T. Tongue base reduction with hyoepiglottoplasty: a treatment for severe obstructive sleep apnea. Laryngoscope 1999;109:1273–1280

99. Chan AS, Lee RW, Cistulli PA. Dental appliance treatment for obstructive sleep apnea. Chest. 2007;132:693–699

100. Chan J, Younes A, Koltari PJ. Occult supraglottic lymphatic malformation presenting as obstructive sleep apnea. Int J Pediatr Otorhinolaryngol 2003;67:293–296

101. Charuzi I, Fraser D, Peiser J, Ovnat A, Lavie P. Sleep apnea syndrome in the morbidly obese undergoing bariatric surgery. Gastroenterol Clin North Am 1987;16: 517–519

102. Charuzi I, Ovnat A, Peiser J, Saltz H, Weitzman S, Lavie P. The effect of surgical weight reduction on sleep quality in obesity-related sleep apnea syndrome. Surgery 1985;97: 535–538

103. Chen JM, Schloss MD, Azouz ME. Antro-choanal polyp: a 10-year retrospective study in the pediatric population with a review of the literature. J Otolaryngol 1989;18:168–172

104. Chen MF, Fang TJ, Lee LA, Li HY, Wang CJ, Chen IH. Huge supraglottic cyst causing obstructive sleep apnea in an adult. Otolaryngol Head Neck Surg 2006;135: 986–988

105. Chen S, Zhang S, Qiu Q, Sheng X, Wang X. The effect of the pillar implant system in the management of snoring and OSAHS patients [in Chinese]. Lin Chung Er Bi Yan Hou Tou Jing Wai Ke Za Zhi 2008;22:539–541

106. Cheney FW, Posner KL, Lee LA, Caplan RA, Domino KB. Trends in Anesthesia-related death and brain damage. A closed claims analysis. Anesthesiology 2006;105: 1081–1086

107. Chervin RD, Ruzicka DL, Giordani BJ, Weatherly RA, Dillon JE, Hodges EK, Marcus CL, Guire KE. Sleep-disordered breathing, behavior, and cognition in children before and after adenotonsillectomy. Pediatrics 2006;117:769–778

108. Chervin RD, Weatherly RA, Garetz SL, Ruzicka DL, Giordani BJ, Hodges EK, Dillon JE, Guire KE. Pediatric sleep questionnaire: prediction of sleep apnea and outcomes. Arch Otolaryngol Head Neck Surg 2007;133:216–222

109. Chetty KG, Kadifa F, Berry RB, Mahutte CK. Acquired laryngomalacia as a cause of obstructive sleep apnea. Chest 1994;106:1898–1899

110. Chisholm E, Kotecha B. Oropharyngeal surgery for obstructive sleep apnoea in CPAP failures. Eur Arch Otorhinolaryngol 2007;264:51–55

111. Choban PS, Flancbaum L. The effect of Roux limb lengths on outcome after Roux-en-Y gastric bypass: a prospective, randomized clinical trial. Obes Surg 2002;12: 540–545

112. Cincik H, Cekin E, Cetin B, Gungor A, Poyrazoglu E. Comparison of uvulopalatopharyngoplasty, laser-assisted uvulopalatoplasty and cautery-assisted uvulopalatoplasty in the treatment of primary snoring. ORL J Otorhinolaryngol Relat Spec 2006;68: 149–155

113. Cline CL. The effects of intra-nasal obstruction on the general health. Med Surg Rep 1892;67:259–260

114. Cohen SR, Lefaivre JF, Burstein FD, Simms C, Kattos AV, Scott PH, Montgomery GL, Graham LR. Surgical treatment of obstructive sleep apnea in neurologically compromised patients. Plast Reconstr Surg 1997;99:638–646

115. Cohen SR, Simms C, Burstein FD, Thomsen J. Alternatives to tracheostomy in infants and children with obstructive sleep apnea. J Pediatr Surg 1999;34:182–187

116. Cohen SR, Suzman K, Simms C, Burstein FD, Riski J, Montgomery G. Sleep apnea surgery versus tracheostomy in children: an exploratory study of the comparative effects on quality of life. Plast Reconstr Surg 1998;102:1855–1864

117. Cohen SR. Craniofacial distraction with a modular internal distraction system: evolution of design and surgical techniques. Plast Reconstr Surg 1999;103: 1592–1607

118. Coleman JA. Laser-assisted uvulopalatoplasty: long-term results with a treatment for snoring. Ear Nose Throat J 1998;77:22–34

119. Coleman SC, Smith TL. Midline radiofrequency tissue reduction of the palate for bothersome snoring and sleep-disordered breathing: a clinical trial. Otolaryngol Head Neck Surg 2000;122:387–394

120. Colen TY, Seidman C, Weedon J, Goldstein NA. Effect of intracapsular tonsillectomy on quality of life for children with obstructive sleep-disordered breathing. Arch Otolaryngol Head Neck Surg 2008;134:124–127

121. Collop N, Hartenbaum N, Rosen I, Phillips B. Paying attention to at-risk commercial vehicle operators. Chest 2006;130:637–639

122. Connolly LA. Anesthetic management of obstructive sleep apnea patients. J Clin Anesth 1991;3:461–469

123. Conradt R, Hochban W, Brandenburg U, Heitmann J, Peter JH. Long-term follow-up after surgical treatment of obstructive sleep apnoea by maxillomandibular advancement. Eur Respir J 1997;10:123–128

124. Conway WA, Victor LD, Magillian DJ, Fujita S, Zorick FJ, Roth T. Adverse effects of tracheostomy for sleep apnea. JAMA 1981;246:347–350

125. Coticchia JM, Yun RD, Nelson L, Koempel J. Temperature-controlled radiofrequency treatment of tonsillar hypertrophy for reduction of upper airway obstruction in pediatric patients. Arch Otolaryngol Head Neck Surg 2006;132:425–430

126. Coughlin S, Mawdsley L, Mugarza JA, Calverley PMA, Wilding JPH. Obstructive sleep apnoea is independently associated with an increased prevalence of metabolic syndrome. Eur Heart J 2004;25:735–741

127. Courey MS, Fomin D, Smith T, Huang S, Sanders D, Reinisch L. Histologic and physiologic effects of electrocautery, CO_2 laser, and radiofrequency injury in the porcine soft palate. Laryngoscope 1999;109:1316–1319

128. Craig TJ, Mende C, Hughes K, Kakumanu S, Lehman EB, Chinchilli V. The effect of topical fluticasone on objective sleep testing and the symptoms of rhinitis, sleep, and daytime somnolence in perennial allergic rhinitis. Allergy Asthma Proc 2003;24: 53–58

129. Crampette L, Mondain M, Rombaux P. Sphenochoanal polyp in children. Diagnosis and treatment. Rhinology 1995;33:43–45

130. Croft CB, Pringle M. Sleep nasendoscopy: a technique of assessment in snoring and obstructive sleep apnoea. Clin Otolaryngol 1991;16:504–509

131. Croft CB, Thomson HG, Samuels MP, Southall DP. Endoscopic evaluation and treatment of sleep-associated upper airway obstruction in infants and young children. Clin Otolaryngol 1990;15:209–216

132. Dagan Y. Rhinoplasty and sleep apnea syndrome. Somnologie 1997;1(Suppl 2): 49

133. Dalmasso F, Prota R. Snoring: analysis, measurement, clinical implications and applications: review. Eur Resp J 1996;9:146–159

134. Darrow DH, Weiss DD. Management of sleep-related breathing disorders in children. Op Tech Otorhinolaryngol 2002;13:111–118

135. Dart RA, Gregoire JR, Guttermann DD, Woolf SH. The association of hypertension and secondary cardiovascular disease with sleep-disordered breathing. Chest 2003;123: 244–260

136. Dattilo DJ, Drooger SA. Outcome assessment of patients undergoing maxillofacial procedures for the treatment of sleep apnea: comparison of subjective and objective results. J Oral Maxillofac Surg 2004;62:164–168

137. Dattilo DJ, Kolodychak MT. The use of the mini anchor system in the hyoid suspension technique for the treatment of obstructive sleep apnea syndrome. J Oral Maxillofac Surg 2000;58:919–920

138. Dayal VS, Phillipson EA. Nasal surgery in the management of sleep apnea. Ann Otol Rhinol Laryngol 1985;94:550–554

139. de la Chaux R, Dreher A, Klemens C, Rasp G, Leunig A. Respiratory sleep disorders: benefit from laser-surgery [in German]. MMW Fortschr Med 2004;146:49–50, 52

140. de la Chaux R, Klemens C, Patscheider M, Reichel O, Dreher A. Tonsillotomy in the treatment of obstructive sleep apnea syndrome in children: polysomnographic results. Int J Pediatr Otorhinolaryngol 2008;72:1411–1417

141. Deitel M, Shahi B, Anand PK, Deitel FH, Cardinell DL. Long-term outcome in a series of jejunoileal bypass patients. Obes Surg 1993;3:247–252

142. Dematteis M, Lévy P, Pépin JL. A simple procedure for measuring pharyngeal sensitivity: a contribution to the diagnosis of sleep apnoea. Thorax 2005;60:418–426

143. den Herder C, Hessel NS, de Vries N. Hyoidthyroidpexia (HTP), a new surgical treatment for sleep apnoea syndrome. Manuscript in preparation

144. den Herder C, Kox D, van Tinteren H, de Vries N. Bipolar radiofrequency induced thermotherapy of the tongue base: its complications, acceptance and effectiveness under local anesthesia. Eur Arch Otorhinolaryngol 2006;263:1031–1040

145. den Herder C, van Tinteren H, de Vries N. Hyoidthyroidpexia: a surgical treatment for sleep apnea syndrome. Laryngoscope 2005;115:740–745

146. den Herder C, van Tinteren H, de Vries N. Sleep endoscopy versus modified Mallampati score in sleep apnea and snoring. Laryngoscope 2005;115:735–739

147. Denny AD, Talisman R, Hanson P, Recinos RF. Mandibular distraction osteogenesis in very young patients to correct airway obstruction. Plast Reconstr Surg 2001;108: 302–311

148. Denoyelle F, Mondain M, Grésillon N, Roger G, Chaudré F, Garabédian EN. Failures and complications of supraglottoplasty in children. Arch Otolaryngol Head Neck Surg 2003;129:1077–1080

149. Densert O, Desai H, Eliasson A, Frederiksen L, Andersson D, Olaison J, Widmark C. Tonsillotomy in children with tonsillar hypertrophy. Acta Otolaryngol 2001;121: 854–858

150. Derkay CS, Darrow DH, Welch C, Sinacori JT. Post-tonsillectomy morbidity and quality of life in pediatric patients with obstructive tonsils and adenoid: microdebrider vs electrocautery. Otolaryngol Head Neck Surg 2006;134:114–120

151. DeRowe A, Günther E, Fibbi A, Lehtimaki K, Vahatalo K, Maurer J, Ophir D. Tongue-base suspension with a soft tissue-to-bone anchor for obstructive sleep apnea: preliminary clinical results of a new minimally invasive technique. Otolaryngol Head Neck Surg 2000;122: 100–103

152. Di Girolamo S, Marinelli L, Galli A, Ottaviani F. Retropharyngeal lipoma causing sleep apnea syndrome. J Oral Maxillofac Surg 1998;56:1003–1004

153. Dindo D, Müller MK, Weber M, Clavien PA. Obesity in general elective surgery. Lancet 2003;361:2032–2035

154. Dixon JB, Schachter LM, O'Brien PE. Polysomnography before and after weight loss in obese patients with severe sleep apnea. Int J Obes (Lond) 2005;29:1048–1054

155. Djupesland G, Lyberg T, Krogstad O. Cephalometric analysis and surgical treatment of patients with obstructive sleep apnea syndrome. Acta Otolaryngol 1987;103: 551–557

156. Djupesland G, Schrader H, Lyberg T, Refsum H, Lilleas F, Godtlibsen OB. Palato-pharyngoglossoplasty in the treatment of patients with obstructive sleep apnea. Acta Otolaryngol 1992;112(Suppl 492): 50–54

157. Djupesland G, Skatvedt O, Borgersen K. Dichtomous physiological effects of noctur-nal external nasal dilution in heavy snorers: the answer to a rhinologic controversy? Am J Rhinol 2001;15:95–103

158. Dobrowski JM, Ahmed M. Positive airway pressure for obstructive sleep apnea. In: Fairbanks DNF, Mickelson SA, Woodson BT (Eds) Snoring and obstructive sleep apnea, 3rd edn. Lippincott Williams & Wilkins, Philadelphia, 2002: pp 95–106

159. Donnelly LF, Surdulescu V, Chini BA, Casper KA, Poe SA, Amin RS. Upper airway motion depicted at cine MR imaging performed during sleep: comparison between young patients with and those without obstructive sleep apnea. Radiology 2003;227: 239–245

160. Dorion D, Praud JP. The larynx and neonatal apneas. Otolaryngol Head Neck Surg 2003;128:463–469

161. Dorn M, Pirsig W, Verse T. Management of patients with severe obstructive sleep apnea following rhinosurgical interventions. A pilot study [in German]. HNO 2001;49: 642–645

162. Drager LF, Bortolotto LA, Figueiredo AC, Krieger EM, Lorenzi GF. Effects of con-tinuous positive airway pressure on early signs of atherosclerosis in obstructive sleep apnea. Am J Respir Crit Care Med 2007;176:706–712

163. Dreher A, de la Chaux R, Grevers G, Kastenbauer E. Influence of nasal obstruction on sleep-associated breathing disorders [in German]. Laryngorhinootologie 1999; 78:313–317

164. Ducic Y, Marsan J, Olberg B, Marsan S, Maclachlan L, Lamothe A. Comparison of laser-assisted uvulopalatopharyngoplasty to electrocautery-assisted uvulopalatophar-yngoplasty: a clinical and pathological correlation in an animal model. J Otolaryngol 1996;25: 234–238

165. Dündar A, Özünlü A, Sahan M, Özgen F. Lingual tonsil hypertrophy producing obstructive sleep apnea. Laryngoscope 1996;106:1167–1169

166. Dyken ME, Sommers VK, Yamada T, Ren ZY, Zimmerman MB. Investigating the relationship between stroke and obstructive sleep apnea. Stroke 1996;27:401–407

167. Elasfour A, Miyazaki S, Itasaka Y, Yamakawa K, Ishikawa K, Togawa K. Evaluation of uvulopalatopharyngoplasty in treatment of obstructive sleep apnea syndrome. Acta Otolaryngol 1998;118(Suppl 537): 52–56

168. Ellis PDM, Williams JE, Shneerson JM. Surgical relief of snoring due to palatal flut-ter: a preliminary report. Ann R Coll Surg Engl 1993;75:286–290

169. Ellis PDM, Harris MLL, Williams JE, Shneerson JM. The relief of snoring by nasal surgery. Clin Otolaryngol 1992;17:525–527

170. Ellis PDM. Laser palatoplasty for snoring due to palatal flutter: a further report. Clin Otolaryngol 1994;19:350–351

171. Elsherif I, Hussein SN. The effect of nasal surgery in snoring. Am J Rhinol 1998; 12:77–79

172. Elwood ET, Burstein FD, Graham L, Williams JK, Paschal M. Midface distraction to alleviate upper airway obstruction in achondroplastic dwarfs. Cleft Palate Craniofac J 2003;40: 100–103

173. Emery BE, Flexon PB. Radiofrequency volumetric tissue reduction of the soft palate: a new treatment for snoring. Laryngoscope 2000;110:1092–1098

174. Ericsson E, Graf J, Hultcrantz E. Pediatric tonsillotomy with radiofrequency technique: long-term follow-up. Laryngoscope 2006;116:1851–1857

175. Ericsson E, Hultcrantz E. Tonsil surgery in youths: good results with a less invasive method. Laryngoscope 2007;117:654–661

176. Ericsson E, Ledin T, Hultcrantz E. Long-term improvement of quality of life as a result of tonsillotomy (with radiofrequency technique) and tonsillectomy in youths. Laryngoscope 2007;117:1272–1279

177. Ericsson E, Wadsby M, Hultcrantz E. Pre-surgical child behavior ratings and pain management after two different techniques of tonsil surgery. Int J Pediatr Otorhinolaryngol 2006;70:1749–1758

178. Erler T, Paditz E. Obstructive sleep apnea syndrome in children: a state-of-the-art review. Treat Respir Med 2004;43:107–122

179. Esteller E, Matino E, Segarra F, Sanz JJ, Adema JM, Estivill E. Adverse effects of continuous positive airway pressure therapy and its relation to the nose [in Spanish]. Acta Otorhinolaringologica Espanola 2004;55:17–22

180. Eun YG, Kim SW, Kwon KH, Byun JY, Lee KH. Single-session radiofrequency tongue base reduction combined with uvulopalatopharyngoplasty for obstructive sleep apnea syndrome. Eur Arch Otorhinolaryngol 2008;265:1495–1500

181. Faber CE, Grymer L, Norregaard O, Hilberg O. Flextube refelectometry for localization of upper airway narrowing – a preliminary study in models and awake subjects. Resp Med 2001;95:639–648

182. Faber CE, Grymer L. Available techniques for objective assessment of upper airway narrowing in snoring and sleep apnea. Sleep Breath 2003;7:77–86

183. Faber CE, Hilberg O, Jensen FT, Norregaard O, Grymer L. Flextube refelectometry for determination of sites of upper airway narrowing in sleeping obstructive sleep apnoea patients. Resp Med 2001;95:639–648

184. Fairbanks DN. Operative techniques of uvulopalatopharyngoplasty. Ear Nose Throat J 1999;78:846–850

185. Fairbanks DN. Predicting the effect of nasal surgery on snoring with a simple test. Ear Nose Throat J 1990;69:847

186. Fairbanks DNF, Fujita S. Snoring and obstructive sleep apnea, 2nd edn. Raven, New York, 1994

187. Fairbanks DNF. Effect of nasal surgery on snoring. South Med J 1985;78: 268–270

188. Fairbanks DNF. Snoring: surgical vs. nonsurgical management. Laryngoscope 1984; 94:1188–1192

189. Farrar J, Ryan J, Oliver E, Gillespie MB. Radiofrequency ablation for the treatment of obstructive sleep apnea: a meta-analysis. Laryngoscope 2008;118:1878–1883

190. Fauroux B, Pigeot J, Polkey MI, Roger G, Boule M, Clement A, Lofaso F. Chronic stridor caused by laryngomalacia in children: work of breathing and effects of noninvasive ventilatory assistance. Am J Respir Crit Care Med 2001;164:1874–1878

191. Faye-Lund H, Djupesland G, Lyberg T. Glossopexia – evaluation of a new surgical method for treating obstructive sleep apnea syndrome. Acta Otolaryngol 1992;112(Suppl 492): 46–49

192. Ferguson KA, Heighway H, Ruby RRF. A randomized trial of laser-assisted uvulo-palatoplasty in the treatment of mild obstructive sleep apnea. Am J Respir Crit Care Med 2003; 167:15–19

193. Ferguson KA, Ono T, Lowe AA, Keenan SP, Fleetham JA. A randomized crossover study of an oral appliance vs nasal-continuous positive airway pressure in the treatment of mild-moderate obstructive sleep apnea. Chest 1996;109:1269–1275

194. Ferguson M, Smith TL, Zanation AM, Yarbrough WG. Radiofrequency tissue volume reduction. Multilesion vs single-lesion treatments for snoring. Arch Otolaryngol Head Neck Surg 2001;127:312–318

195. Fernandez AZ Jr, Demaria EJ, Tichansky DS, Kellum JM, Wolfe LG, Meador J, Sugerman HJ. Multivariate analysis of risk factors for death following gastric bypass for treatment of morbid obesity. Ann Surg 2004;239:698–702

196. Fibbi A, Ameli F, Brocchetti F, Peirano M, Garaventa G, Presta A, Baricalla F. Combined genioglossus advancement (ACMG): inferior sagittal mandibular osteotomy with genioglossus advancement and stabilization with suture in patients with OSAS. Preliminary clinical results [in Italian]. Acta Otorhinolaryngol Ital 2002; 22:153–157

197. Finkelstein Y, Shapiro-Feinberg M, Stein G, Ophir D. Uvulopalatopharyngoplasty vs. laser-assisted uvulopalatoplasty. Arch Otolaryngol Head Neck Surg 1997;123: 265–276

198. Finkelstein Y, Stein G, Ophir D, Berger R, Berger G. Laser-assisted uvulopalatoplasty for the management of obstructive sleep apnea. Myths and facts. Arch Otolaryngol Head Neck Surg 2002;128:429–434

199. Finkelstein Y, Talmi Y, Zohar Y. Readaptation of the velopharyngeal valve following the uvulopalatopharyngoplasty operation. Plast Reconstr Surg 1988;82:20–30

200. Fischer J, Mayer G, Hermann J, Riemann D, Sitter H. Untersuchungsstandards im medizinischen Zentrum [in German]. Somnologie 2001;5(Suppl 3): 41–59

201. Fischer Y, Khan M, Mann WJ. Multilevel temperature-controlled radiofrequency therapy of soft palate, base of tongue, and tonsils in adults with obstructive sleep apnea. Laryngoscope 2003;113:1786–1791

202. Fjermedal O, Saunte C, Pedersen S. Septoplasty and/or submucosal resection? 5 years nasal septum operations. J Laryngol Otol 1988;102:796–798

203. Fletcher EC. Recurrence of sleep apnea syndrome following tracheostomy. A shift from obstructive to central apnea. Chest 1989;96:205–209

204. Flum DR, Dellinger EP. Impact of gastric bypass operation on survival: a population-based analysis. J Am Coll Surg 2004;199:543–551

205. Foltán R, Hoffmannová J, Pretl M, Donev F, Vlk M. Genioglossus advancement and hyoid myotomy in treating obstructive sleep apnoea syndrome – a follow-up study. J Craniomaxillofac Surg 2007;35:246–251

206. Fontaine KR, Redden DT, Wang C, Westfall AO, Allison DB. Years of life lost due to obesity. JAMA 2003;289:187–193

207. Francois J, Manaligod JM. Upper airway abnormalities in Canavan disease. Int J Pediatr Otorhinolaryngol 2002;66:303–307

208. Freedman DS, Khan LK, Serdula MK, Galuska DA, Dietz WH. Trends and correlates of class 3 obesity in the United States from 1990 through 2000. JAMA 2002;288:1758–1761

209. Friedman BC, Hendeles-Amitai A, Kozminsky E, Leiberman A, Friger M, Tarasiuk A, Tal A. Adenotonsillectomy improves neurocognitive function in children with obstructive sleep apnea syndrome. Sleep 2003;26:999–1005

210. Friedman M. Response to: "adenotonsillectomy and obstructive sleep apnea in children:a prospective survey. Otolaryngol Head Neck Surg 2007;137:527; author reply 527–528

211. Friedman M, Duggal P, Joseph NJ. Revision uvulopalatoplasty by Z-palatoplasty. Otolaryngol Head Neck Surg 2007;136:638–643

212. Friedman M, Ibrahim H, Lee G, Joseph NJ. Combined uvulopalatopharyngoplasty and radiofrequency tongue base reduction for treatment of obstructive sleep apnea/hypopnea syndrome. Otolaryngol Head Neck Surg 2003;129:611–621

213. Friedman M, Ibrahim HZ, Vidyasagar R, Pomeranz J, Joseph NJ. Z-palatoplasty (ZPP): a technique for patients without tonsils. Otolaryngol Head Neck Surg 2004;131:89–100

214. Friedman M, Lin HC, Gurpinar B, Joseph NJ. Minimally invasive single-stage multi-level treatment for obstructive sleep apnea/hypopnea syndrome. Laryngoscope 2007;117:1859–1863

215. Friedman M, LoSavio P, Ibrahim H, Ramakrishnan V. Radiofrequency tonsil reduction: safety, morbidity, and efficacy. Laryngoscope 2003;113:882–887

216. Friedman M, Schalch P, Joseph NJ. Palatal stiffening after failed uvulopalatopharyngoplasty with the pillar implant system. Laryngoscope 2006;116:1956–1961

217. Friedman M, Schalch P, Lin HC, Kakodkar KA, Joseph NJ, Mazloom N. Palatal implants for the treatment of snoring and obstructive sleep apnea/hypopnea syndrome. Otolaryngol Head Neck Surg 2008;138:209–216

218. Friedman M, Soans R, Gurpinar B, Lin HC, Joseph N. Evaluation of submucosal minimally invasive lingual excision technique for treatment of obstructive sleep apnea/hypopnea syndrome. Otolaryngol Head Neck Surg 2008;139:378–384

219. Friedman M, Soans R, Joseph N, Kakadkar S, Friedman J. The effect of multilevel upper airway surgery on continuous positive airway pressure therapy in obstructive sleep apnea/hypopnea syndrome. Laryngoscope 2009;119:193–196

220. Friedman M, Tanyeri H, La Rosa M, Landsberg R, Vaidyanathan K, Pieri S, Caldarelli D. Clinical predictors of obstructive sleep apnea. Laryngoscope. 1999;109: 1901–1907

221. Friedman M, Tanyeri H, Lim JW, Landsberg R, Vaidyanathan K, Caldarelli D. Effect of improved nasal breathing on obstructive sleep apnea. Otolaryngol Head Neck Surg 2000;122:71–74

222. Friedman M, Vidyasagar R, Bliznikas D, Joseph NJ. Patient selection and efficacy of pillar implant technique for treatment of snoring and obstructive sleep apnea/hypopnea syndrome. Otolaryngol Head Neck Surg 2006;134:187–196

223. Fritscher LG, Canani S, Mottin CC, Fritscher CC, Berleze D, Chapman K, Chatkin JM. Bariatric surgery in the treatment of obstructive sleep apnea in morbidly obese patients. Respiration 2007;74:647–652

224. Fujita S, Conway W, Zorick F. Surgical correction of anatomic abnormalities in obstructive sleep apnea syndrome: uvulopalatopharyngoplasty. Otolaryngol Head Neck Surg 1981;89: 923–934

225. Fujita S, Woodson BT, Clark JL, Wittig R. Laser midline glossectomy as a treatment for the obstructive sleep apnea. Laryngoscope 1991;101:805–809

226. Fujita S. Obstructive sleep apnea syndrome: pathophysiology, upper airway evaluation and surgical treatment. Ear Nose Throat J 1993;72:67–72

227. Fujita S. Pharyngeal surgery for obstructive sleep apnea and snoring. In: Fairbanks DNF (Ed) Snoring and obstructive sleep apnea. Raven, New York, 1987: pp 101–128

228. Fuso L, Maiolo C, Tramaglino LM, Benedetto RT, Russo AR, Spadaro S, Pagliari G. Orolaryngeal sarcoidosis presenting as obstructive sleep apnoea. Sarcoidosis Vasc Diffuse Lung Dis 2001;18:85–90

229. Garetz SL. Behavior, cognition, and quality of life after adenotonsillectomy for pediatric sleep-disordered breathing: summary of the literature. Otolaryngol Head Neck Surg 2008; 138(1 Suppl): S19-S26

230. George CF. Sleep apnea, alertness, and motor vehicle crashes. Am J Respir Crit Care Med 2007;176:954–956

231. Giannoni C, Sulek M, Friedman EM, Duncan NO. Acquired nasopharyngeal stenosis: a warning and a review. Arch Otolaryngol Head Neck Surg 1998;124:163–167

232. Gillespie MB, Flint PW, Smith PL, Eisele DW, Schwartz AR. Diagnosis and treatment of obstructive sleep apnea of the larynx. Arch Otolaryngol Head Neck Surg 1995;121: 335–339

233. Goessler UR, Hein G, Verse T, Stuck BA, Hörmann K, Maurer JT. Soft palate implants as a minimally invasive treatment for mild to moderate obstructive sleep apnea. Acta Otolaryngol 2007;127:527–531

234. Goh YH, Lim KA. Modified maxillomandibular advancement for the treatment of obstructive sleep apnea: a preliminary report. Laryngoscope 2003;113:1577–1582

235. Goh YH, Mark I, Fee WE Jr. Quality of life 17 to 20 years after uvulopalatopharyngoplasty. Laryngoscope 2007;117:503–506

236. Goldstein SJ, Shprintzen RJ, Wu RH, Thorpy MJ, Haham SY, Marion R, Sher AE, Saenger P. Achondroplasia and obstructive sleep apnea: correction of apnea and abnormal sleep-entrained growth hormone release by tracheostomy. Birth Defects Orig Artic Ser 1985;21: 93–101

237. Golz A, Goldenberg D, Netzer A, Westerman ST, Joachims HZ. Epiglottic carcinoma presenting as obstructive sleep apnea. J Otolaryngol 2001;30:58–59

238. Gong W, Wang E, Zhang B, Da J. A retropharyngeal lipoma causing obstructive sleep apnea in a child. J Clin Sleep Med 2006;2:328–329

239. Görür K, Döven O, Ünal M, Akkus N, Özcan C. Preoperative and postoperative cardiac and clinical findings in patients with adenotonsillar hypertrophy. Int J Pediatr Otorhinolaryngol 2001;59:41–46

240. Gozal D, Crabtree VM, Sans Capdevila O, Witcher LA, Kheirandish-Gozal L. C-reactive protein, obstructive sleep apnea, and cognitive dysfunction in school-aged children. Am J Respir Crit Care Med 2007;176:188–193

241. Griffen WO Jr, Bivins BA, Bell RM. The decline and fall of the jejunoileal bypass. Surg Gynecol Obstet 1983;157:301–308

242. Gronau S, Fischer Y. Tonsillotomy [in German]. Laryngorhinootologie 2005;84: 685–690

243. Grontved A, Jorgensen K, Petersen SV. Results of uvulopalatopharyngoplasty in snoring. Acta Otolaryngol (Stockh) 1992; (Suppl 492): 11–14

244. Gross ND, Cohen JI, Andersen PE, Wax MK. Defatting tracheostomy in morbidly obese patients. Laryngoscope 2002;112:1940–1944

245. Grymer LF, Illum P, Hilberg O. Bilateral inferior turbinoplasty in chronic nasal obstruction. Rhinol 1996;34:50–53

246. Guardiano S, Scott JA, Ware JC, Schechner SA. The longterm results of gastric bypass on indexes of sleep apnea. Chest 2003;124:1615–1619

247. Guilleminault C, Korobkin R, Winkle R. A review of 50 children with obstructive sleep apnea syndrome. Lung 1981;159:275–287

248. Guilleminault C, Lee JH, Chan A. Pediatric obstructive sleep apnea syndrome. Arch Pediatr Adolesc Med 2005;159:775–785

249. Guilleminault C, Li KK, Khramtsov A, Pelayo R, Martinez S. Sleep disordered breathing: surgical outcomes in prepubertal children. Laryngoscope 2004;114:132–137

250. Guilleminault C, Li KK, Quo S, Inouye RN. A prospective study on the surgical outcomes of children with sleep-disordered breathing. Sleep 2004;27:95–100

251. Guilleminault C, Partinen M, Praud JP, Quera-Salva MA, Powell N, Riley R. Morphometric facial changes and obstructive sleep apnea in adolescents. J Pediatr 1989;114:997–999

252. Guilleminault C, Simmons FB, Motta J, Cummiskey J, Rosekind M, Schroeder JS, Dement WC. Obstructive sleep apnea syndrome and tracheostomy. Arch Intern Med 1981;141: 985–988

253. Guilleminault C, van den Hoed J, Mitler MM. The sleep apnea syndrome and its symptoms. In: Guilleminault C, Dement WC (Eds). Sleep apnea syndromes. Alan R Liss, New York, 1978, pp 1–12

254. Guimaraes CV, Kalra M, Donnelly LF, Shott SR, Fitz K, Singla S, Amin RS. The frequency of lingual tonsil enlargement in obese children. AJR Am J Roentgenol 2008;190:973–975

255. Gupta RM, Parvizi J, Hanssen AD, Gay PC. Postoperative complications in patients with obstructive sleep apnea syndrome undergoing hip or knee replacement: a case-control study. Mayo Clin Proc 2001;76:897–905

256. Haapaniemi JJ, Laurikainen EA, Halme P, Antila J. Long-term results of tracheostomy for severe obstructive sleep apnea syndrome. ORL J Otorhinolaryngol Relat Spec 2001;63: 131–136

257. Haavisto L, Suonpaa J. Complications of uvulopalatoplasty. Clin Otolaryngol 1994;19: 243–247

258. Haentjens P, Van Meerhaeghe A, Moscariello A, De Weerdt S, Poppe K, Dupont A, Velkeniers B. The impact of continuous positive airway pressure on blood pressure in patients with obstructive sleep apnea syndrome: evidence from a meta-analysis of placebo-controlled randomized trials. Arch Intern Med 2007;167:757–764

259. Hagert B, Wahren LK, Wikblad K, Ödkvist L. Patients´and cohabitants reports on snoring and daytime sleepiness, 1–8 years after surgical treatment of snoring. ORL J Otolaryngol Relat Spec 1999;61:19–24

260. Haines KL, Nelson LG, Gonzalez R, Torrella T, Martin T, Kandil A, Dragotti R, Anderson WM, Gallagher SF, Murr MM. Objective evidence that bariatric surgery improves obesity-related obstructive sleep apnea. Surgery 2007;141:354–358

261. Halbower AC, Ishman SL, McGinley BM. Childhood obstructive sleep-disordered breathing. A clinical update and discussion of technological innovations and challenges. Chest 2007;132:2030–2041

262. Han F, Song W, Zhang L, Dong X, He Q. Influence of UPPP surgery on tolerance to subsequent continuous positive airway pressure in patients with OSAHS. Sleep Breath 2006; 10:37–42

263. Hanada T, Furuta S, Tateyama T, Uchizono A, Seki D, Ohyama M. Laser-assisted uvulopalatoplasty with Nd:YAG laser for sleep disorders. Laryngoscope 1996;106: 1531–1533

264. Harada K, Higashinakagawa M, Omura K. Mandibular lengthening by distraction osteogenesis for treatment of obstructive sleep apnea syndrome: a case report. J Craniomand Prac 2003;21:61–67

265. Haraldsson PO, Carenfelt C, Lysdahl M, Tingvall C. Does uvulopalatopharyngoplasty inhibit automobile accidents? Laryngoscope 1995;105:657–661

266. Haraldsson PO, Carenfelt C, Persson HE, Sachs C, Tornros J. Simulated long-term driving performance before and after uvulopalatopharyngoplasty. ORL J Otorhinolaryngol Relat Spec 1991;53:106–110

267. Harper J, Madan AK, Ternovits CA, Tichansky DS. What happens to patients who do not follow-up after bariatric surgery? Am Surg 2007;73:181–184

268. Hartenbaum N, Collop N, Rosen IM, Phillips B, George CF, Rowley JA, Freedman N, Weaver TE, Gurubhagavatula I, Strohl K, Leaman HM, Moffitt GL; American College of Chest Physicians; American College of Occupational and Environmental Medicine; National Sleep Foundation. Sleep apnea and commercial motor vehicle operators: statement from the joint task force of the American College of Chest Physicians, the American College of Occupational and Environmental Medicine, and the National Sleep Foundation. Chest 2006;130:902–905

269. Haslam DW, James WPT. Obesity. Lancet 2005;366:1197–1209

270. Hassid S, Afrapoli AH, Decaaestecker C, Choufani G. UPPP for snoring: long-term results and patient satisfaction. Acta Otorhinolaryngol Belg 2002;56:157–162

271. He J, Kryger MH, Zorick FJ, Conway W, Roth T. Mortality and apnea index in obstructive sleep apnea: experience in 385 male patients. Chest 1988;94:9–14

272. Heimer D, Scharf S, Liebermann A, Lavie P. Sleep apnoea syndrome treated by repair of deviated nasal septum. Chest 1983;84:184–185

273. Hein H, Magnussen H. Wie steht es um die medikamentöse Therapie bei schlafbezogenen Atmungsstörungen [in German]? Somnologie 1998;2:77–88

274. Helling K, Abrams J, Bertram WK, Hohner S, Scherer H. Laser tonsillectomy in tonsillar hyperplasia of early childhood [in German]. HNO 2002;50:470–478

275. Hendler BH, Costello BJ, Silverstein K, Yen D, Goldberg A. A protocol for uvulopalatoplasty, mortised genioplasty, and maxillomandibular advancement in patients with obstructive sleep apnea: an analysis of 40 cases. J Oral Maxillofac Surg 2001; 59:892–897

276. Herlihy JP, Whitlock WL, Dietrich RA, Shaw T. Sleep apnea syndrome after irradiation of the neck. Arch Otolaryngol Head Neck Surg 1989;115:1467–1469

277. Hessel NS, de Vries N. Diagnostic work up of socially unacceptable snoring. I. History or sleep registration. Eur Arch Otorhinolaryngol 2002;259:154–157

278. Hessel NS, de Vries N. Diagnostic work-up of socially unacceptable snoring. II. Sleep endoscopy. Eur Arch Otorhinolaryngol 2002;259:158–161

279. Hessel NS, de Vries N. Increase of the apnoea-hypopnoea index after uvulopalatopharyngoplasty: analyis of failure. Clin Otolaryngol 2004;29:682–685

280. Hewitt RJ, Dasgupta A, Singh A, Dutta C, Kotecha BT. Is sleep nasendoscopy a valuable adjunct to clinical examination in the evaluation of upper airway obstruction? Eur Arch Otorhinolaryngol 2009;266:691–697

281. Hibbert J, Stell P. Adenoidectomy. An evaluation of the indications. Arch Dis Child 1978; 53:910–911

282. Hicklin LA, Tostevin P, Dasan S. Retrospective survey of long-term results and patient satisfaction with uvulopalatopharyngoplasty for snoring. J Laryngol Otol 2000;114: 675–681

283. Ho WK, Wei WI, Chung KF. Managing disturbing snoring with palatal implants: a pilot study. Arch Otolaryngol Head Neck Surg 2004;130:753–758

284. Hochban W, Conradt R, Brandenburg U, Heitmann J, Peter JH. Surgical maxillofacial treatment of obstructive sleep apnea. Plast Reconstr Surg 1997;99:619–626

285. Hockstein NG, Anderson TA, Moonis G, Gustafson KS, Mirza N. Retropharyngeal lipoma causing obstructive sleep apnea: case report including five-year follow-up. Laryngoscope 2002;112:1603–1605

286. Hoffstein V, Mateika S, Metes A. Effect of nasal dilation on snoring and apneas during different stages of sleep. Sleep 1993;16:360–365

287. Hoffstein V, Taylor R. Rapid development of obstructive sleep apnea following hemidiaphragmatic and unilateral vocal cord paralysis as a complication of mediastinal surgery. Chest 1985;88:145–147

288. Hoffstein V. Snoring. Chest 1996;109:201–222

289. Hofmann T, Schwantzer G, Reckenzaun E, Koch H, Wolf G. Radiofrequency tissue volume reduction of the soft palate and UPPP in the treatment of snoring. Eur Arch Otorhinolaryngol 2006;263:164–170

290. Holinger PH, Johnson KC, Schiller F. Congenital anomalies of the larynx. Ann Otol Rhinol Laryngol 1954;63:581–606

291. Hoolsema EM. Cautery-assisted palatal stiffening operation and nasalance of speech. Ann Otol Rhinol Laryngol 1999;108:705–707

292. Hörmann K, Baisch A. The hyoid suspension. Laryngoscope 2004;114:1677–1679

293. Hörmann K, Erhardt T, Hirth K, Maurer JT. Modified uvula flap in therapy of sleep-related breathing disorders [in German]. HNO 2001;49:361–366

294. Hörmann K, Hirth K, Erhardt T, Maurer JT, Verse T. Modified hyoid suspension for therapy of sleep related breathing disorders. operative technique and complications [in German]. Laryngorhinootologie 2001;80:517–521

295. Hörmann K, Maurer JT, Baisch A. Snoring/sleep apnea–surgically curable [in German]. HNO 2004;52:807–813

296. Hörmann K, Maurer JT. Klinische Untersuchungen (Nase, Nasennebenhöhlen, Naso-, Oro-, Hypopharynx, Larynx) [in German]. In: Schulz H (Ed) Kompendium Schlafmedizin. Ecomed, Landsberg/Lech, 1997: pp 1–3; XIV – 7.1.2

297. Houghton DJ, Camilleri AE, Stone P. Adult obstructive sleep apnoea syndrome and tonsillectomy. J Laryngol Otol 1997;111:829–832

298. Hsieh TH, Fang TJ, Li HY, Lee SW. Simultaneous midline laser glossectomy with palatopharyngeal surgery for obstructive sleep apnoea syndrome. Int J Clin Pract 2005;59:501–503

299. Hsu PP, Brett RH. Multiple level pharyngeal surgery for obstructive sleep apnoea. Singapore Med J 2001;42:160–164

300. Huang MHS, Lee ST, Rajendran K. Structure of the musculus uvulae: functional and surgical implications of an anatomic study. Cleft Palate Craniofac J 1997;34:466–474

301. Huang TW, Cheng PW. Microdebrider-assisted extended uvulopalatoplasty: an effective and safe technique for selected patients with obstructive sleep apnea syndrome. Arch Otolaryngol Head Neck Surg 2008;134:141–145

302. Huber K, Sadick H, Maurer JT, Hörmann K, Hammerschmitt N. Tonsillotomy with the argon-supported monopolar needle–first clinical results [in German]. Laryngorhinootologie 2005;84:671–675

303. Hudgel DW, Harasick T, Katy RL, Witt WJ, Abelson TI. Uvulopalatopharyngoplasty in obstructive sleep apnea. Value of preoperative localization of site of upper airway narrowing during sleep. Am Rev Respir Dis 1991;143:942–946

304. Hudgel DW. Variable site of airway narrowing among obstructive sleep apnea patients. J Appl Physiol 1986;61:1403–1409

305. Hukins C, Mitchell IC, Hillman DR. Radiofrequency tissue volume reduction of the soft palate in simple snoring. Arch Otolaryngol Head Neck Surg 2000;126:602–606

306. Hultcrantz E, Ericsson E. Pediatric tonsillotomy with the radiofrequency technique: less morbidity and pain. Laryngoscope 2004;114:871–877

307. Hultcrantz E, Johansson K, Bengtson H. The effect of uvulopalatopharyngoplasty without tonsillectomy using local anaesthesia: a prospective long-term follow-up. J Laryngol Otol 1999;113:542–547

308. Hultcrantz E, Linder A, Markström A. Long-term effects of intracapsular partial tonsillectomy (tonsillotomy) compared with full tonsillectomy. Int J Pediatr Otorhinolaryngol 2005; 69:463–469

309. Hultcrantz E, Linder A, Markström A. Tonsillectomy or tonsillotomy? – A randomized study comparing postoperative pain and long-term effects. Int J Pediatr Otorhinolaryngol 1999;51:171–176

310. Hultcrantz E, Svanholm H. Down syndrome and sleep apnea – a therapeutic challenge. Int J Pediatr Otorhinolaryngol 1991;21:263–268

311. Hung J, Whitford EG, Parsons RW, Hillman DR. Association of sleep apnoea with myocardial infarction in men. Lancet 1990;336:261–264

312. Hüttenbrink KB, Wrede H, Lagemann S, Schleicher E, Hummel T. Endonasal measurement of mucociliary clearance at various locations in the nose: a new diagnostic tool for nasal function [in German]? Laryngorhinootologie 2006;85:24–31

313. Ievers-Landis CE, Redline S. Pediatric sleep apnea: implications of the epidemic of childhood overweight. Am J Respir Crit Care Med 2007;175:436–441

314. Ikematsu T. Study of snoring. Therapy [in Japanese]. J Jpn Otol Rhinol Laryngol Soc 1964; 64:434–435

315. Ilgen F. Laser-assisted tonsillotomy in children with obstructive sleep apnea and adenotonsillary hyperplasia–experiences as an outpatient procedure [in German]. Laryngorhinootologie 2005;84:665–670

316. Illum P. Septoplasty and compensatory inferior turbinate hypertrophy: long-term results after randomized turbinoplasty. Eur Arch Otorhinolaryngol 1997;254 (Suppl 1):S89–S92

317. Iseri M, Balcioglu O. Radiofrequency versus injection snoreplasty in simple snoring. Otolaryngol Head Neck Surg 2005;133:224–228

318. Israel Y, Cervantes O, Abrahão M, Ceccon FP, Marques Filho MF, Nascimento LA, Zonato AI, Tufik S. Obstructive sleep apnea in patients undergoing supracricoid horizontal or frontolateral vertical partial laryngectomy. Otolaryngol Head Neck Surg 2006;135: 911–916

319. Izadi K, Yellon R, Mandell DL, Smith M, Song SY, Bidic S, Bradley JP. Correction of upper airway obstruction in the newborn with internal mandibular distraction osteogenesis. J Craniofac Surg 2003;14:493–499

320. Jacobowitz O. Palatal and tongue base surgery for surgical treatment of obstructive sleep apnea: a prospective study. Otolaryngol Head Neck Surg 2006;135:258–264

321. Jäger L, Günther E, Gauger J, Nitz W, Kastenbauer E, Reiser M. Functional MRI of the pharynx in obstructive sleep apnea using rapid 2D FLASH sequences [in German]. Radiologe 1996;36:245–253

322. Jahnke K. Laser-tonsillotomy, state of the art and open questions [in German]. Laryngorhinootologie 2005;84:651–652

323. Jain A, Sahni JK. Polysomnographic studies in children undergoing adenoidectomy and/or tonsillectomy. J Laryngol Otol 2002;116:711–715

324. Jakubikova J, Zitnan D, Batorova A. An unusual reason for obstructive sleep apnea in a boy with hemophilia B: supraglottic papilloma. Int J Pediatr Otorhinolaryngol 1996;34:165–169

325. James PT, Rigby N, Leach R. The obesity epidemic, metabolic syndrome and future prevention strategies. Eur J Cardiovasc Prev Rehabil 2004;11:3–8

326. Janson C, Gislason T, Bengtsson H, Eriksson G, Lindberg E, Lindholm CE, Hultcrantz E, Hetta J, Boman G. Long-term follow-up of patients with obstructive sleep apnea treated with uvulopalatopharyngoplasty. Arch Otolaryngol Head Neck Surg 1997;123:257–262

327. Janson C, Hillerdal G, Larsson L, Hultcrantz E, Lindholm CE, Bengtsson H, Hetta J. Excessive daytime sleepiness and fatigue in nonapnoeic snorers: improvement after UPPP. Eur Respir J 1994;7:845–849

328. Janson C, Nöges E, Svedberg-Brandt S, Lindberg E. What characterizes patients who are unable to tolerate continuous positive airway pressure (CPAP) treatment? Resp Med 2000; 94:145–149

329. Jecker P, Orloff LA, Mann WJ. Extraesophageal reflux and upper aerodigestive tract diseases. ORL J Otorhinolaryngol Relat Spec 2005;67:185–191

330. Jenkinson C, Davies RJO, Stradling JR. Comparison of therapeutic and subtherapeutic nasal continuous positive airway pressure for obstructive sleep apneoea: a randomised prospective parallel trial. Lancet 1999;353:2100–2105

331. Jennum P, Hein HO, Suadicani P, Gyntelberg F. Cardiovascular risk factors in snorers. A cross sectional study of 3323 men aged 54 to 74 years: the Copenhagen Mal Study. Chest 1992;102:1371–1376

332. Johal A, Hector MP, Battagel JM, Kotecha BT. Impact of sleep nasendoscopy on the outcome of mandibular advancement splint therapy in subjects with sleep-related breathing disorders. J Laryngol Otol 2007;121:668–675

333. Johnson JT, Braun TW. Preoperative, intraoperative, and postoperative management of patients with obstructive sleep apnea syndrome. Otolaryngol Clin North Am 1998;31: 1025–1030

334. Johnson NT, Chinn J. Uvulopalatopharyngoplasty and inferior sagittal mandibular osteotomy with genioglossus advancement for treatment of obstructive sleep apnea. Chest 1994;105: 278–283

335. Jokic R, Klimaszewski A, Crossley M, Sridhar G, Fitzpatrick MF. Positional treatment vs continuous positive airway pressure in patients with positional obstructive sleep apnea syndrome. Chest 1999;115:771–781

336. Kacker A, Honrado C, Martin D, Ward R. Tongue reduction in Beckwith-Wiedemann syndrome. Int J Pediatr Otorhinolaryngol 2000;53:1–7

337. Kalarchian MA, Marcus MD, Levine MD Courcoulas AP, Pilkonis PA, Ringham RM, Soulakova JN, Weissfeld LA, Rofey DL. Psychiatric disorders among bariatric surgery candidates: relationship to obesity and functional health status. Am J Psychiatry 2007;164:328–334

338. Kaluskar SK, Kaul GH. Long-term results of KTP/532 laser uvulopalatopharyngoplasty. Rev Laryngol Otol Rhinol 2000;121:59–62

339. Kamami YV. Laser CO_2 for snoring: preliminary results. Acta Otorhinolaryngol Belg 1990;44:451–456

340. Kamami YV. Outpatient treatment of snoring and sleep apnea syndrome with CO_2 laser: laser-assisted uvulopalatoplasty. In: Clayman L (Ed) Lasers in maxillofacial surgery and dentistry. Thieme, New York, 1998: pp 111–116

341. Kania RE, Schmitt E, Petelle B, Meyer B. Radiofrequency soft palate procedure in snoring: influence of energy delivered. Otolaryngol Head Neck Surg 2004;130: 67–72

342. Kapas L, Hong L, Cady AB, Opp MR, Postlethwaite AE, Seyer JM, Krueger JM. Somnogenic, pyrogenic, and anorectic activities of tumor necrosis factor-a and TNFa fragments. Am J Physiol 1992;263:708–715

343. Karakasis DT, Michaelides CM, Tsara V. Mandibular distraction combined with tongue-base traction for treatment of obstructive sleep apnea syndrome. Plast Reconstr Surg 2001;108:1673–1676
344. Katsantonis GP, Friedman WH, Krebs FJ, Walsh JK. Nasopharyngeal complications following uvulopalatopharyngoplasty. Laryngoscope 1987;97:309–314
345. Katsantonis GP. Limitations, pitfalls, and risk management in uvulopalatopharyngoplasty. In Fairbanks DNF, Fujita S (Eds) Snoring and obstructive sleep apnea, 2 edn. Raven, New York, 1994; 147–162
346. Kavey NB, Whyte J, Blitzer A, Gidro-Frank S. Sleep-related laryngeal obstruction presenting as snoring or sleep apnea. Laryngoscope 1989;99:851–854
347. Kawano K, Usui N, Kanazawa H, Hara I. Changes in nasal and oral respiratory resistance before and after uvulopalatopharyngoplasty. Acta Otolaryngol 1996; (Suppl 523): 236–238
348. Kaya N. Sectioning the hyoid bone as a therapeutic approach for obstructive sleep apnea. Sleep 1984;7:77–78
349. Keenan SP, Burt H, Ryan CF, Fleetham JA. Long-term survival of patients with obstructive sleep apnea treated by uvulopalatopharyngoplasty or nasal CPAP. Chest 1994;105:155–159
350. Kern RC, Kutler DI, Reid KJ, Conley DB, Herzon GD, Zee P. Laser-assisted uvulopalatoplasty and tonsillectomy for the management of obstructive sleep apnea syndrome. Laryngoscope 2003;113:1175–1181
351. Kerr P, Millar T, Buckle P, Kryger M. The importance of nasal resistance in obstructive sleep apnea syndrome. J Otolaryngol 1992;21:189–195
352. Kerschner JE, Lynch JB, Kleiner H, Flanary VA, Rice TB. Uvulopalatopharyngoplasty with tonsillectomy and adenoidectomy as a treatment for obstructive sleep apnea in neurologically impaired children. Int J Pediatr Otorhinolaryngol 2002;62:229–235
353. Kerstens HC, Tuinzing DB, van der Kwast WA. Temporomandibular joint symptoms in orthognathic surgery. J Craniomaxillofac Surg 1989;17:215–218
354. Kezirian EJ, Goldberg AN. Hypopharyngeal surgery in obstructive sleep apnea: an evidence-based medicine review. Arch Otolaryngol Head Neck Surg 2006; 132:206–213
355. Kezirian EJ, Powell NB, Riley RW, Hester JE. Incidence of complications in radiofrequency treatment of the upper airway. Laryngoscope. 2005;115:1298–1304
356. Kezirian EJ, Weaver EM, Yueh B, Deyo RA, Khuri SF, Daley J, Henderson W. Incidence of serious complications after uvulopalatopharyngoplasty. Laryngoscope 2004;114:450–453
357. Kezirian EJ, Weaver EM, Yueh B, Khuri SF, Daley J, Henderson WG. Risk factors for serious complication after uvulopalatopharyngoplasty. Arch Otolaryngol Head Neck Surg 2006;132:1091–1098
358. Khalifa MS, Kamel RH, Abu Zikry M, Kandil TM. Effect of enlarged adenoids on arterial blood gases in children. J Laryngol Otol 1991;105:436–438
359. Kiely JL, Nolan P, McNicholas WT. Intranasal corticosteroid therapy for obstructive sleep apnea in patients with co-existing rhinitis. Thorax 2004;59:50–55
360. Kim SH, Eisele DW, Smith PL, Schneider H, Schwartz AR. Evaluation of patients with sleep apnea after tracheotomy. Arch Otolaryngol Head Neck Surg 1998;124: 996–1000

361. Kim ST, Choi JH, Jeon HG, Cha HE, Kim DY, Chung YS. Polysomnographic effects of nasal surgery for snoring and obstructive sleep apnea. Acta Otolaryngol 2004; 124:297–300

362. Koempel JA, Solares CA, Koltai PJ. The evolution of tonsil surgery and rethinking the surgical approach to obstructive sleep-disordered breathing in children. J Laryngol Otol 2006;120:993–1000

363. Koltai PJ, Solares CA, Koempel JA, Hirose K, Abelson TI, Krakovitz PR, Chan J, Xu M, Mascha EJ. Intracapsular tonsillar reduction (partial tonsillectomy): reviving a historical procedure for obstructive sleep disordered breathing in children. Otolaryngol Head Neck Surg 2003;129:532–538

364. Konno A, Hoshino T, Togawa K. Influence of upper airway obstruction by enlarged tonsils and adenoids upon recurrent infection of the lower airway in childhood. Laryngoscope 1980;90:1709–1716

365. Kosko JR, Derkay CS. Uvulopalatopharyngoplasty: treatment of obstructive sleep apnea in neurologically impaired pediatric patients. Int J Pediatr Otorhinolaryngol 1995;32:241–246

366. Kotecha B, Paun S, Leong P, Croft CB. Laser-assisted uvulopalatoplasty: an objective evaluation of the technique and results. Clin Otolaryngol 1998;23:354–359

367. Koutsourelakis I, Georgoulopoulos G, Perraki E, Vagiakis E, Roussos C, Zakynthinos SG. Randomised trial of nasal surgery for fixed nasal obstruction in obstructive sleep apnoea. Eur Resp J 2008;31:110–117

368. Krespi YP, Kacker A. Hyoid suspension for obstructive sleep apnea. Oper Techn Otolaryngol Head Neck Surg 2002;13:144–149

369. Krespi YP, Kacker A. Management of nasopharyngeal stenosis after uvulopalatoplasty. Otolaryngol Head Neck Surg 2000;123:692–695

370. Krespi YP, Kacker A. Management of nasopharyngeal stenosis following uvulopalatoplasty. Oper Tech Otolaryngol 2002;13:161–165

371. Krespi YP, Keidar A, Khosh MM, Pearlman SJ, Zammit G. The efficacy of laser-assisted uvulopalatoplasty in the management of obstructive sleep apnea syndrome and upper airway resistance syndrome. Oper Tech Otolaryngol Head Neck Surg 1994;5:235–243

372. Krieg R. Resection der Cartilago quadrangularis septi narium zur Heilung der Scoliosis septi. Medicinisches Correspondez- Blatt Württemberg ärztl Landesvereins Stuttgart 1886; 56:209–213

373. Krishna S, Hughes LF, Lin SY. Postoperative hemorrhage with nonsteroidal anti-inflammatory drug use after tonsillectomy. Arch Otolaryngol Head Neck Surg 2003;129:1086–1089

374. Kubo I. Ueber die eigentliche Ursprungsstelle und die Radikaloperation der solitaeren Choanalpolypen [in German]. Arch Laryngol Rhinol 1909;21:82–99

375. Kuehn DP, Templeton PJ, Maynard JA. Muscle spindles in the velopharyngeal musculature of humans. J Speech Hear Res 1990;33:488–493

376. Kuhlo W, Doll E, Franck MC. Successful management of Pickwickian syndrome using long-term tracheostomy [in German]. Dtsch Med Wschr 1969;94:1286–1290

377. Kühnel TS, Hein G, Hohenhorst W, Maurer JT. Soft palate implants: a new option for treating habitual snoring. Eur Arch Otorhinolaryngol 2005;262:277–280

378. Kuo PC, West RA, Bloomquist DS, McNeil RW. The effect of mandibular osteotomy in three patients with hypersomnia sleep apnea. Oral Surg Oral Med Oral Pathol 1979;48:385–392

379. Kurth BM, Schaffrath Rosario A. The prevalence of overweight and obese children and adolescents living in Germany. Results of the German Health Interview and Examination Survey for Children and Adolescents (KiGGS). BundesgesundheitsblGesundheitsforsch Gesundheitsschutz 2007;50:736–743

380. Kyrmizakis DE, Chimona TS, Papadakis CE, Bizakis JG, Velegrakis GA, Schiza S, Siafakas NM, Helidonis ES. Laser-assited uvulopalatoplasty for the treatment of snoring and mild obstructive sleep apnea syndrome. J Otolaryngol 2003;32:174–179

381. Kyrmizakis DE, Papadakis CE, Bizakis JG, Velegrakis GA, Siafakas NM, Helidonis ES. Sucralfate alleviating post-laser-assisted uvulopalatoplasty pain. Am J Otolaryngol 2001;22:55–58

382. Lam YY, Chan EY, Ng DK, Chan CH, Cheung JM, Leung SY, Chow PY, Kwok KL. The correlation among obesity, apnea-hypopnea index, and tonsil size in children. Chest 2006;130:1751–1756

383. Laranne J, Matsune S, Shima T, Ohyama M, Courey MS, Fomin D, Smith T, Huang S, Sanders D, Reinisch L. Histological changes in elastic components of soft palate scars after CO_2 and contact Nd:YAG laser incisions in the dog as an experimental model. Eur Arch Otorhinolaryngol 1996;253:454–459

384. Larrosa F, Hernandez L, Morello A, Ballester E, Quinto L, Montserrat JM. Laser-assisted uvulopalatoplasty for snoring: does it meet the expectations? Eur Respir J 2004;24: 66–70

385. Larsson LH, Carlsson-Nordlander B, Svanborg E. Four-year follow-up after uvulo-palatopharyngoplasty in 50 unselected patients with obstructive sleep apnea syndrome. Laryngoscope 1994;104:1362–1368

386. Lauretano AM, Khosla RK, Richardson G, Matheson J, Weiss JW, Graham C, Fried MP. Efficacy of laser-assisted uvulopalatoplasty. Lasers Surg Med 1997;21:109–116

387. Laurikainen E, Aitasalo K, Erkinjuntti M, Wanne O. Sleep apnea syndrome in children – secondary to adenotonsillar hypertrophy. Acta Otolaryngol 1992; (Suppl 492): 38–41

388. Lavie P, Zomer J, Eliaschar I, Joachim Z, Halpern E, Rubin AH, Alroy G. Excessive daytime sleepiness and insomnia. Association with deviated nasal septum and nocturnal breathing disorders. Arch Otolaryngol 1982;108:373–377

389. Ledereich PS, Thorpy MJ, Glovinsky PK, Burack B, McGregor P, Rozycki DL, Sher AE. Five year follow-up of daytime sleepiness and snoring after tracheotomy in patients with obstructive sleep apnea. In: Chouard CH (Ed) Chronic rhonchopathy. Proceedings of the First International Congress on Chronic Rhonchopathy. John Libbey Eurotext, Paris, 1988: pp 354–357

390. Lee NR, Givens CD, Wilson J, Robins RB. Staged surgical treatment of obstrcutive sleep apnea syndrome: a review of 35 patients. J Oral Maxillofac Surg 1999;57: 382–385

391. Leiberman A, Stiller-Timor L, Tarasiuk A, Tal A. The effect of adenotonsillectomy on children suffering from obstructive sleep apnea syndrome (OSAS): the Negev perspective. Int J Pediatr Otorhinolaryngol 2006;70:1675–1682

392. Leong AC, Davis JP. Morbidity after adenotonsillectomy for paediatric obstructive sleep apnoea syndrome: waking up to a pragmatic approach. J Laryngol Otol 2007;121:809–817

393. Levin BC, Becker GD. Uvulopalatopharyngoplasty for snoring: long-term results. Laryngoscope 1994;104:1150–1152

394. Levinus Lemnious. The touchstone of complexions. London 1581

395. Lewis MR, Ducic Y. Genioglossus muscle advancement with the genioglossus bone advancement technique for base of tongue obstruction. J Otolaryngol 2003;32: 168–173

396. Li HY, Chen NH, Lee LA, Shu YH, Fang TJ, Wang PC. Use of morphological indicators to predict outcomes of palatopharyngeal surgery in patients with obstructive sleep apnea. ORL J Otorhinolaryngol Relat Spec 2004;66:119–123

397. Li HY, Chen NH, Shu YH, Wang PC. Changes in quality of life and respiratory disturbance after extended uvulopalatal flap surgery in patients with obstructive sleep apnea. Arch Otolaryngol Head Neck Surg 2004;130:195–200

398. Li HY, Huang YS, Chen NH, Fang TJ, Liu CY, Wang PC. Mood improvement after surgery for obstructive sleep apnea. Laryngoscope 2004;114:1098–1102

399. Li HY, Li KK, Chen NH, Wang CJ, Liao YF, Wang PC. Three-dimensional computed tomography and polysomnography findings after extended uvulopalatal flap surgery for obstructive sleep apnea. Am J Otolaryngol 2005;26:7–11

400. Li HY, Li KK, Chen NH, Wang PC. Modified uvulopalatopharyngoplasty: the extended uvulopalatal flap. Am J Otolaryngol 2003;24:311–316

401. Li HY, Wang PC, Hsu CY, Chen NH, Lee LA, Fang TJ. Same-stage palatopharyngeal and hypopharyngeal surgery for severe obstructive sleep apnea. Acta Otolaryngol 2004;124: 820–826

402. Li KK, Guilleminault C, Riley RW, Powell NB. Obstructive sleep apnea and maxillomandibular advancement: an assessment of airway changes using radiographic and nasopharyngoscopic examinations. J Oral Maxillofac Surg 2002;60:526–530

403. Li KK, Powell NB, Riley RW, Guilleminault C. Distraction osteogenesis in adult obstructive sleep apnea surgery: a preliminary report. J Oral Maxillofac Surg 2002; 60:6–10

404. Li KK, Powell NB, Riley RW, Guilleminault C. Temperature-controlled radiofrequency tongue base reduction for sleep-disordered breathing: long-term outcomes. Otolaryngol Head Neck Surg 2002;127:230–234

405. Li KK, Powell NB, Riley RW, Troell RJ, Guilleminault C. Long-term results of maxillomandibular advancement surgery. Sleep Breath 2000;4:137–139

406. Li KK, Powell NB, Riley RW, Troell RJ, Guilleminault C. Radiofrequency volumetric tissue reduction for treatment of turbinate hypertrophy: a pilot study. Otolaryngol Head Neck Surg 1998;119:569–573

407. Li KK, Powell NB, Riley RW, Troell RJ, Guilleminault C. Radiofrequency volumetric tissue reduction of the palate: an extended follow-up study. Otolaryngol Head Neck Surg 2000;122:410–414

408. Li KK, Powell NB, Riley RW, Zonato A, Gervacio L, Guilleminault C. Morbidly obese patients with severe obstructive sleep apnea: is airway reconstructive surgery a viable treatment option? Laryngoscope 2000;110:982–987

409. Li KK, Riley RW, Powell NB, Guilleminault C. Maxillomandibular advancement for persistent obstructive sleep apnea after phase I surgery in patients without maxillo-mandibular deficiency. Laryngoscope 2000;110:1684–1688

410. Li KK, Riley RW, Powell NB, Troell RJ. Obstructive sleep apnea surgery: genioglossus advancement revisited. J Oral Maxillofac Surg 2001;59:1181–1184

411. Li KK, Riley RW, Powell NB, Zonato A, Troell R, Guilleminault C. Postoperative findings after maxillomandibular advancement for obstructive sleep apnea syndrome. Laryngoscope 2000;110:325–327

412. Li KK, Troell RJ, Riley RW, Powell NB, Koester U, Guilleminault C. Uvulopalatopharyngoplasty, maxillomandibular advancement, and the velopharynx. Laryngoscope 2001;111:1075–1078

413. Li KK. Hyoid suspension/advancement. In: Fairbanks DNF, Mickelson SA, Woodson BT (Eds) Snoring and obstructive sleep apnea, 3rd edn. Lippincott Williams & Wilkins, Philadelphia, 2003: pp. 178–182

414. Lim DJ, Kang SH, Kim BH, Kim HG. Treatment of primary snoring using radiofrequency-assisted uvulopalatoplasty. Eur Arch Otorhinolaryngol 2007;264:761–767

415. Lim J, McKean M. Adenotonsillectomy for obstructive sleep apnoea in children. Cochrane Database Syst Rev 2003; (1): CD 003136; update in 2009; (2): CD 003136

416. Lin HS, Prasad AS, Pan CJ, Rowley JA. Factors associated with noncompliance to treatment with positive airway pressure. Arch Otolaryngol Head Neck Surg 2007;133:69–72

417. Lin SW, Chen NH, Li HY, Fang TJ, Huang CC, Tsai YH, Lee CH. A comparison of the long-term outcome and effects of surgery or continuous positive airway pressure on patients with obstructive sleep apnea syndrome. Laryngoscope 2006;116: 1012–1016

418. Lister MT, Cunningham MJ, Benjamin B, Williams M, Tirrell A, Schaumberg DA, Hartnick CJ. Microdebrider tonsillotomy vs electrosurgical tonsillectomy: a randomized, double-blind, paired control study of postoperative pain. Arch Otolaryngol Head Neck Surg 2006; 132:599–604

419. Littner M, Kushida CA, Hartse K, McDowell Anderson W, Davila D, Johnson SF, Wise MS, Hirshkowitz M, Woodson BT (Standards of Practice Committee, American Academy of Sleep Medicine). Practice parameters for the use of laser-assisted uvulopalatoplasty: an update for 2000. Sleep 2001;24:603–619

420. Liu SA, Li HY, Tsai WC, Chang KM. Associated factors to predict outcomes of uvulopharyngopalatoplasty plus genioglossal advancement for obstructive sleep apnea. Laryngoscope 2005;115:2046–2050

421. Lobstein T, Baur L, Uauy R. Obesity in children and young people: a crisis in public health. Obes Rev 2004;5(Suppl 1): 4–104

422. Lobstein T, Jackson-Leach R. Child overweight and obesity in the USA: prevalence rates according to IOTF definitions. Int J Pediatr Obes 2007;2:62–64

423. Lobstein T, Millstone E. Context for the PorGrow study: Europe's obesity crisis. Obes Rev 2007;8(Suppl 2): 7–16

424. Loke D, Ghosh S, Panarese A, Bull PD. Endoscopic division of the ary-epiglottic folds in severe laryngomalcia. Int J Pediatr Otorhinolaryngol 2001;60:59–63

425. Low WK. Can snoring relief after nasal septal surgery be predicted? Clin Otolaryngol 1994; 19:142–144

426. Lu SJ, Chang SY, Shiao GM. Comparison between short-term and long-term post-operative evaluation of sleep apnea after uvulopalatopharyngoplasty. J Laryngol Otol 1995; 109:308–312

427. Lugaresi E, Cirignotta F, Gerardi R, Montagna P. Snoring and sleep apnea: natural history of heavy snorers disease. In: Guilleminault C, Partinen M (Eds) Obstructive sleep apnea syndrome: clinical research and treatment. Raven, New York, 1990: pp 25–36

428. Lujan JAFM, Hernandez Q, Liron R, Cuenca JR, Valero G, Parrilla P. Laparoscopic versus open gastric by pass in the treatment of morbid obesity: a randomized prospective study. Ann Surg 2004;239:433–437

429. Lysdahl M, Haraldsson PO. Long-term survival after uvulopalatopharyngoplasty in nonobese heavy snorers: a 5- to 9-year follow-up of 400 consecutive patients. Arch Otolaryngol Head Neck Surg 2000;126:1136–1140

430. Lysdahl M, Haraldsson PO. Uvulopalatopharyngoplasty versus laser uvulopalato-plasty: prospective long-term follow-up of self-reported symptoms. Acta Otolaryngol 2002;122: 752–757

431. Macdonald A, Drinnan M, Johnston A, Reda M, Griffiths C, Wilson J, Gibson GJ. Evaluation of potential predictors of outcome of laser-assisted uvulopalatoplasty for snoring. Otolaryngol Head Neck Surg. 2006;134:197–203

432. Macnab T, Blokmanis A, Dickson RI. Long-term results of uvulopalatopharyngo-plasty for snoring. J Otolaryngol 1992;21:350–354

433. Mair EA, Day RH. Cautery-assisted palatal stiffening operation. Otolaryngol Head Neck Surg 2000;122:547–555

434. Manni R, Ottolini A, Cerveri I, Bruschi C, Zoia MC, Lanzi G, Tartara A. Breathing patterns and HbSaO$_2$ changes during nocturnal sleep in patients with Duchenne muscular dystrophy. J Neurol 1989;236:391–394

435. Marais J. The value of sedation nasendoscopy: a comparison between snoring and non-snoring patients. Clin Otolaryngol 1998;23:74–76

436. Marcus CL, Keens TG, Bautista DB, von Pechmann WS, Ward SL. Obstructive sleep apnea in children with Down syndrome. Pediatrics 1991;88:132–139

437. Margardino TM, Tom LWC. Surgical management of obstructive sleep apnea in children with cerebral palsy. Laryngoscope 1999;109:1611–1615

438. Marrone O, Bonsignore MR. Pulmonary hemodynamics in obstructive sleep apnoea. Sleep Med Rev 2002;6:175–193

439. Martin F. Treatment of snoring and some obstructive sleep apnea syndrome by combined nasal and palatopharyngeal surgery [in German]. Laryngorhinootologie 1986;65:562–565

440. Martinho FL, Zonato AI, Bittencourt LR, Soares MC, Silva RF, Gregório LC, Tufik S. Obese obstructive sleep apnea patients with tonsil hypertrophy submitted to tonsil-lectomy. Braz J Med Biol Res 2006;39:1137–1142

441. Masdon JL, Magnuson JS, Youngblood G. The effects of upper airway surgery for obstructive sleep apnea on nasal continuous positive airway pressure settings. Laryngoscope 2004;114:205–207

442. Masters IB, Chang AB, Harris M, O'Neil MC. Modified nasopharyngeal tube for upper airway obstruction. Arch Dis Child 1999;80:186–187

443. Mathus-Vliegen EM, Tytgat GN. Intragastric balloon for treatment-resistant obesity: safety, tolerance, and efficacy of 1-year balloon treatment followed by a 1-year balloon-free follow-up. Gastrointest Endosc 2005;61:19–27

444. Mattila PS, Hammarén-Malmi S, Tarkkanen J, Saxen H, Pitkäniemi J, Karvonen M, Tuomilehto J. Adenoidectomy during early life and the risk of asthma. Pediatr Allergy Immunol 2003;14:358–362

445. Maturo SC, Mair EA. Submucosal minimally invasive lingual excision: an effective, novel surgery for pediatric tongue base reduction. Ann Otol Rhinol Laryngol 2006;115:624–630

446. Maurer JT, Eichler C, Hörmann K, Stuck BA. Videoendoscopy under sedation in sleep apnea patients – does treatment recommendation change? gms Ger Med Sci, 2008. http://www.egms.de/en/meetings/hno2008/08hno93.shtml

447. Maurer JT, Hein G, Stuck BA, Verse T, Hörmann K. Treatment of obstructive sleep apnea with a new vest preventing the supine position [in German]. DMW 2003;128: 71–75

448. Maurer JT, Hein G, Verse T, Hörmann K, Stuck BA. Long-term results of palatal implants for primary snoring. Otolaryngol Head Neck Surg 2005;133:573–578

449. Maurer JT, Verse T, Stuck BA, Hörmann K, Hein G. Palatal implants for primary snoring: short-term results of a new minimally invasive surgical technique. Otolaryngol Head Neck Surg 2004;132:125–131

450. Maurer JT. Update on surgical treatments for sleep apnea. Swiss Med Weekly 2009; 139: 624–629

451. Maw AR, Jeans WD, Cable HR. Adenoidectomy. A prospective study to show clinical and radiological changes two years after operation. J Laryngol Otol 1983;97: 511–518

452. Mayer-Brix J, Becker H, Peter JH. Nasal high pressure ventilation in obstructive sleep apnea syndrome. Theoretical and practical otorhinolaryngologic aspects [in German]. Laryngorhinootologie 1989;68:295–298

453. McArdle N, Dervereux G, Heidarnejad H, Engleman HM, Mackay TW, Douglas NJ. Long-term use of CPAP therapy for sleep apnea/hypopnea syndrome. Am J Respir Crit Care Med 1999;159:1108–1114

454. McCarthy JG, Schreiber J, Karp N, Thorne CH, Grayson BH. Lengthening the human mandible by gradual distraction. Plast Reconstr Surg 1992;89:1–10

455. McColley SA, April MM, Caroll JL, Naclerio RM, Loughlin GM. Respiratory compromise after adenotonsillectomy in children with obstructive sleep apnea. Arch Otolaryngol Head Neck Surg 1992;118:940–943

456. McGuirt WF Jr, Johnson JT, Sanders MH. Previous tonsillectomy as prognostic indicator for success of uvulopalatopharyngoplasty. Laryngoscope 1995;105:1253–1255

457. McSwiney PF, Cavannagh NP, Languth P. Outcome in congenital stridor (laryngomalacia). Arch Dis Child 1977;52:215–218

458. Meling TR, Tveten S, Due-Tønnessen BJ, Skjelbred P, Helseth E. Monobloc and midface distraction osteogenesis in pediatric patients with severe syndromal craniosynostosis. Pediatr Neurosurg 2000;33:89–94

459. Mendelson WB. Use of sleep laboratory in suspected sleep apnea syndrome: is one night enough? Cleve Clin J Med 1994;61:299–303

460. Meoli AL, Rosen CL, Kristo D, Kohrman M, Gooneratne N, Aguillard RN, Fayle R, Troell R. Nonprescription treatments of snoring or obstructive sleep apnea: an evaluation of products with limited scientific evidence. Sleep 2003;26:619–624

461. Metes A, Hoffstein V, Mateika S, Cole P, Haight JSJ. Site of airway obstruction in patients with obstructive sleep apnea before and after uvuloplatopharyngoplasty. Laryngoscope 1991;101:1102–1108

462. Meyer TJ, Eveloff SE, Kline LR, Millman RP. One negative polysomnogram does not exclude obstructive sleep apnea. Chest 1993;103:756–760

463. Mickelson SA, Ahuja A. Short-term objective and long-term subjective results of laser-assisted uvulopalatoplasty for obstructive sleep apnea. Laryngoscope 1999;109: 362–367

464. Mickelson SA, Hakim I. Is postoperative intensive care monitoring necessary after uvuloplatopharyngoplasty? Otolaryngol Head Neck Surg 1998;119:352–356

465. Mickelson SA, Rosenthal L. Midline glossectomy and epiglottidectomy for obstructive sleep apnea syndrome. Laryngoscope 1997;107:614–619

466. Mickelson SA. Laser-assisted uvulopalatoplasty for obstructive sleep apnea. Laryngoscope 1996;106:10–13

467. Miller FR, Watson D, Boseley M. The role of genial bone advancement trephine system in conjunction with uvulopalatopharyngoplasty in the multilevel management of obstructive sleep apnea. Otolaryngol Head Neck Surg 2004;130:73–79

468. Miller FR, Watson D, Malis D. Role of the tongue base suspension suture with The Repose System bone screw in the multilevel surgical management of obstructive sleep apnea. Otolaryngol Head Neck Surg 2002;126:392–398

469. Mintz SM, Ettinger AC, Geist JR, Geist RY. Anatomic relationship of the genial tubercles to the dentition as determined by cross-sectional tomography. J Oral Maxillofac Surg 1995;53:1324–1326

470. Mitchell RB, Kelly J. Behavior, neurocognition and quality-of-life in children with sleep-disordered breathing. Int J Pediatr Otorhinolaryngol 2006;70:395–406

471. Mitchell RB, Kelly J. Behavorial changes in children with mild sleep-disordered breathing or obstructive sleep apnea after adenotonsillectomy. Laryngoscope 2007;117:1685–1688

472. Mitchell RB, Kelly J. Outcome of adenotonsillectomy for obstructive sleep apnea in obese and normal-weight children. Otolaryngol Head Neck Surg 2007;137:43–48

473. Mitchell RB, Kelly J. Outcomes and quality of life following adenotonsillectomy for sleep-disordered breathing in children. ORL J Otorhinolaryngol Relat Spec 2007;69: 345–348

474. Miyazaki S, Itasaka Y, Tada H, Ishikawa K, Togawa K. Effectiveness of tonsillectomy in adult sleep apnea syndrome. Psychiatry Clin Neurosci 1998;52:222–223

475. Mofid MM, Manson PN, Robertson BC, Tufaro AP, Elias JJ, Vander Kolk CA. Craniofacial distraction osteogenesis: a review of 3278 cases. Plast Reconstr Surg 2001;108:1103–1114

476. Mognol P, Chosidow D, Marmuse JP. Laparoscopic gastric bypass versus laparoscopic adjustable gastric banding in the super-obese: a comparative study of 290 patients. Obes Surg 2005;15:76–81

477. Montgomery-Downs HE, Crabtree VM, Gozal D. Cognition, sleep and respiration in at-risk children treated for obstructive sleep apnoea. Eur Resp J 2005;25:336–342

478. Montgomery-Downs HE, Crabtree VM, Sans Capdevila O, Gozal D. Infant-feeding methods and childhood sleep-disordered breathing. Pediatrics 2007;120:1030–1035

479. Moore K. Site specific versus diffuse treatment/presenting severity of obstructive sleep apnea. Sleep Breath 2000;4:145–146

480. Moore MH, Guzman-Stein G, Proudman TW, Abbott AH, Netherway DJ, David DJ. Mandibular lengthening by distraction for airway obstruction in Treacher-Collins syndrome. J Craniofac Surg 1994;5:22–25

481. Morar P, Nandapalan V, Lesser THJ, Swift AC. Mucosal-strip/uvulectomy by the CO_2 laser as a method of treating simple snoring. Clin Otolaryngol 1995;20:308–311

482. Morgan WE, Friedmann EM, Duncan NO, Sulek M. Surgical management of macroglossia in children. Arch Otolaryngol Head Neck Surg 1996;122:326–329

483. Morovic CG, Monasterio L. Distraction osteogenesis for obstructive apneas in patients with congenital craniofacial malformations. Plast Reconstr Surg 2000;105: 2324–2330

484. Mortimore I, Marshall I, Wraith PK, Sellar RJ, Douglas NJ. Neck and total body fat deposition in nonobese and obese patients with sleep apnea compared with that in control subjects. Am J Respir Crit Care Med 1998;157:280–283

485. Mortimore IL, Bradley PA, Murray JA, Douglas NJ. Uvulopalatopharyngoplasty may compromise nasal CPAP therapy in sleep apnea syndrome. Am J Respir Crit Care Med 1996;154:1759–1762

486. Moser RJ, Rajagopal KR. Obstructive sleep apnea in adults with tonsillar hypertrophy. Arch Intern Med 1987;147:1265–1267

487. Must A, Spadano J, Coakley EH, Field AE, Colditz G, Dietz WH. The disease burden associated with overweight and obesity. JAMA 1999;282:1523–1529

488. Nahmias JS, Karetzky MS. Treatment of the obstructive sleep apnea syndrome using a nasopharyngeal tube. Chest 1988;94:1142–1147

489. Nakata S, Miyazaki S, Ohki M, Morinaga M, Noda A, Sugiura T, Sugiura M, Teranishi M, Katayama N, Nakashima T. Reduced nasal resistance after simple tonsillectomy in patients with obstructive sleep apnea. Am J Rhinol 2007;21:192–195

490. Nakata S, Noda A, Yagi H, Yanafi E, Mimura T, Okada T, Misawa H, Nakashima T. Nasal resistance for determinant factor of nasal surgery in CPAP failure patients with obstructive sleep apnea syndrome. Rhinology 2005;44:296–299

491. Nakata S, Noda A, Yanagi E, Suzuki K, Yamamoto H, Nakashima T. Tonsil size and body mass index are important factors for efficacy of simple tonsillectomy in obstructive sleep apnoea syndrome. Clin Otolaryngol 2006;31:41–45

492. Näslund E, Kral JG. Patient selection and the physiology of gastrointestinal antiobesity operations. Surg Clin North Am 2005;85:725–740

493. Nelson LM, Barrera JE. High energy single session radiofrequency tongue treatment in obstructive sleep apnea surgery. Otolaryngol Head Neck Surg. 2007;137: 883–888

494. Nelson LM. Combined temperature-controlled radiofrequency tongue reduction and UPPP in apnea surgery. Ear Nose Throat J 2001;80:640–644

495. Nelson LM. Radiofrequency treatment for obstructive tonsillar hypertrophy. Arch Otolaryngol Head Neck Surg 2000;126:736–740

496. Nelson LM. Temperature-controlled radiofrequency tonsil reduction: extended follow-up. Otolaryngol Head Neck Surg 2001;125:456–461

497. Nelson LM. Temperature-controlled radiofrequency tonsil reduction in children. Arch Otolaryngol Head Neck Surg 2003;129:533–537

498. Neruntarat C. Genioglossus advancement and hyoid myotomy under local anesthesia. Otolaryngol Head Neck Surg 2003;129:85–91

499. Neruntarat C. Genioglossus advancement and hyoid myotomy: short-term and long-term results. J Laryngol Otol 2003;117:482–486

500. Neruntarat C. Hyoid myotomy with suspension under local anesthesia for obstructive sleep apnea syndrome. Eur Arch Otorhinolaryngol 2003;260:286–290

501. Neruntarat C. Laser-assisted uvulopalatoplasty: short-term and long-term results. Otolaryngol Head Neck Surg 2001;124:90–93

502. Neruntarat C. Uvulopalatal flap for snoring on an outpatient basis. Otolaryngol Head Neck Surg 2003;129:353–359

503. Newman J. Snare uvulectomy for upper airway resistance syndrome. Oper Techn Otolaryngol Head Neck Surg 2002;13:178–181

504. Nguyen AT, Jobin V, Payne R, Beauregard J, Naor N, Kimoff RJ. Laryngeal and velopharyngeal sensory impairment in obstructive sleep apnea. Sleep 2005;28: 585–593

505. Nguyen NT, Goldman C, Rosenquist CJ, Arango A, Cole CJ, Lee SJ, Wolfe BM. Laparoscopic versus open gastric bypass: a randomized study of outcomes, quality of life, and costs. Ann Surg 2001;234:279–291

506. Nguyen NT, Paya M, Stevens CM, Mayandadi S, Zainabadi K, Wilson SE. The relationship between hospital volume and outcome in bariatric surgery at academic medical centers. Ann Surg 2004;240:586–593

507. Nieminen P, Tolonen U, Löpponen H. Snoring and obstructive sleep apnea in children. Arch Otolaryngol Head Neck Surg 2000;126:481–486

508. NIH: National Institutes of Health Conference. Gastrointestinal surgery for severe obesity: consensus development conference statement. Am J Clin Nutr 1992;55:615S-619S

509. Nishimura B, Tabuchi K, Aoyagi Y, Tobita T, Wada T, Kohanawa R, Nagata C, Morishita Y, Hara A. Epiglottic cyst in an infant. Auris Nasus Larynx 2008;35: 282–284

510. Nixon GM, Brouillette RT. Obstructive sleep apnea in children: do intranasal corticosteroids help? Am J Respir Med 2002;1:159–166

511. Nordgard S, Hein G, Stene BK, Skjøstad KW, Maurer JT. One-year results: palatal implants for the treatment of obstructive sleep apnea. Otolaryngol Head Neck Surg 2007;136: 818–822

512. Nordgard S, Stene BK, Skjostad KW, Bugten V, Wormdal K, Hansen NV, Nilsen AH, Midtlyng TH. Palatal implants for the treatment of snoring: long-term results. Otolaryngol Head Neck Surg 2006;134:558–564

513. Nordgard S, Stene BK, Skjøstad KW. Soft palate implants for the treatment of mild to moderate obstructive sleep apnea. Otolaryngol Head Neck Surg 2006;134: 565–570

514. Nordgard S, Wormdal K, Bugten V, Stene BK, Skjøstad KW. Palatal implants: a new method for the treatment of snoring. Acta Otolaryngol 2004;124:970–975

515. North American Association for the Study of Obesity (NAASO) and the National Heart. Clinical guide- lines on the identification, evaluation, and treatment of

overweight and obesity in adults: the evidence report. National Institutes of Health, Bethesda, MD, 1998. NIH publication 98–4083

516. North American Association for the Study of Obesity and the National Heart, Lung, and Blood Institute. The practical guide: identification, evaluation, and treatment of overweight and obesity in adults. National Institutes of Health, Bethesda, MD, 2000. NIH publication 00–4084

517. O´Brien PE, Dixon JB, Lap-Band: outcomes and results. J Laparoendosc Adv Surg Tech A 2003;13:265

518. Obwegeser H. Fortschritte und Schwerpunkte der orthopädischen Kiefer -und Gesichtschirurgie. In: Fortschr Kiefer Gesichtschir 1976; 21:54–60

519. Obwegeser H. In: Zur Operationstechnik bei der Progenie und anderer Unterkieferanomalien [in German]. Dtsch Zahn Mund Kieferheilk 1955; 23:1–2

520. O'Connor-Reina C, Garcia-Iriarte MT, Gomez Angel D, Rodríguez-Diaz A. Bipolar radiofrequency uvulopalatoplasty combined with injection snoreplasty: a reasonable option for the problem of snoring. ORL J Otorhinolaryngol Relat Spec 2009;71: 105–111

521. Oeverland B, Akre H, Kvaerner KJ et al. Patient discomfort in polysomnography with esophageal pressure measurements. Eur Arch Otorhinolaryngol 2005;262:241–245

522. Olsen KD, Suh KW, Staats BA. Surgically correctable causes of sleep apnea syndrome. Otolaryngol Head Neck Surg 1981;89:726–731

523. Oluwasanmi AF, Mal RK. Diathermy epiglottectomy: endoscopic technique. J Laryngol Otol 2001;115:289–292

524. Omur M, Ozturan D, Elez F, Unver C, Derman S. Tongue base suspension combined with UPPP in severe OSA patients. Otolaryngol Head Neck Surg 2005;133:218–223

525. Orliaguet O, Pepin JL, Veale D, Kelkel E, Pinel N, Levy P. Hunter`s syndrome and associated sleep apnoea cured by CPAP and surgery. Eur Respir J 1999;13:1195–1197

526. Orr WC, Martin RJ. Obstructive sleep apnea associated with tonsillar hypertrophy in adults. Arch Intern Med 1981;141:990–992

527. Ortiz-Monasterio F, Drucker M, Molina F, Ysunza A. Distraction osteogenesis in Pierre Robin sequence and related respiratory problems in children. J Craniofac Surg 2002;13: 79–83

528. Orvidas LJ, Beatty CW, Weaver AL. Antrochoanal polyps in children. Am J Rhinol 2001;15: 321–325

529. Osborne JE, Osman EZ, Hill PD, Lee BV, Sparkes C. A new acoustic method of differentiating palatal from non-palatal snoring. Clin Otolaryngol 1999;24:130–133

530. Osman EZ, Abo-Khatwa, Hill PD, Lee BWV, Osborne J. Palatal surgery for snoring: objective long-term evaluation. Clin Otolaryngol 2003;28:257–261

531. Osman EZ, Osborne JE, Hill PD, Lee BWV, Hammad Z. Uvulopalatopharyngoplasty versus laser assisted uvulopalatoplasty for the treatment of snoring: an objective randomized clinical trial. Clin Otolaryngol 2000;25:305–310

532. Osman EZ, Osborne JE, Hill PD, Lee BWV. Snoring assessment: do home studies and hospital studies give different results? Clin Otolaryngol 1998;23:524–527

533. Osnes T, Rollheim J, Hartmann E. Effect of UPPP with respect to site of pharyngeal obstruction in sleep apnoea: follow-up at 18 months by overnight recording of airway pressure and flow. Clin Otolaryngol Allied Sci 2002;27:38–43

534. Overweight, obesity, and health risk national task force on the prevention and treatment of obesity. Arch Intern Med 2000;160:898–904

535. Oxford Centre for Evidence-based Medicine Levels of Evidence. May 2001. www.cebm.net

536. Paavonen EJ, Strang-Karlsson S, Räikkönen K, Heinonen K, Pesonen AK, Hovi P, Andersson S, Järvenpää AL, Eriksson JG, Kajantie E. Very low birth weight increases risk for sleep-disordered breathing in young adulthood: the Helsinki Study of very low birth weight adults. Pediatrics 2007;120:778–784

537. Pack AI, Maislin G, Staley B, Pack FM, Rogers WC, George CF, Dinges DF. Impaired performance in commercial drivers: role of sleep apnea and short sleep duration. Am J Respir Crit Care Med 2006;174:446–454

538. Paditz E, Knauth H, Baerthold W. Effect of adenotomy on mental performance of children with adenoid vegetations [in German]. Wien Med Wochenschr 1996; 146:327–328

539. Pang KP, Terris DJ. Modified cautery-assisted palatal stiffening operation: new method for treating snoring and mild obstructive sleep apnea. Otolaryngol Head Neck Surg 2007;136: 823–826

540. Pang KP, Woodson BT. Expansion sphincter pharyngoplasty: a new technique for the treatment of obstructive sleep apnea. Otolaryngol Head Neck Surg 2007;137: 110–114

541. Pang KP. Identifying patients who need close monitoring during and after upper airway surgery for obstructive sleep apnoea. J Laryngol Otol 2006;120:655–660

542. Pantin CC, Hillman DR, Tennant M. Dental side effects of an oral device to treat snoring and obstructive sleep apnea. Sleep 1999;22:237–240

543. Paoli JR, Lauwers F, Lacassagne L, Tiberge M. Treatment of obstructive sleep apnea syndrome by mandibular elongation using osseous distraction followed by a Le Fort I advancement osteotomy: case report. J Oral Maxillofac Surg 2001;59:216–219

544. Paradise JL, Blustone CD, Bachmann RZ, Colborn DK, Bernard BS, Taylor FH, Rogers KD, Schwarzbach RH, Stool SE, Friday GA et al. Efficacy of tonsillectomy for recurrent throat infection in severely affected children. N Engl J Med 1984;310:674–683

545. Partinen M, Guilleminault C, Quera-Salva MA, Jamieson A. Obstructive sleep apnea and cephalometric roentgenograms: the role of upper airway abnormalities in the definition of abnormal breathing during sleep. Chest 1988;93:1199–1205

546. Partinen M, Jamieson A, Guilleminault C. Long-term outcome for obstructive sleep apnea syndrome patients. Chest 1988;94:1200–1204

547. Pasche P, Pellanda A, Jaques B. Obstructive sleep apnea syndrome and snoring: what is the role of surgery? Otorhinolaryngol Nova 2000;10:127–137

548. Patton TJ, Thawley SE, Water RC, Vandermeer PJ, Ogura JH. Expansion hyoidplasty: a potential surgical procedure designed for selected patients with obstructive sleep apnea syndrome. Experimental canine results. Laryngoscope 1983;93: 1387–1396

549. Pavone M, Paglietti MG, Petrone A, Crinò A, De Vincentiis GC, Cutrera R. Adenotonsillectomy for obstructive sleep apnea in children with Prader-Willi syndrome. Pediatr Pulmonol 2006;41:74–79

550. Payne RJ, Kost KM, Frenkiel S, Zeitouni AG, Sejean G, Sweet RC, Naor N, Hernandez L, Kimoff RJ. Laryngeal inflammation assessed using the reflux finding score in obstructive sleep apnea. Otolaryngol Head Neck Surg 2006;134:836–842

551. Pazos G, Mair EA. Complications of radiofrequency ablation in the treatment of sleep-disordered breathing. Otolaryngol Head Neck Surg 2001;125:462–466

552. Peiser J, Lavie P, Ovnat A, Charuzi I. Sleep apnea syndrome in the morbidly obese as an indication for weight reduction surgery. Ann Surg 1984;199:112–115

553. Pellnitz D. Über den durch das Altern bedingten Gestaltswandel der menschlichen Epiglottis [in German]. Arch Ohr Nas Kehlk Heilk 1961;178:350–354

554. Peppard P, Young T, Palta M, Dempsey J, Skatrud J. Longitudinal study of moderate weight change and sleep-disordered breathing. JAMA 2000;284:3015–3021

555. Peppard P, Young T, Palta M, Skatrud J. Prospective study of the association between sleep disordered breathing and hypertension. N Engl J Med 2000;342:1378–1384

556. Perello-Scherdel E, Quesada P, Lorente J, Lao J, Prades J. Long-term follow-up of partial resection of the palate as a surgical treatment for obstructive sleep apnea syndrome. In: Tos M, Thomsen J, Balle V (Eds) Rhinology – a state of the art. Kugler, Amsterdam, New York, 1995: pp 261–262

557. Pérez-Rodrigo C, Aranceta Bartrina J, Serra Majem L, Moreno B, Delgado Rubio A. Epidemiology of obesity in Spain. Dietary guidelines and strategies for prevention. Int J Vitam Nutr Res 2006;76:163–171

558. Perlyn CA, Schmelzer RE, Sutera SP, Kane AA, Govier D, Marsh JL. Effect of distraction osteogenesis of the mandible on upper airway volume and resistance in children with micrognathia. Plast Reconstr Surg 2002;109:1809–1818

559. Petri N, Suadicani P, Wildschiodtz G, Bjorn-Jorgensen J. Predictive value of Mueller maneuver, cephalometry and clinical features for the outcome of uvulopalatopharyngoplasty. Acta Otolaryngol (Stockh) 1994;114:565–571

560. Pfaar O, Spielhaupter M, Schirkowski A, Wrede H, Mösges R, Hörmann K, Klimek L. Treatment of hypertrophic palatine tonsils using bipolar radiofrequency-induced thermotherapy (RFITT). Acta Otolaryngol 2007;127:1176–1181

561. Phillipson EA. Control of breathing during sleep. Am Rev Respir Dis 1978;118:909–939

562. Piccin O, Sorrenti G. Adult obstructive sleep apnea related to nasopharyngeal obstruction: a case of retropharyngeal lipoma and pathogenetic considerations. Sleep Breath 2007;11:305–307

563. Pillar G, Peled R, Lavie P. Recurrence of sleep apnea without concomitant weight reduction increase 7.5 years after weight reduction surgery. Chest 1994;106:1702–1704

564. Pinczower EF. Globus sensation after laser-assisted uvulopalatoplasty. Am J Otolaryngol 1998;19:107–108

565. Pirsig W, Schäfer J, Yildiz F, Nagel J. Uvulopalatopharyngoplasty without complications: a Fujita modification [in German]. Laryngorhinootologie 1989;68:585–590

566. Pirsig W, Verse T. Long-term results in the therapy of obstructive sleep apnea. Eur Arch Otorhinolaryngol 2000;257:570–577

567. Pirsig W. Diagnostics in sleep apnea [in German]. HNO 1995;43:333–335

568. Pirsig W. There is no rationale for radical UPPP. Somnologie 1997;1(Suppl 1): 48

569. Pirsig W. Uvulopalatopharyngoplasty. In: Kountakis SE, Önerci M (Eds) Rhinologic and sleep apnea surgical techniques. Springer, Heidelberg, 2007: pp 323–330

570. Poirier P, Giles TD, Bray GA, Hong Y, Stern JS, Pi-Sunyer FX, Eckel RH; American Heart Association; Obesity Committee of the Council on Nutrition, Physical Activity, and Metabolism. Obesity and cardiovascular disease: pathophysiology, evaluation, and effect of weight loss: an update of the 1997 American Heart Association Scientific Statement on Obesity and Heart Disease from the Obesity Committee of the Council on Nutrition, Physical Activity, and Metabolism. Circulation 2006;113:898–918

571. Polonovski JM, Contencin P, Francois M, Viala P, Narcy P. Aryepiglottic fold excision for the treatment of severe laryngomalacia. Ann Otol Rhinol Laryngol 1990;99: 625–627

572. Poulose BK, Griffin MR, Moore DE, Zhu Y, Smalley W, Richards WO, Wright JK, Melvin W, Holzman MD. Risk factors for post-operative mortality in bariatric surgery. J Surg Res 2005;127:1–7

573. Powell N, Riley R, Guilleminault C, Troell R. A reversible uvulopalatal flap for snoring and sleep apnea syndrome. Sleep 1996;19:593–599

574. Powell NB, Riley RW, Guilleminault C, Nino-Murcia G. Obstructive sleep apnea, continuous positive airway pressure, and surgery. Otolaryngol Head Neck Surg 1988;99:362–369

575. Powell NB, Riley RW, Guilleminault C. Radiofrequency tongue base reduction in sleep-disordered breathing: a pilot study. Otolaryngol Head Neck Surg 1999;120: 656–664

576. Powell NB, Riley RW, Troell RJ, Blumen MB, Guilleminault C. Radiofrequency volumetric reduction of the tongue. A porcine pilot study for the treatment of obstructive sleep apnea syndrome. Chest 1998;111:1348–1355

577. Powell NB, Riley RW, Troell RJ, Li K, Blumen MB, Guilleminault C. Radiofrequency volumetric tissue reduction of the palate in subjects with sleep disordered breathing. Chest 1998;113:1163–1174

578. Powell NB, Zonato AI, Weaver EM, Li K, Troell R, Riley RW, Guilleminault C. Radiofrequency treatment of turbinate hypertrophy in subjects using continuous positive airway pressure: a randomized, double-blind, placebo-controlled clinical pilot trial. Laryngoscope 2001;111:1783–1790

579. Poyrazoglu E, Dogru S, Saat B, Güngör A, Cekin E, Cincik H. Histologic effects of injection snoreplasty and radiofrequency in the rat soft palate. Otolaryngol Head Neck Surg 2006;135:561–564

580. Pribitkin EA, Schutte SL, Keane WM, Mao V, Cater JR, Doghramji K, Youakim JM, Rosen MR, Breuninger W. Efficacy of laser-assisted uvulopalatoplasty in obstructive sleep apnea. Otolaryngol Head Neck Surg 1998;119:643–647

581. Prinsell JR. Maxillomandibular advancement (MMA) in a site-specific treatment approach for obstructive sleep apnea: a surgical algorithm. Sleep Breath 2000;4: 147–154

582. Prinsell JR. Maxillomandibular advancement surgery in a site-specific treatment approach for obstructive sleep apnea in 50 consecutive patients. Chest 1999;116: 1519–1529

583. Puhan MA, Suarez A, Lo Cascio C, Zahn A, Heitz M, Braendli O. Didgeridoo playing as alternative treatment for obstructive sleep apnoea syndrome: randomised controlled trial. BMJ 2006;332:266–270

584. Punjabi NM, Polotsky VY. Disorders of glucose metabolism in sleep apnea. J Appl Physiol 2005;99:1998–2007

585. Purser S, Irving L, Marty D. Redundant supraglottic mucosa in association with obstructive sleep epnea. Laryngoscope 1994;104:114–116

586. Quinn SJ, Daly N, Ellis PD. Observation of the mechanism of snoring using sleep nasendoscopy. Clin Otolaryngol 1995;20:360–364

587. Ramirez SG, Loube DI. Inferior sagittal osteotomy with hyoid bone suspension for obese patients with sleep apnea. Arch Otolaryngol Head Neck Surg 1996;122: 953–957

588. Randerath W, Bauer M, Blau A, Fietze I, Galetke W, Hein H, Maurer JT, Orth M, Rasche K, Rühle KH, Sanner B, Stuck BA, Verse T. Taskforce der Arbeitsgruppe Apnoe der DGSM. Are there alternative therapeutical options other than CPAP in the treatment of the obstructive sleep apnea syndrome [in German]. Pneumologie 2007; 61:458–466

589. Randerath WJ, Galetke W, Domanski U, Weitkunat R, Ruhle KH. Tongue-muscle training by intraoral electrical neurostimulation in patients with obstructive sleep apnea. Sleep 2004;27:254–259

590. Rappai M, Collop N, Kemp S, de Shazo R. The nose and sleep disordered breathing. What we know and what we do not know. Chest 2003;124:2309–2323

591. Rasheid S, Banasiak M, Gallagher SF, Lipska A, Kaba S, Ventimiglia D, Anderson WM, Murr MM. Gastric bypass is an effective treatment for obstructive sleep apnea in patients with clinically significant obesity. Obes Surg 2003;13:58–61

592. Reda M, Sims AJ, Collins MM, McKee GJ, Marshall H, Kelly PJ, Wilson JA. Morphological assessment of the soft palate in habitual snoring using image analysis. Laryngoscope 1999;109:1655–1660

593. Reddy DK, Matt BH. Unilateral vs. bilateral supraglottoplasty for severe laryngomalacia in children. Arch Otolaryngol Head Neck Surg 2001;127:694–699

594. Reeder MK, Goldman MD, Loh L, Muir AD, Casey KR, Gitlin DA. Postoperative obstructive sleep apnea: hemodynamic effects of treatment with nasal CPAP. Anesthesia 1991;46: 849–853

595. Remacle M, Betsch C, Lawson G, Jamart J, Eloy P. A new technique for laser-assisted uvulopalatoplasty: decision-tree analysis and results. Laryngoscope 1999;109:763–768

596. Remmers JE, de Groot WJ, Sauerland EK, Anch AM. Pathogenesis of the upper airway occlusion during sleep. J Appl Physiol 1978;44:931–938

597. Rennotte M, Baele P, Aubert G, Rodenstein DO. Nasal continuous positive airway pressure in the perioperative management of patients with obstructive sleep apnea submitted to surgery. Chest 1995;107:367–374

598. Renquist K, Jeng G, Mason EE. Calculating follow-up rates. Obes Surg 1992;2:361–367

599. Reyes BG, Arnold JE, Brooks LJ. Congenital absence of the epiglottis and its potential role in obstructive sleep apnea. Int J Pediatr Otorhinolaryngol 1994;30:223–226

600. Richard W, Kox D, den Herder C, van Tinteren H, de Vries N. One stage multilevel surgery (uvulopalatopharyngoplasty, hyoid suspension, radiofrequent ablation of the tongue base with/without genioglossus advancement), in obstructive sleep apnea syndrome. Eur Arch Otorhinolaryngol 2007;264:439–444

601. Riley R, Guilleminault C, Herran J, Powell NB. Cephalometric analysis and flow-volume loops in obstructive sleep apnea patients. Sleep 1983;6:303–311

602. Riley R, Guilleminault C, Powell N, Simmons FB. Palatopharyngoplasty failure, cephalometric roentgenograms and obstructive sleep apnea. Otolaryngol Head Neck Surg 1985;93:1199–1205

603. Riley RW, Powell NB, Guilleminault C, Nino-Murcia G. Maxillary, mandibular, and hyoid advancement: an alternative to tracheostomy in obstructive sleep apnea syndrome. Otolaryngol Head Neck Surg 1986;94:584–588

604. Riley RW, Powell NB, Guilleminault C, Ware W. Obstructive sleep anpnea syndrome following surgery for mandibular prognathism. J Oral Maxillofac Surg 1987;45: 450–452

605. Riley RW, Powell NB, Guilleminault C. Inferior mandibular osteotomy and hyoid myotomy suspension for obstructive sleep apnea: a review of 55 patients. J Oral Maxillofac Surg 1989; 47:159–164

606. Riley RW, Powell NB, Guilleminault C. Inferior sagittal osteotomy of the mandible with hyoid myotomy-suspension: a new procedure for obstructive sleep apnea. Otolaryngol Head Neck Surg 1986;94:589–593

607. Riley RW, Powell NB, Guilleminault C. Maxillofacial surgery and nasal CPAP. A comparison of treatment for obstructive sleep apnea syndrome. Chest 1990;98: 1421–1425

608. Riley RW, Powell NB, Guilleminault C. Obstructive sleep apnea and the hyoid: a revised surgical procedure. Otolaryngol Head Neck Surg 1994;111:717–721

609. Riley RW, Powell NB, Guilleminault C. Obstructive sleep apnea syndrome: a review of 306 consecutively treated surgical patients. Otolaryngol Head Neck Surg 1993;108: 117–125

610. Riley RW, Powell NB, Li KK, Troell RJ, Guilleminault C. Surgery and obstructive sleep apnea: long-term clinical outcomes. Otolaryngol Head Neck Surg 2000;122: 415–421

611. Riley RW, Powell NB, Li KK, Weaver EM, Guilleminault C. An adjunctive method of radiofrequency volumetric tissue reduction of the tongue for OSAS. Otolaryngol Head Neck Surg 2003;129:37–42

612. Ripberger R, Pirsig W. Long-term compliance with nasal CPAP treatment for obstructive sleep apnoea: prospective study in 50 patients [in German]. Laryngorhinootologie 1994;73: 581–585

613. Ritter CT, Trudo FJ, Goldberg AN, Welch KC, Maislin G, Schwab RJ. Quantitative evaluation of the upper airway during nasopharyngoscopy with the Müller maneuver. Laryngoscope 1999;109:954–963

614. Robinson S, Ettema SL, Brusky L, Woodson BT. Lingual tonsillectomy using bipolar radiofrequency plasma excision. Otolaryngol Head Neck Surg 2006;134:328–330

615. Robinson S, Lewis R, Norton A, McPeake S. Ultrasound-guided radiofrequency submucosal tongue-base excision for sleep apnoea: a preliminary report. Clin Otolaryngol Allied Sci 2003;28:341–345

616. Robinson S. External submucosal glossectomy. In: Friedman M (Ed) Sleep apnea and snoring: surgical and non-surgical therapy. Saunders Elsevier, Philadelphia, 2009: pp 292–300
617. Robinson S. Minimally invasive submucosal glossectomy. In: Friedman M (Ed) Sleep apnea and snoring: surgical and non-surgical therapy. Saunders Elsevier, Philadelphia, 2009: pp 248–257
618. Rodgers GK, Chan KH, Dahl RE. Antral choanal polyp presenting as obstructive sleep apnea syndrome. Arch Otolaryngol Head Neck Surg 1991;117:914–916
619. Roger G, Morriseau-Durand MP, Abbeele van den T, Nicollas R, Triglia JM, Narcy P, Abadie V, Manac'h Y, Garabedian EN. The CHARGE association. The role of tracheotomy. Arch Otolaryngol Head Neck Surg 1999;125:33–38
620. Rojewski TE, Schuller DE, Clark RW, Schmidt HS, Potts RE. Synchronous video recording of the pharyngeal airway and polysomnograph in patients with obstructive sleep apnea. Laryngoscope 1982;92:246–250
621. Rollheim J, Tvinnereim M, Sitek J, Osnes T. Repeatability of sites of sleep-induced upper airway obstruction. A 2-night study based on recordings of airway pressure and flow. Eur Arch Otorhinolaryngol 2001;258:259–264
622. Romanow JH, Catalano PJ. Initial U.S. pilot study: palatal implants for the treatment of snoring. Otolaryngol Head Neck Surg 2006;134:551–557
623. Rombaux P, Hamoir M, Bertrand B, Aubert G, Liistro G, Rodenstein D. Postoperative pain and side effects after uvulopalatopharyngoplasty, laser-assisted uvulopalatoplasty, and radiofrequency tissue volume reduction in primary snoring. Laryngoscope 2003;113:2169–2173
624. Rombaux P, Hamoir M, Plouin-Gaudon I, Liistro G, Aubert G, Rodenstein D. Obstructive sleep apnea syndrome after reconstructive laryngectomy for glottic carcinoma. Eur Arch Otorhinolaryngol 2000;257:502–506
625. Rombaux P, Liistro G, Hamoir M, Bertrand B, Aubert G, Verse T, Rodenstein D. Nasal obstruction and its impact on sleep-related breathing disorders: a review. Rhinology 2005;43:242–250
626. Rosen GM, Muckle RP, Mahowald MW, Goding GS, Ullevig C. Postoperative respiratory compromise in children with obstructive sleep apnea syndrome: can it be anticipated? Pediatrics 1994;93:784–788
627. Rosenfeld RM, Green RP. Tonsillectomy and adenoidectomy: changing trends. Ann Otol Rhinol Laryngol 1990;99:187–191
628. Rothschild MA, Catalano P, Biller HF. Ambulatory pediatric tonsillectomy and the identification of high-risk subgroups. Otolaryngol Head Neck Surg 1994;110:203–210
629. Rubin AH, Eliaschar I, Joachim Z, Alroy G, Lavie P. Effects of nasal surgery and tonsillectomy on sleep apnea. Bull Eur Physiopathol Respir 1983;19:612–615
630. Rubinstein I, Colapinto N, Rotstein LE, Brown IG, Hoffstein V. Improvement in upper airway function after weight loss in patients with obstructive sleep apnea. Am Rev Respir Dis 1988;138:1192–1195
631. Ruboyianes JM, Cruz RM. Pediatric adenotonsillectomy for obstructive sleep apnea. Ear Nose Throat J 1996;75:430–433
632. Ruff ME, Oakes WJ, Fisher SR, Spock A. Sleep apnea and vocal cord paralysis secondary to type I Chiari malformation. Pediatrics 1987;80:231–234

633. Ryan CF, Love LL. Unpredictable results of laser assisted uvulopalatoplasty in the treatment of obstructive sleep apnoea. Thorax 2000;55:399–404

634. Ryan CM, Bradley TD. Pathogenesis of obstructive sleep apnea. J Appl Physiol 2005;99: 2440–2450

635. Rybak LP, Maisel RH. Endoscopic findings in sleep apnea syndrome. J Otolaryngol 1979;8: 487–493

636. Sadaoka T, Kakitsuba N, Fujiwara Y, Kanai R, Takahashi H. The value of sleep nasendoscopy in the evaluation of patients with suspected sleep-related breathing disorders. Clin Otolaryngol Allied Sci 1996;21:485–489

637. Said B, Strome M. Long-term results of radiofrequency volumetric tissue reduction of the palate for snoring. Ann Otol Laryngol 2003;112:276–279

638. Salib RJ, Sadek SA, Dutt SN, Pearman K. Antrochoanal polyp presenting with obstructive sleep apnoea and cachexia. Int J Pediatr Otorhinolaryngol 2000;54: 163–166

639. Samuels MP, Stebbens VA, Davies SC, Picton-Jones E, Southall DP. Sleep related upper airway obstruction and hypoxaemia in sickle cell disease. Arch Dis Child 1992;67:925–929

640. Sanders JC, King MA, Mitchell RB, Kelly JP. Perioperative complications of adenotonsillectomy in children with obstructive sleep apnea syndrome. Anesth Analg 2006;103: 1115–1121

641. Sandler NA, Braun TW. Hyoid myotomy and suspension for obstructive sleep apnea syndrome. J Oral Maxillofac Surg 1997;55:656

642. Satoh K, Tsutsumi K, Tosa Y, Mikawa M, Hosaka Y. Le Fort III distraction osteogenesis of midface-retrusion in a case of Hajdu Cheny syndrome. J Craniofac Surg 2002;13:298–302

643. Saunders NC, Tassone P, Wood G, Norris A, Harries M, Kotecha B. Is acoustic analysis of snoring an alternative to sleep nasendoscopy? Clin Otolaryngol Allied Sci 2004;29:242–246

644. Schäfer J. How can one recognize a velum snorer [in German]? Laryngorhinootologie 1989; 68:290–294

645. Schäfer J. Spektralanalyse pathologischer schlafabhängiger Atemgeräusche der oberen Luftwege unter besonderer Berücksichtigung der Diagnostik und Therapie des obstruktiven Schlafapnoe-Syndroms und chronischer Rhonchopathien [in German]. University of Ulm, Ulm, Germany, 1990, Thesis

646. Schäfer J. Surgery of the upper airway: can surgical outcome be predicted? Sleep 1993; 16(Suppl 8): S98-S99

647. Scheuller M, Weider D. Bariatric surgery for treatment of sleep apnea syndrome in 15 morbidly obese patients: long-term results. Otolaryngol Head Neck Surg 2001;125: 299–302

648. Schierle HP, Schliephake H, Dempf R. Distraktionsosteogenese im Rahmen der Therapie peripherer Atemwegsobstruktionen im Säuglingsalter [in German]. Dtsch Zahnärztl Z 2000; 55:44–48

649. Schlieper J, Brinkmann B, Karmeier A, Pakusa T. Success rate and complications in primary laser-assisted uvulopalatoplasty (LAUP) for patients with rhonchopathy [in German]. Mund Kiefer Gesichts Chir 2002;6:146–152

650. Schmitz JP, Bitonti DA, Lemke RR. Hyoid myotomy and suspension for obstructive sleep apnea syndrome. J Oral Maxillofac Surg 1996;54:1339–1345

651. Schwaab M, Hansen S, Gurr A, Dazert S. Significance of blood tests prior to adenoidectomy [in German]. Laryngorhinootologie 2008;87:100–106

652. Schwab R. Pro/con editorials. Pro: sleep apnea is not an anatomic disorder. Am J Respir Crit Care Med 2003;168:270–273

653. Schwartz AR, Schubert N, Rothman W, Godley F, Marsh B, Eisele D, Nadeau J, Permutt L, Gleadhill I, Smith PL. Effect of uvulopalatopharyngoplasty on upper airway collapsibility in obstructive sleep apnea. Am Rev Respir Dis 1992;145: 527–532

654. Scott DB. Endotracheal intubation: friend or foe. BMJ 1986;292:157–158

655. Seemann RP, DiToppa JC, Holm MA, Hanson J. Does laser-assisted uvulopalatoplasty work? An objective analysis using pre- and postoperative polysomnographic studies. J Otolaryngol 2001;30:212–215

656. Seid AB, Park SM, Kearns MJ, Gugenheimer S. Laser division of the aryepiglottic folds for severe laryngomalacia. Int J Pediatr Otorhinolaryngol 1985;10:153–158

657. Senders CW, Navarrete EG. Laser supraglottoplasty for laryngomalacia: are specific anatomical defects more influential than associated anomalies on outcome? Int J Pediatr Otorhinolaryngol 2001;57:235–244

658. Sériès F, Pierre S St, Carrier G. Effects of surgical correction of nasal obstruction in the treatment of obstructive sleep apnea. Am Rev Respir Dis 1992;146:1261–1265

659. Sériès F, Pierre S St, Carrier G. Surgical correction of nasal obstruction in the treatment of mild sleep apnoea: importance of cephalometry in predicting outcome. Thorax 1993;48: 360–363

660. Shah RN, Mills PR, George PJ, Wedzicha JA. Upper airway sarcoidosis presenting as obstructive sleep apnoea. Thorax 1998;53:232–233

661. Sharp HR, Mitchell DB. Long-term results of laser-assisted uvulopalatoplasty for snoring. J Laryngol Otol 2001;115:897–900

662. Shehab ZP, Robin PE. Comparison of the effectiveness of uvulopalatopharyngoplasty and laser palatoplasty for snoring. Clin Otolaryngol 1997;22:158–161

663. Shepard JW, Thawley SE. Localization of upper airway collapse during sleep in patients with obstructive sleep apnea. Am Rev Respir Dis 1990;141:1350–1355

664. Sher AE, Flexon PB, Hillman D, Emery B, Swieca J, Smith TL, Cartwright R, Dierks E, Nelson L. Temperature-controlled radiofrequency tissue volume reduction in the human soft palate. Otolaryngol Head Neck Surg 2001;125:312–318

665. Sher AE, Schechtman KB, Piccirillo JF. The efficacy of surgical modifications of the upper airway in adults with obstructive sleep apnea syndrome. Sleep 1996;19:156–177

666. Sher AE, Thorpy MJ, Shprintzen RJ, Spielman AJ, Burack B, McGregor PA. Predictive value of Mueller maneuver in selection of patients for uvulopalatopharyngoplasty. Laryngoscope 1985;95:1483–1487

667. Shibata N, Nishimura T, Hasegawa K, Hattori C, Suzuki K. Influence of sleep respiratory disturbance on nocturnal blood pressure. Acta Otolaryngol 2003; (Suppl 550): 32–35

668. Shine NP, Coates HL, Lannigan FJ. Obstructive sleep apnea, morbid obesity, and adenotonsillar surgery: a review of the literature. Int J Pediatr Otorhinolaryngol. 2005;69:1475–1482

669. Shine NP, Lannigan FJ, Coates HL, Wilson A. Adenotonsillectomy for obstructive sleep apnea in obese children: effects on respiratory parameters and clinical outcome. Arch Otolaryngol Head Neck Surg 2006;132:1123–1127

670. Shine NP, Lewis RH. The "Propeller" incision for transpalatal advancement pharyngoplasty: a new approach to reduce post-operative oronasal fistulae. Auris Nasus Larynx 2008;35: 397–400

671. Shintani T, Asakura K, Kataura A. The effect of adenotonsillectomy in children with OSA. Int J Pediatr Otorhinolaryngol 1998;44:51–58

672. Shott SR, Amin R, Chini B, Heubi C, Hotze S, Akers R. Obstructive sleep apnea: should all children with Down syndrome be tested? Arch Otolaryngol Head Neck Surg 2006;132: 432–436

673. Sidman J, Wood RE, Poole M, Potsma DS. Management of plexiform neurofibroma of the larynx. Ann Otol Rhinol Laryngol 1987;96:53–55

674. Sidman JD, Sampson D, Templeton B. Distraction osteogenesis of the mandible for airway obstruction in children. Laryngoscope 2001;111:1137–1146

675. Simmons FB, Guilleminault C, Dement WC, Tilkian AG, Hill M. Surgical management of airway obstruction during sleep. Laryngoscope 1977;87:326–338

676. Simmons FB, Guilleminault C, Silvestri R. Snoring and some obstructive sleep apnea, can be cured by oropharyngeal surgery. Palatopharyngoplasty. Arch Otolaryngol 1983;109: 503–507

677. Simmons FB, Hill MW. Hypersomnia caused by upper airway obstruction. Ann Otol Rhinol Laryngol 1974;83:670–673

678. Simmons FB. Tracheotomy in obstructive sleep apnea patients. Laryngoscope 1979; 89: 1702–1703

679. Singh A, Al-Reefy H, Hewitt R, Kotecha B. Evaluation of ApneaGraph in the diagnosis of sleep-related breathing disorders. Eur Arch Otorhinolaryngol 2008;265: 1489–1494

680. Sirotnak J, Brodsky L, Pizzuto M. Airway obstruction in the Crouzon syndrome: case report and review of literature. Int J Pediatr Otorhinolaryngol 1995;31:235–246

681. Sivan Y, Ben-Ari J, Schonfeld TM. Laryngomalacia: a cause for early near miss for SIDS. Int J Pediatr Otorhinolaryngol 1991;21:59–64

682. Sjostrom L, Lindroos AK, Peltonen M, Torgerson J, Bouchard C, Carlsson B, Dahlgren S, Larsson B, Narbro K, Sjöström CD, Sullivan M, Wedel H; Swedish Obese Subjects Study Scientific Group. Lifestyle, diabetes, and cardio vascular risk factors 10 years after bariatric surgery. N Engl J Med 2004;351:2683–2693

683. Skatvedt O, Akre H, Godtlibsen OB. Continuous pressure measurements in the evaluation of patients for laser-assisted uvulopalatoplasty. Eur Arch Otorhinolaryngol 1996;253:390–394

684. Skatvedt O, Akre H, Godtlibsen OB. Nocturnal polysomnography with and without continuous pharyngeal and esophageal pressure measurements. Sleep 1996;19:485–490

685. Skatvedt O. Continuous measurements in the pharynx and esophagus during sleep in patients with obstructive sleep apnea syndrome. Laryngoscope 1992;102:1275–1280

686. Skatvedt O. Continuous pressure measurements during sleep to localize obstruction in the upper airways in heavy snorers and patients with obstructive sleep apnea syndrome. Eur Arch Otorhinolaryngol 1995;252:11–14

687. Skatvedt O. Laser-assisted uvulopalatoplasty. Description of the technique and pre- and postoperative evaluation of subjective symptoms. ORL J Otolaryngol Relat Spec 1996;58: 243–247

688. Skjostad KW, Stene BK, Norgard S. Consequences of increased rigidity in palatal implants for snoring: a randomized controlled study. Otolaryngol Head Neck Surg 2006;134:63–66

689. Smith E, Wenzel S, Rettinger G, Fischer Y. Quality of life in children with obstructive sleeping disorder after tonsillectomy, tonsillotomy or adenotomy [in German]. Laryngorhinootologie 2008;87:490–497

690. Smith I, Lasserson T, Wright J. Drug therapy for obstructive sleep apnoea in adults. Cochrane Database Syst Rev 2006; (2): CD 003002, 2002, (2)

691. Smith SL, Pereira KD. Tonsillectomy in children: indications, diagnosis and complications. ORL J Otorhinolaryngol Relat Spec 2007;69:336–339

692. Sobol SE, Wetmore RF, Marsh RR, Stow J, Jacobs IN. Postoperative recovery after microdebrider intracapsular or monopolar electrocautery tonsillectomy: a prospective, randomized, single-blinded study. Arch Otolaryngol Head Neck Surg 2006; 132:270–274

693. Sohn H, Rosenfeld RM. Evaluation of sleep-disordered breathing in children. Otolaryngol Head Neck Surg 2003;128:344–352

694. Solares CA, Koempel JA, Hirose K, Abelson TI, Reilly JS, Cook SP, April MM, Ward RF, Bent JP III, Xu M, Koltai PJ. Safety and efficacy of powered intracapsular tonsillectomy in children: a multi-center retrospective case series. Int J Pediatr Otorhinolaryngol 2005;69: 21–26

695. Sörensen H, Solow B, Greve E. Assessment of the nasopharyngeal airway. A rhinomanometric and radiographic study in children with adenoids. Acta Otolaryngol 1980;89:227–232

696. Sorin A, Bent JP, April MM, Ward RF. Complications of microdebrider-assisted powered intracapsular tonsillectomy and adenoidectomy. Laryngoscope 2004;114: 297–300

697. Sorrenti G, Piccin O, Latini G, Scaramuzzino G, Mondini S, Rinaldi Ceroni A. Tongue suspension technique in obstructive sleep apnea: personal experience [in Italian]. Acta Otorhinolaryngol Ital 2003;23:274–280

698. Sorrenti G, Piccin O, Scaramuzzino G, Mondini S, Cirignotta F, Ceroni AR. Tongue base reduction with hyoepiglottoplasty for the treatment of severe OSA. Acta Otorhinolaryngol Ital 2004;24:204–210

699. Souter MA, Stevenson S, Sparks B, Drennan C. Upper airway surgery benefits patients with obstructive sleep apnoea who cannot tolerate nasal continuous positive airway pressure. J Laryngol Otol 2004;118:270–274

700. Spilsbury JC, Storfer-Isser A, Kirchner HL, Nelson L, Rosen CL, Drotar D, Redline S. Neighborhood disadvantage as a risk factor for pediatric obstructive sleep apnea. J Pediatr 2006;149:342–347

701. Statham MM, Elluru RG, Buncher R, Kalra M. Adenotonsillectomy for obstructive sleep apnea syndrome in young children: prevalence of pulmonary complications. Arch Otolaryngol Head Neck Surg 2006;132:476–480

702. Steinschneider A, Weinstein SL, Diamond E. The sudden infant death syndrome and apnea/obstruction during neonatal sleep and feeding. Pediatrics 1982;70:858–863

703. Stern TP, Auckley D. Obstructive sleep apnea following treatment of head and neck cancer. Ear Nose Throat J 2007;86:101–103

704. Stevenson EW, Turner GT, Sutton FD, Doekel RC, Pegram V, Hernandez J. Prognostic significance of age and tonsillectomy in uvulopalatopharyngoplasty. Laryngoscope 1990;100: 820–823

705. Steward DL, Huntley TC, Woodson BT, Surdulescu V. Palate implants for obstructive sleep apnea: multi-institution, randomized, placebo-controlled study. Otolaryngol Head Neck Surg 2008;139:506–510

706. Steward DL, Weaver EM, Woodson BT. A comparison of radiofrequency treatment schemes for obstructive sleep apnea syndrome. Otolaryngol Head Neck Surg 2004; 130:579–585

707. Steward DL, Weaver EM, Woodson BT. Multilevel temperature-controlled radiofrequency for obstructive sleep apnea: extended follow-up. Otolaryngol Head Neck Surg 2005;132: 630–635

708. Steward DL. Effectiveness of multilevel (tongue and palate) radiofrequency tissue ablation for patients with obstructive sleep apnea syndrome. Laryngoscope 2004;114: 2073–2084

709. Stocker DJ. Management of the bariatric surgery patient. Endocrinol Metab Clin North Am 2003;32:437–457

710. Stoohs R, Guilleminault C. Obstructive sleep apnea syndrome or abnormal upper airway resistance during sleep? J Clin Neurophysiol 1990;7:83–92

711. Stradling JR, Thomas G, Earley ARH, Williams P, Freeland A. Effect of adenotonsillectomy on nocturnal hypoxaemia, sleep disturbance, and symptoms in snoring children. Lancet 1990;335:249–253

712. Stripf EA, Kühnemund M, Selivanova O, Mann WJ. Practicability of a surgical multilevel therapy in patients with obstructive sleep apnea [in German]. HNO 2007; 55(Suppl 1): E1-E6

713. Strohl K. Pro/con editorials. Con: sleep apnea is an anatomic disorder. Am J Respir Crit Care Med 2003;168:270–273

714. Strome M. Obstructive sleep apnea in Down syndrome children: a surgical approach. Laryngoscope 1986;96:1340–1342

715. Stuck BA, Genzwürker HV. Tonsillectomy in children: preoperative evaluation of risk factors [in German]. Anaesthesist 2008;57:499–504

716. Stuck BA, Köpke J, Maurer JT, Verse T, Eckert A, Bran G, Düber C, Hörmann K. Lesion formation in radiofrequency surgery of the tongue base. Laryngoscope 2003; 113:1572–1576

717. Stuck BA, Köpke J, Maurer JT, Verse T, Eckert A, Düber C, Hörmann K. Magnetic resonance imaging in the evaluation of temperature-controlled radiofrequency volumetric tissue reduction [in German]. HNO 2003;51:717–720

718. Stuck BA, Maurer JT, Hein G, Hörmann K, Verse T. Radiofrequency surgery of the soft palate in the treatment of snoring – a review of the literature. Sleep 2004;27: 551–555

719. Stuck BA, Maurer JT, Hörmann K, Baisch A. Tongue-advancement – erste Ergebnisse einer neuen Technik zur chirurgischen Therapie der retrolingualen Obstruktion [in German]. Somnology (Abstract) 2007;11(Suppl 1): 33

720. Stuck BA, Maurer JT, Verse T, Hörmann K. Tongue base reduction with temperature-controlled radiofrequency volumetric tissue reduction for treatment of obstructive sleep apnea syndrome. Acta Otolaryngol 2002;122:531–536

721. Stuck BA, Neff W, Hörmann K, Verse T, Bran G, Baisch A, Düber C, Maurer JT. Anatomic changes after hyoid suspension for obstructive sleep apnea: an MRI study. Otolaryngol Head Neck Surg 2005;133:397–402

722. Stuck BA, Sauter A, Hörmann K, Verse T, Maurer JT. Radiofrequency surgery of the soft palate in the treatment of snoring. A placebo-controlled trial. Sleep 2005;28:847–850

723. Stuck BA, Starzak K, Hein G, Verse T, Hörmann K, Maurer JT. Combined radiofrequency surgery of the tongue base and soft palate in obstructive sleep apnoea. Acta Otolaryngol 2004;124:827–832

724. Stuck BA, Starzak K, Verse T, Hörmann K, Maurer JT. Complications of temperature controlled radiofrequency volumetric tissue reduction for sleep disordered breathing. Acta Otolaryngol 2003;123:532–535

725. Sugerman HJ, Fairman RP, Sood RK, Engle K, Wolfe L, Kellum JM. Long-term effects of gastric surgery for treating respiratory insufficiency of obesity. Am J Clin Nutr 1992;55 (2 Suppl): 597S–601S

726. Sugerman HJ, Starkey JV, Birkenhauer R. A randomized prospective trial of gastric bypass versus vertical banded gastroplasty for morbid obesity and their effects on sweets versus non-sweets eaters. Ann Surg 1987;205:613–624

727. Sugiura T, Noda A, Nakata S, Yasuda Y, Soga T, Miyata S, Nakai S, Koike Y. Influence of nasal resistance on initial acceptance of continuous positive airway pressure in treatment for obstructive sleep apnea syndrome. Respiration 2007;74:56–60

728. Sullivan CE, Issa FG, Berthon-Jones M, Eves L. Reversal of obstructive sleep apnoea by continuous positive airway pressure applied through the nares. Lancet 1981;1:862–865

729. Summers CL, Stradling JR, Baddeley RM. Treatment of sleep apnoea by vertical gastroplasty. Br J Surg 1990;77:1271–1272

730. Suratt PM, Barth JT, Diamond R, D'Andrea L, Nikova M, Perriello VA Jr, Carskadon MA, Rembold C. Reduced time in bed and obstructive sleep-disordered breathing in children are associated with cognitive impairment. Pediatrics 2007;119:320–329

731. Suratt PM, Dee P, Atkinson RL, Armstrong P, Wilhoit SC. Fluoroscopic and computed tomographic features of the pharyngeal airway in obstructive sleep apnea. Am Rev Respir Dis 1983;127:487–492

732. Swift AC. Upper airway obstruction, sleep disturbance and adenotonsillectomy in children. J Laryngol Otol 1988;102:419–422

733. Tait AR, Voepel-Lewis T, Burke C, Kostrzewa A, Lewis I. Incidence and risk factors for perioperative adverse respiratory events in children who are obese. Anesthesiology 2008; 108:375–380

734. Tatla T, Sandhu G, Croft CB, Kotecha B. Celon radiofrequency thermo-ablative palatoplasty for snoring – a pilot study. J Laryngol Otol 2003;117:801–806

735. Tauman R, Gulliver TE, Krishna J, Montgomery-Downs HE, O'Brien LM, Ivanenko A, Gozal D. Persistence of obstructive sleep apnea syndrome in children after adenotonsillectomy. J Pediatr 2006;149:803–808

736. Teitelbaum J, Diminutto M, Comiti S, Pépin JL, Deschaux C, Raphaël B, Bettega G. Lateral cephalometric radiography of the upper airways for evaluation of surgical treatment of obstructive sleep apnea syndrome [in French]. Rev Stomatol Chir Maxillofac 2007;1081: 13–20

737. Teran-Santos J, Jimenez-Gomez A, Cordero-Guevara J. The association between sleep apnea and the risk of traffic accidents. Cooperative Group Burgos-Santander. N Engl J Med 1999; 340:847–851

738. Terris DJ, Chen V. Occult mucosal injuries with radiofrequency ablation of the palate. Otolaryngol Head Neck Surg 2001;125:468–472

739. Terris DJ, Clerk AA, Norbash AM, Troell RJ. Characterization of postoperative edema following laser-assisted uvulopalatoplasty using MRI and polysomnography: implications for the outpatient treatment of obstructive sleep apnea syndrome. Laryngoscope 1996;106: 124–128

740. Terris DJ, Coker JF, Thomas AJ, Chavoya M. Preliminary fndings from a prospective, randomized trial of two palatal operations for sleep-disordered breathing. Otolaryngol Head Neck Surg 2002;127:315–323

741. Terris DJ, Kunda LD, Gonella MC. Minimally invasive tongue base surgery for obstructive sleep apnoea. J Laryngol Otol 2002;116:716–721

742. Thatcher GW, Maisel RH. The long-term evaluation of tracheostomy in the management of severe obstructive sleep apnea. Laryngoscope 2003;113:201–204

743. Thomas AJ, Chavoya M, Terris DJ. Preliminary findings from a prospective, randomized trial of two tongue-base surgeries for sleep-disordered breathing. Otolaryngol Head Neck Surg 2003;129:539–546

744. Thorneman G, Kervall JA. Pain treatment after tonsillectomy: advantages of analgetics regularly given compared with analgetics on demand. Acta Otolaryngol 2000; 120:986–989

745. Togawa K, Konno A, Miyazaki S, Yamakawa K, Okawa M. Obstructive sleep dyspnea. Acta Otolaryngol 1988;458:167–173

746. Toh ST, Hsu PP, Ng YH, Teo TW, Tan KL, Lu KS. Incidence of complications after temperature-controlled radiofrequency treatment for sleep-disordered breathing: a Singapore sleep centre experience. J Laryngol Otol 2008;122:490–494

747. Toynton SC, Saunders MW, Bailey CM. Aryepiglottoplasty for laryngomalacia: 100 consecutive cases. J Laryngol Otol 2001;115:35–38

748. Troell RJ, Powell NB, Riley RW, Li KK, Guilleminault C. Comparison of postoperative pain between laser-assisted uvulopalatoplasty, uvulopalatopharyngoplasty, and radiofrequency volumetric tissue reduction of the palate. Otolaryngol Head Neck Surg 2000;122:402–409

749. Trotter MI, D'Souza AR, Morgan DW. Medium-term outcome of palatal surgery for snoring using the Somnus™ unit. J Laryngol Otol 2002;116:116–118

750. Tunkel DE, McColley SA, Baroody FM, Marcus CL, Carrol JL, Loughlin GM. Polysomnography in the evaluation of readiness for decannulation in children. Arch Otolatyngol Head Neck Surg 1996;122:721–724

751. Tvinnereim M, Cole P, Haight JS, Hoffstein V. Diagnostic airway pressure recording in sleep apnea syndrome. Acta Otolaryngol 1995;115:449–454

752. Tvinnereim M, Mateika S, Cole P, Haight JSJ, Hoffstein V. Diagnosis of obstructive sleep apnea using portable transducer catheter. Am Rev Respir Dis 1995;127: 487–492

753. Tvinnereim M, Mitic S, Hansen RK. Plasma radiofrequency preceded by pressure recording enhances success for treating sleep-related breathing disorders. Laryngoscope 2007;117: 731–736

754. Tzifa KT, Shehab ZP, Robin PE. The relation between tonsillectomy and snoring. Clin Otolaryngol 1998;23:148–151

755. Uemura T, Hayashi T, Satoh K, Mitsukawa N, Yoshikawa A, Jinnai T, Hosaka Y. A case of improved obstructive sleep apnea by distraction osteogenesis for midface hypoplasia of an infantile Crouzon's syndrome. J Craniofac Surg 2001;12:73–77

756. Unkel C, Lehnerdt G, Metz K, Jahnke K, Dost P. Long-term results of laser-tonsillotomy in obstructive tonsillar hyperplasia [in German]. Laryngorhinootologie 2004;83: 466–469

757. Uppal S, Nadig S, Jones C, Nicolaides AR, Coatesworth AP. A prospective single-blind randomized-controlled trial comparing two surgical techniques for the treatment of snoring: laser palatoplasty versus uvulectomy with punctate palatal diathermy. Clin Otolaryngol Allied Sci 2004;29:254–263

758. Urschitz MS, Guenther A, Eggebrecht E, Wolf J, Urschitz-Duprat PM, Schlaud M, Poets CF. Snoring, intermittent hypoxia and academic performance in primary school children. Am J Respir Crit Care Med 2003;168:464–468

759. Utley DS, Goode RL, Hakim I. Radiofrequency energy tissue ablation for the treatment of nasal obstruction secondary to turbinate hypertrophy. Laryngoscope 1999; 109:683–686

760. Utley DS, Shin EJ, Clerk AA, Terris DJ. A cost-effective and rational surgical approach to patients with snoring, upper airway resistance syndrome, or obstructive sleep apnea syndrome. Laryngoscope 1997;107:726–734

761. Valencia-Flores M, Orea A, Herrera M, Santiago V, Rebollar V, Castaño VA, Oseguera J, Pedroza J, Sumano J, Resendiz M, García-Ramos G. Effect of bariatric surgery on obstructive sleep apnea and hypopnea syndrome, electrocardiogram, and pulmonary arterial pressure. Obes Surg 2004;14:755–762

762. van de Graf WB, Gottfried SB, Mitra J, van Lunteren E, Cherniack NS, Strohl KP. Respiratory function of hyoid muscles and hyoid arch. J Appl Physiol 1984;57: 197–204

763. van den Broek E, Richard W, van Tinteren H, de Vries N. UPPP combined with radiofrequency thermotherapy of the tongue base for the treatment of obstructive sleep apnea syndrome. Eur Arch Otorhinolaryngol 2008;265:1361–1365

764. van Gemert WG, van Wersch MM, Greve JW, Soeters PB. Revisional surgery after failed vertical banded gastroplasty: restoration of vertical banded gastroplasty or conversion to gastric bypass. Obes Surg 1998;8:21–28

765. Verhulst SL, Schrauwen N, Haentjens D, Rooman RP, Van Gaal L, De Backer WA, Desager KN. Sleep-disordered breathing and the metabolic syndrome in overweight and obese children and adolescents. J Pediatr 2007;150:608–512

766. Verse T, Baisch A, Hörmann K. Multi-level surgery for obstructive sleep apnea. Preliminary objective results [in German]. Laryngorhinootologie 2004;83:516–522

767. Verse T, Baisch A, Maurer JT, Stuck BA, Hörmann K. Multilevel surgery for obstructive sleep apnea: short-term results. Otolaryngol Head Neck Surg 2006;134: 571–477

768. Verse T, de la Chaux R, Dreher A, Fischer Y, Grundmann T, Hecksteden K, Hörmann K, Hohenhorst W, Ilgen F, Kühnel T, Mahl N, Maurer JT, Pirsig W, Roth B, Siegert R, Stuck BA. ArGe Schlafmedizin der Deutschen Gesellschaft für Hals-Nasen-Ohren-Heilkunde, Kopf- und Hals-Chirurgie. Guideline: treatment of adult obstructive sleep apnea [in German]. Laryngorhinootologie 2008;87:192–204

769. Verse T, Kroker B, Pirsig W, Brosch S. Tonsillectomy for treatment of obstructive sleep apnea in adults with tonsillar hypertrophy. Laryngoscope 2000;110:1556–1559

770. Verse T, Maurer JT, Pirsig W. Effect of nasal surgery on sleep related breathing disorders. Laryngoscope 2002;112:64–68

771. Verse T, Pirsig W, Kroker BA. Obstructive sleep apnea and nasal polyps [in German]. Laryngorhinootologie 1998;77:150–152

772. Verse T, Pirsig W, Zimmermann E. Obstructive sleep apnea in older patients after the closure of a tracheostoma [in German]. Dtsch Med Wochenschr 2000;125:137–141

773. Verse T, Pirsig W. Age-related changes in the epiglottis causing failure of nasal continuous positive airway pressure therapy. J Laryngol Otol 1999;113:1022–1025

774. Verse T, Pirsig W. Indications for performing uvulopalatopharyngoplasty and laser-assisted uvulopalatopharyngoplasty [in German]. HNO 1998;46:553–561

775. Verse T, Pirsig W. Laser-assisted uvulopalatoplasty. A metanalysis. In: Fabiani M, Saponara M (Eds) Surgery for snoring and obstructive sleep apnea syndrome. Kugler, Amsterdam, 2003: pp 463–474

776. Verse T, Pirsig W. Meta-analysis of laser-assisted uvulopalatopharyngoplasty. What is clinically relevant up to now [in German]? Laryngorhinootolgie 2000;79:273–284

777. Verse T, Pirsig W. Pharyngeal pressure measurements in topodiagnosis of obstructive sleep apnea [in German]. HNO 1997;45:898–904

778. Verse T, Pirsig W. The impact of nasal surgery on obstructive sleep apnea. Sleep Breath 2003;7:63–76

779. Verse T, Schwalb J, Hörmann K, Stuck BA, Maurer JT. Submental transcutaneous electrical stimulation for obstructive sleep apnea [in German]. HNO 2003;51: 966–970

780. Vgontzas AN, Bixler EO, Chrousos GP. Sleep apnea is a manifestation of the metabolic syndrome. Sleep Med Rev 2005;9:211–224

781. Vicente E, Marín JM, Carrizo S, Naya MJ. Tongue-base suspension in conjunction with uvulopalatopharyngoplasty for treatment of severe obstructive sleep apnea: long-term follow-up results. Laryngoscope 2006;116:1223–1227

782. Vilaseca I, Morello A, Montserrat JM, Santamaria J, Iranzo A. Usefulness of uvulo-palatopharyngoplasty with genioglossus and hyoid advancement in the treatment of obstructive sleep apnea. Arch Otolaryngol Head Neck Surg 2002;128:435–440

783. Villani S, Brevi B, Sesenna E. Distraction osteogenesis in a newborn infant with Pierre-Robin sequence [in German]. Mund Kiefer Gesichtschir 2002;6:197–201

784. Villareal A, Hudgel D, Roth T. Improvement of obstructive sleep apnea after radiation therapy of vocal cord carcinoma. Sleep Med 2007;9:96–97

785. Virkkula P, Bachour A, Hytönen M, Salmi T, Malmberg H, Hurmerinta K, Maasilta P. Snoring is not relieved by nasal surgery despite improvement in nasal resistance. Chest 2006;129: 81–87

786. Vlastos IM, Parpounas K, Economides J, Helmis G, Koudoumnakis E, Houlakis M. Tonsillectomy versus tonsillotomy performed with scissors in children with tonsillar hypertrophy. Int J Pediatr Otorhinolaryngol 2008;72:857–863

787. Vukovic L, Hutchings J. Patient evaluation of laser-assisted uvulopalatoplasty. J Otolaryngol (Toronto) 1996;25:404–407

788. Waite PD, Wooten V, Lachner J, Guyette RF. Maxillomandibular advancement surgery in 23 patients with obstructive sleep apnea syndrome. J Oral Maxillofac Surg 1989;47: 1256–1261

789. Waldhorn RE, Herrick TW, Nguyen MC, O'Donnell AE, Sodero J, Potolicchio SJ. Long-term compliance with nasal continuous positive airway pressure therapy of obstructive sleep apnea. Chest 1990;97:33–38

790. Walker RP, Gatti WM, Poirier N, Davis JS. Objective assessment of snoring before and after laser-assisted uvulopaplatoplasty. Laryngoscope 1996;106:1372–1377

791. Walker RP, Grigg-Damberger MM, Gopalsami C, Totten MC. Laser-assisted uvulopalatoplasty for snoring and obstructive sleep apnea: results in 170 patients. Laryngoscope 1995;105:938–943

792. Walker RP, Grigg-Damberger MM, Gopalsami C. Laser-assisted uvulopalatopharyngoplasty for the treatment of mild, moderate, and severe obstructive sleep apnea. Laryngoscope 1999; 109:79–85

793. Walker RP, Grigg-Damberger MM, Gopalsami C. Uvulopalatopharyngoplasty versus laser-assisted uvulopalatoplasty for the treatment of obstructive sleep apnea. Laryngoscope 1997; 107:76–82

794. Walker RP, Levine HL, Hopp ML, Greene D, Pang K. Palatal implants: a new approach for the treatment of obstructive sleep apnea. Otolaryngol Head Neck Surg 2006;135:549–554

795. Walker RP, Levine HL, Hopp ML, Greene D. Extended follow-up of palatal implants for OSA treatment. Otolaryngol Head Neck Surg 2007;137:822–827

796. Walsh P, Smith D, Coakeley D, Dunne B, Timon C. Sleep apnoea of unusual origin. J Laryngol Otol 2002;116:138–139

797. Wang X, Wang XX, Liang C, Yi B, Lin Y, Li ZL. Distraction osteogensis in correction of micrognathia accompanying obstructive sleep apnea syndrome. Plast Reconstr Surg 2003;112: 1549–1557

798. Wang Z, Rebeiz EE, Shapshay SM. Laser soft palate "stiffening": an alternative to uvulopalatopharyngoplasty. Lasers Surg Med 2002;30:40–43

799. Ward SL, Marcus CL. Obstructive sleep apnea in infants and young children. J Clin Neurophysiol 1996;13:610–618

800. Wassmuth Z, Mair E, Loube D, Leonhard D. Cautery-assisted palatal stiffening operation for the treatment of obstructive sleep apnea syndrome. Otolaryngol Head Neck Surg 2000;122: 547–555

801. Weber M, Müller MK, Bucher T, Wildi S, Dindo D, Horber F, Hauser R, Clavien PA. Laparoscopic gastric bypass is superior to laparoscopic gastric banding for treatment of morbid obesity. Ann Surg 2004;240:975–983

802. Weber M, Müller MK, Michel JM, Belal R, Horber F, Hauser R, Clavien PA. Laparoscopic Roux-en-Y gastric by pass, but not rebanding, should be proposed as rescue procedure for patients with failed laparoscopic gastric banding. Ann Surg 2003;238:827–834

803. Wedman J, Miljeteig H. Treatment of simple snoring using radio waves for ablation of uvula and soft palate: a day-case surgery procedure. Laryngoscope 2002;112: 1256–1259

804. Weiner R, Blanco-Engert R, Weiner S, Matkowitz R, Schaefer L, Pomhoff I. Outcome after laparoscopic adjustable gastric banding – 8 years experience. Obes Surg 2003;13: 427–434

805. Welinder R, Cardell LO, Uddman R, Malm L. Reduced nasal airway resistance following uvulopalatopharyngoplasty. Rhinology 1997;35:16–18

806. Weller WE, Hannan EL. Relationship between provider volume and postoperative complications for bariatric procedures in New York State. J Am Coll Surg 2006;202: 753–761

807. Wells WA. Some nervous and mental manifestations occurring in connection with nasal disease. Am J Med Sci 1898;116:677–692

808. Welt S, Maurer JT, Hörmann K, Stuck BA. Radiofrequency surgery of the tongue base in the treatment of snoring–a pilot study. Sleep Breath 2007;11:39–43

809. Wennmo C, Olsson P, Flisberg K, Paulsson B, Luttrup S. Treatment of snoring- with and without carbon dioxide laser. Acta Otolaryngol (Stockh) 1992; (492 Suppl): 152–155

810. Werle AH, Nicklaus PJ, Kirse DJ, Bruegger DE. A retrospective study of tonsillectomy in the under 2-year-old child: indications, perioperative management, and complications. Int J Pediatr Otorhinolaryngol 2003;67:453–460

811. Westling A, Gustavsson S. Laparoscopic vs open Roux-en-Y gastric by pass: a prospective, randomized trial. Obes Surg 2001;11:284–292

812. Wetmore SJ, Scrima L, Hiller FC. Sleep apnea in epistaxis patients treated with nasal packs. Otolaryngol Head Neck Surg 1988;98:596–599

813. Whinney DJ, Williamson PA, Bicknell PG. Punctate diathermy of the soft palate: a new approach in the surgical management of snoring. J Laryngol Otol 1995;109: 849–852

814. White CS, Dilwick MF. Prevalence and variance of temporomandibular dysfunction in orthognathic surgery patients. Int J Adult Orthodon Orthognath Surg 1992;7:7–14

815. Giles TL, Lasserson TJ, Smith BH, White J, Wright J, Cates CJ. Continuous positive airway pressure for obstructive sleep apnoea in adults. Cochrane Database Syst Rev 2006;(1):CD 001106

816. Wiest GH, Ficker JH, Lehnert G, Hahn EG. Secondary obstructive sleep apnoea syndrome in a patient with tracheal stenosis and bilateral recurrent nerve palsy [in German]. Dtsch Med Wochenschr 1998;123:522–526

817. Williams AJ, Arand D, Yan-Go F, Clark G, Miller T. Adjuvant therapies for obstructive sleep apnea. Am Rev Respir Dis 1991;143: A590

818. Williams JK, Maull D, Grayson BH, Longaker MT, McCarthy JG. Early decannulation with bilateral mandibular distraction for tracheostomy-dependent patients. Plast Reconstr Surg 1999;103:48–57

819. Windfuhr JP, Chen YS. Post-tonsillectomy and -adenoidectomy hemorrhage in nonselected patients. Ann Otol Rhinol Laryngol 2003;112:63–70

820. Woo P. Aquired laryngomalacia: epiglottis prolapse as a cause of airway obstruction. Ann Otol Rhinol Laryngol 1992;101:314–320

821. Woodhead CJ, Allen MB. Nasal surgery for snoring. Clin Otolaryngol 1994;19: 41–44

822. Woodson BT, deRowe A, Hawke M, Wenig B, Ross EB, Katsantonis GP, Mickelson SA, Bonham RE, Benbadis S. Pharyngeal suspension suture with repose bone screw for obstructive sleep apnea. Otolaryngol Head Neck Surg 2000;122:395–401

823. Woodson BT, Fujita S. Clinical experience with lingualplasty as part of the treatment of severe obstructive sleep apnea. Otolaryngol Head Neck Surg 1992;107:40–48

824. Woodson BT, Hanson PR, Melugin MB, Dama AA. Sequential upper airway changes during mandibular distraction for obstructive sleep apnea. Otolaryngol Head Neck Surg 2003;128: 142–144

825. Woodson BT, Naganuma H. Comparison of methods of airway evaluation in obstructive sleep apnea syndrome. Otolaryngol Head Neck Surg 1999;120:460–463

826. Woodson BT, Nelson L, Mickelson S, Huntley T, Sher A. A multi-institutional study of radiofrequency volumetric tissue reduction for OSAS. Otolaryngol Head Neck Surg 2001; 125:303–311

827. Woodson BT, Robinson S, Lim HJ. Transpalatal advancement pharyngoplasty outcomes compared with uvulopalatopharyngoplasty. Otolaryngol Head Neck Surg 2005;133: 211–217

828. Woodson BT, Steward DL, Weaver EM, Javaheri S. A randomized trial of temperature-controlled radiofrequency, continuous positive airway pressure, and placebo for obstructive sleep apnea syndrome. Otolaryngol Head Neck Surg 2003;128: 848–861

829. Woodson BT, Toohill RJ. Transpalatal advancement pharyngoplasty for obstructive sleep apnea. Laryngoscope 1993;103:269–276

830. Woodson BT, Wooten MR. Comparison of upper-airway evaluations during wakefulness and sleep. Laryngoscope 1994;104:821–828

831. Woodson BT, Wooten MR. Manometric and endoscopic localization of airway obstruction after ululopalatopharyngoplasty. Otolaryngol Head Neck Surg 1994;111: 38–43

832. Woodson BT. A tongue suspension suture for obstructive sleep apnea and snorers. Otolaryngol Head Neck Surg 2001;124:297–303

833. Woodson BT. Acute effects of palatopharyngoplasty on airway collapsibility. Otolaryngol Head Neck Surg 1999;121:82–86

834. Woodson BT. Changes in airway characteristics after transpalatal advancement pharyngoplasty compared to uvulopalatopharyngoplasty (UPPP). Sleep 1996;19(Suppl 10): S291-S293

835. Woodson BT. Retropalatal airway characteristics in uvulopalatopharyngoplasty compared with transpalatal advancement pharyngoplasty. Laryngoscope 1997;107: 735–740

836. World Health Organization. World Health Report 2002. Available at: http://www.who.int/whr/en/index.html. Accessed Jan 4, 2009

837. Wright S, Haight J, Zamel N, Hoffstein V. Changes in pharyngeal properties after uvulopalatopharyngoplasty. Laryngoscope 1989;99:62–65

838. Xu Z, Cheuk DK, Lee SL. Clinical evaluation in predicting childhood obstructive sleep apnea. Chest 2006;130:1765–1771

839. Xu Z, Jiaqing A, Yuchuan L, Shen K. A case-control study of obstructive sleep apnea-hypopnea syndrome in obese and nonobese Chinese children. Chest 2008; 133:684–689

840. Yin SK, Yi HL, Lu WY, Guan J, Wu HM, Cao ZY. Genioglossus advancement and hyoid suspension plus uvulopalatopharyngoplasty for severe OSAHS. Otolaryngol Head Neck Surg 2007;136:626–631

841. Young T, Palat M, Dempsey J, Skatrud J, Weber S, Badr S. The occurrence of sleep-disordered breathing among middle-aged adults. N Engl J Med 1993;328:1230–1235

842. Zafereo ME, Taylor RJ, Pereira KD. Supraglottoplasty for laryngomalacia with obstructive sleep apnea. Laryngoscope 2008;118:1873–1877

843. Zalzal GH, Anon JB, Cotton RT. Epiglottoplasty for the treatment of laryngomalacia. Ann Otol Laryngol 1987;96:72–76

844. Zitsch RP. Continuous positive airway pressure. Use in bilateral vocal cord paralysis. Arch Otolaryngol Head Neck Surg 1992;118:875–876

845. Zonato AI, Bittencourt LR, Martinho FL, Gregório LC, Tufik S. Upper airway surgery: the effect on nasal continuous positive airway pressure titration on obstructive sleep apnea patients. Eur Arch Otorhinolaryngol 2006;263:481–486

846. Zonato AI, Bittencourt LR, Martinho FL, Júnior JF, Gregório LC, Tufik S. Association of systematic head and neck physical examination with severity of obstructive sleep apnea-hypopnea syndrome. Laryngoscope 2003;113:973–980

847. Zonato AI, Martinho FL, Bittencourt LR, de Oliveira Camponês Brasil O, Gregório LC, Tufik S. Head and neck physical examination: comparison between nonapneic and obstructive sleep apnea patients. Laryngoscope 2005;115:1030–1034

Index

A

Adenotonsillectomy (ATE)
  children, 41–44
  OSA, 41–43
  simple snoring, 41
Adult laryngeal obstructive sleep apnea
  floppy epiglottis, 199
  indications and contraindications, 201–202
  postoperative care and complications, 201
  SDB efficiency, 200–201
Adult sleep disordered breathing, 13
Anesthesiologic airway management
  Bonfils intubation fiberscope, 234
  extubating the difficult airway, 237–238
  face mask ventilation, 233
  fibreoptic bronchoscope, 233
  intubation strategies, 232–236
  invasive airway management avoidance, 232
  laryngeal tube suction (LTS II), 235, 236
  life-threatening situations, 236–237
  negative pressure pulmonary edema, 238
  OSA, 231–233
  postoperative care, 238
  supraglottic airway devices, 235
Antral choanal polyps (ACP), 33
Apnea hypopnea index (AHI), 11–13
Apparative treatment
  CPAP ventilation therapy, 7–8
  electrostimulation, 8
  oral appliances, 8
Arytenoidoplasty, 195

B

Backward, upward, rightward pressure
      (BURP), 234
Bariatric surgery

adjustable gastric banding, 222, 223
  intragastric balloon, 224
  jejunal bypass, 224, 225
  malabsorptive procedures, 224
  sleeve gastrectomy, 223
  vertical banded gastroplasty, 222, 223
Bilateral sagittal split osteotomy (BSSO), 177
Biliopancreatic diversion, 221
Body mass index (BMI), 13, 209
Bonfils intubation fiberscope, 234

C

Cautery-assisted palatal stiffening operation
      (CAPSO), 123
Conservative treatment
  drug therapy, 6–7
  sleeping hygiene, 6
  supine position avoidance, 6
  weight reduction, 6
Continuous narrowing, upper airway
  indications, SDB severity, 12, 13
  levels of evidence, 17
  obstruction site, 12
  primary surgical treatment, 11–12
Continuous positive airway pressure (CPAP)
      therapy, 30–31, 178
Corticosteroids, 34

D

Distraction osteogenesis (DOG)
  mandibular distraction osteogenesis,
      184–185
  maxillary-midfacial distraction
      osteogenesis, 186–191
Down's syndrome, 153, 154

E

Epiglottopexy, 195, 196
Epworth sleepiness scale (ESS), 138
Evidence-based medicine (EBM), 13–17
Extended uvulopalatal flap (EUPF), 206

F

Fast fourrier transfer (FFT) analysis, 22
Fibreoptic bronchoscope, 233
Finkelstein test, 68
Flexible endoscopy, 21

G

Gastric banding, 221–223
Genioglossus advancement (GA)
    copious irrigation, 170
    genial tubercle incorporation, 169
    indications and contraindications, 172
    mucosal incision, 170
    OSA, 171, 172
    postoperative care and complications,
        171–172
    surgical technique, 170–172
Glan Clwyd snoring box, 22
Glossopexy technique, 161–163

H

Hörmann's modification
    dermal incision, 147
    Langenbeck retractor, 148
    redon drainage, 148
    redundant fat resection, 147, 148
    thyroid cartilage transfixing, 148, 149
Hyoid suspension (HS)
    first modification, 145–147
    genioglossal advancement (GA), 144
    hörmann's modification, 147–149
    hyoidthyroidpexia, 144
    indications and contraindications, 151–152
    postoperative care and complications, 151
    SDB effectiveness, 150
    sedated endoscopy, 144
    surgical technique, 145–149
Hyoidthyroidpexia, 144, 145, 151

I

Injection snoreplasty
    complications, 128
    indications, 128
    OSA, 128
    postoperative care, 128

    simple snoring, 127
    surgical technique, 126–127
Interstitial radiofrequency treatment (RFT)
    active electrodes, 135
    bipolar application, 52
    Celon system, 53, 134
    complications, 55–56, 139–141, 141
    contraindications, 41, 56, 109–110
    indications, 56, 109–110, 141
    mean postoperative pain scores, 139
    OSA, 107–108, 137, 138
    postoperative care, 55–56, 139–141
    postoperative complications, 108–109
    principle of, 52–53
    punctate diathermy, 103, 104
    SDB, 54–55
    simple snoring, 106–107, 136–137
    Somnus system, 53
    surgical technique, 53–54, 103–106, 133–136
    sutter system, 134
    tissue necrosis and perifocal edema, 52
    tongue ulceration, 140
Intragastric balloons, 221, 224
Intubating laryngeal mask airway.
        See LMA-Fastrach ™

J

Jejunal bypass, 221, 224, 225

L

Langenbeck retractor, 148
Laryngeal obstructive sleep apnea
    adult, 199–202
    pediatric, 193–198
Laryngeal tube suction (LTS II), 235, 236
Laser lingual tonsillectomy (LLT), 206
Laser-assisted uvulopalatoplasty (LAUP)
    American Academy of Sleep Medicine
        (AASM), 99–100
    anesthesia, 98
    contraindications, 100
    indications, 99–100
    long-term complications, 97
    Mannheim/Ulm/Hamburg technique, 91
    modifiied Kamami technique, 88–89
    nasopharyngeal incompetence, 97–98
    nasopharyngeal stenosis, 97, 98
    one-stage-LAUP, 89
    OSA, 94–96
    pain, 99
    postoperative care and complications, 96–99
    radiocephalometric examination, 99

simple snoring, 90, 92–94
surgical techniques, 88–90
Lingual tonsil hypertrophy, 157
Lingualplasty, 155
LMA-Fastrach ™, 235

M
Mandibular osteotomy (MO), 169
Maxillary-midfacial distraction osteogenesis
  complications and postoperative
    care, 188–189
  indications and counter indication, 189–191
  Le-Fort I level, 186
  midfacial distraction, 187
  OSA efficiency, 187–188
  surgical technique, 186–187
  zygomatic arch transition, 186
Maxillomandibular advancement (MMA)
  indications and contraindications, 180–182
  lower jaw surgery, 177–178
  OSA, 178–179
  postoperative care and complications,
    179–180
  stanford 2 phase concept, 175
  surgical technique, 176–178
  upper jaw surgery, 176–177
Midline partial glossectomy (MLP), 179
Multilevel surgery
  body mass index (BMI), 13, 209
  children, 212–213
  divergent concepts, 206
  hypopharyngeal constriction, 211
  mild to moderate OSA effectiveness,
    204–205
  moderate to severe OSA
    effectiveness, 206, 209
  postoperative care and complications,
    210–211
  staged concepts, 209
  tongue muscles partial resection, 211
  UPPP and tonsillectomy, 211

N
Nager syndrome, 184, 188
Nasal surgery
  complications, 28–29
  conservative treatment, 26
  continuous positive airway pressure
    (CPAP), 30–31
  contraindications, 29
  indications, 29
  OSA, 27–28

postoperative care, 28–29
simple snoring, 26–27
Nasopharyngeal surgery
  complications, 35
  contraindications, 36
  indications, 36
  intranasal corticosteroids, 34
  nasopharyngeal tubes, 34–35
  postoperative care, 35
  surgical treatment, 35
  treatment effectiveness, 34–35
Negative pressure pulmonary
    edema (NPPE), 238
Nonsteroidal anti-inflammatory drugs
    (NSAID), 45

O
Obesity, 6
Obstruction site identification
  acoustic reflectometry, 22–23
  flexible endoscopy, 21
  pressure measurements, 20
  radiocephalometry, 22
  respiratory sound analysis, 22
  upper airway narrowing, 23
Obstructive sleep apnea (OSA), 215
  adenotonsillectomy (ATE), 41–43
  anesthesiologic airway management,
    231–233
  antral choanal polyps (ACP), 33
  ATE effect, children, 42
  genioglossus advancement (GA), 171, 172
  injection snoreplasty, 128
  interstitial radiofrequency treatment (RFT),
    107–108, 137, 138
  laryngeal OSA (*see* Laryngeal obstructive
    sleep apnea)
  laser-assisted uvulopalatoplasty
    (LAUP), 94–96
  maxillary-midfacial distraction
    osteogenesis, 187–188
  maxillomandibular advancement
    (MMA), 178–179
  nasal surgery, 27–28
  nasopharyngeal surgery
    (*see* Nasopharyngeal surgery)
  palatal stiffening operation, 125
  pediatric OSA, 2–3
  pharyngeal muscle tone loss, 2
  Pillar® implant, 118
  prevalence, 3
  retropharyngeal lipoma, 34

risk factors, 2
symptoms, 2
TE effect, adults, 45
tongue base resection, 158–159
tongue suspension, 164
tonsillotomy (TT), 48–49
tracheotomy, 216–217
uvulopalatopharyngoplasty (UPPP), 65–66

P

Palatal implants
   complications, 119, 120
   indications and contraindications, 119–120
   OSA, 117–118
   postoperative care, 119, 120
   simple snoring, 116–117
   surgical technique, 115–116
Palatal stiffening operation
   complications, 125–126
   indications, 125
   LAUP, 123
   OSA, 125
   postoperative care, 126
   simple snoring, 124–125
   surgical technique, 122–124
Paryngeal muscle tone loss, 2
Pediatric laryngeal obstructive sleep apnea
   aryepiglottal fold shortening, 195
   arytenoidoplasty, 195
   complex malformation syndromes, 193
   epiglottis partial resection, 194
   indications and contraindications, 198
   laryngomalacia, 194
   partial laser epiglottidectomy, 195
   postoperative care and
          complications, 197–198
   SDB efficiency, 197
   suction test, 195
   surgical techniques, 194–195
Pediatric SDB, 8–9
Pfeiffer syndrome, 184
Pierre–Robin sequence, 34, 188
Pillar® implant
   effectiveness, OSA, 118
   efficacy, simple snoring, 118
   extrusions, 120
Posterior airway space (PAS), 146
Pressure probes, 20

R

Radiocephalometry, 22
Radiofrequency surgery

interstitial radiofrequency treatment (RFT)
      (*see* Interstitial radiofrequency
      treatment (RFT))
   radiofrequency-UPP (RF-UPP) (*see*
      Radiofrequency-UPP (RF-UPP))
Radiofrequency treatment (RFT), 172
Radiofrequency-UPP (RF-UPP)
   contraindications, 114
   indications, 114
   OSA, 112–113
   postoperative care and complications,
          113–114
   simple snoring, 112, 113
   surgical technique, 111–112
Retropharyngeal lipoma, 34
Roux-en-Y gastric bypass, 221

S

Sagittal osteotomy, 178
Sedated endoscopy, 144
Shy-drager syndrome, 199
Simple snoring
   adenotonsillectomy (ATE), 41
   injection snoreplasty, 127
   interstitial radiofrequency treatment
          (RFT), 106–107
   laser-assisted uvulopalatoplasty
          (LAUP), 90, 92
   nasal surgery, 26–27
   palatal stiffening, 124
   pediatric tonsillar surgery, 40
   Pillar® implant, 118
   tonsillotomy (TT), 48
   uvulopalatopharyngoplasty (UPPP), 63–64
Sleep videoendoscopy, 21
Sleeve gastrectomy, 221, 223
Soft palate (SP), 203–206, 210, 211
Stanford 2 phase concept, 175
Stickler syndrome, 188
Supraglottoplasty, 195

T

Tongue base resection
   additional lateral wedge resection, 155
   coblation®, 156, 157
   Down's syndrome, 153, 154
   indications and contraindications, 160
   lingual tonsil excision, 154
   lingual tonsil hypertrophy, 157
   midline resection, 155
   OSA effectiveness, 158–159

postoperative care and complications,
159–160
surgical technique, 154–157
transcollar tongue base resection, 157
Tongue base suspension (TBS), 206
Tongue suspension
anatomical abnormalities, 161
indications and contraindications, 165–166
OSA efficiency, 164
postoperative care and
complications, 164–165
principle, 161
simple snoring efficiency, 163–164
surgical technique, 161–163
Tonsillectomy (TE)
adults, 44–46
children, 40–44
indications and contraindications, 43–44, 45
OSA, 41–45
postoperative care and complications, 43,
44–45
simple snoring, 40–41, 44
Tonsillotomy (TT)
complications, 49
contraindications, 50
indications, 50
OSA, 48–49
postoperative care, 49
simple snoring, 48
surgical technique, 47–48
Tracheotomy
indications and contraindications, 218–219
obstructive sleep apnea (OSA), 215
OSA effectiveness, 216–217
postoperative care and complications,
217–218
surgical technique, 215–216
tracheostomy tube, 216
weight reduction, 216
Transcollar tongue base resection, 157
Transpalatal advancement
pharyngoplasty (TAP)

postoperative care, 129
surgical principle, 128–129
vs. uvulopalatopharyngoplasty (UPPP), 129
Treacher-collins syndrome (TC-S), 188
Treatment decision
adult SDB, 13
criteria, 9
daytime symptoms, 9
obstruction sites, 10
Oxford Centre for evidence-based medicine
levels of evidence, 13–17
patient expectations, 10
pediatric SDB, 8–9
SDB severity, 10–11

U
Upper airway obstruction (UAO), 238
Uvulectomy, 121–122
Uvulopalatopharyngoplasty (UPPP), 20
exclusion criteria, 72
indications and contraindications, 71–73
late-term complications, 70
moderate to severe OSA, 211
multilevel surgery in children, 212–213
nasopharyngeal stenosis, 69–70
OSA, 65–66
pain, 67
severe sleep apneics, 206
simple snoring, 63–64
surgical technique, 60–63
velopharyngeal incompetence, 68
visual analogue scale patients, 70–71

V
Velocardiofacial syndrome, 184
Vertical banded gastroplasty, 221–2223
Visual analogue scale, 139

W
Weight reduction, 6

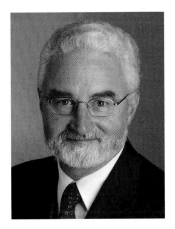

Karl Hörmann is Professor of Otorhinolaryngology, Head and Neck Surgery at the University of Heidelberg, Germany. He is head of the Department of Otorhinolaryngology, Head and Neck Surgery of University Hospital Mannheim, Germany. He is President of the German Academy of Otorhinolaryngolgy and a past president of the German Society of Otorhinolaryngology, Head and Neck Surgery. He has published over 200 scientific articles. He lives with his wife and four children in Mannheim.

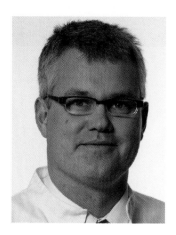

Thomas Verse is Associate Professor of Otorhinolaryngology, Head and Neck Surgery and Director of the Department of Otorhinolaryngology, Head and Neck Surgery of Asklepios Clinic Harburg. He is the head of the task force "Sleep Medicine" of the German Society of Otorhinolaryngology, Head and Neck Surgery. He has published extensive papers in the field of sleep medicine. He lives with his wife and three sons in Hamburg, Germany.